1,000,000 Books

are available to read at

Forgotten Books

www.ForgottenBooks.com

Read online
Download PDF
Purchase in print

ISBN 978-1-334-77481-2
PIBN 10677665

This book is a reproduction of an important historical work. Forgotten Books uses state-of-the-art technology to digitally reconstruct the work, preserving the original format whilst repairing imperfections present in the aged copy. In rare cases, an imperfection in the original, such as a blemish or missing page, may be replicated in our edition. We do, however, repair the vast majority of imperfections successfully; any imperfections that remain are intentionally left to preserve the state of such historical works.

Forgotten Books is a registered trademark of FB &c Ltd.
Copyright © 2018 FB &c Ltd.
FB &c Ltd, Dalton House, 60 Windsor Avenue, London, SW19 2RR.
Company number 08720141. Registered in England and Wales.

For support please visit www.forgottenbooks.com

1 MONTH OF FREE READING

at
www.ForgottenBooks.com

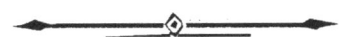

By purchasing this book you are eligible for one month membership to ForgottenBooks.com, giving you unlimited access to our entire collection of over 1,000,000 titles via our web site and mobile apps.

To claim your free month visit:
www.forgottenbooks.com/free677665

* Offer is valid for 45 days from date of purchase. Terms and conditions apply.

English
Français
Deutsche
Italiano
Español
Português

www.forgottenbooks.com

Mythology Photography **Fiction** Fishing Christianity **Art** Cooking Essays Buddhism Freemasonry Medicine **Biology** Music **Ancient Egypt** Evolution Carpentry Physics Dance Geology **Mathematics** Fitness Shakespeare **Folklore** Yoga Marketing **Confidence** Immortality Biographies Poetry **Psychology** Witchcraft Electronics Chemistry History **Law** Accounting **Philosophy** Anthropology Alchemy Drama Quantum Mechanics Atheism Sexual Health **Ancient History Entrepreneurship** Languages Sport Paleontology Needlework Islam **Metaphysics** Investment Archaeology Parenting Statistics Criminology **Motivational**

Reproduced by DUOPAGE process

in the United States of America

MICRO PHOTO INC.
Cleveland 12, Ohio

THE HISTORY OF NURSING IN
THE BRITISH EMPIRE

THE HISTORY OF NURSING

IN

THE BRITISH EMPIRE

BY

SARAH A. TOOLEY

AUTHOR OF THE "LIFE OF FLORENCE NIGHTINGALE," ETC.

WITH 57 ILLUSTRATIONS

"She was oft by them that were sick, and she laid the pillows aright and in point; and she rubbed their feet and boiled water to wash them; and it seemed to her that the less she did to the sick in service, so much the less service did she to God."

LONDON
S. H. BOUSFIELD & CO., LTD.
12, PORTUGAL STREET, W.C.
1906

·PUBLIC HEALTH LIB.

Ref 382817

PRINTED BY
WILLIAM CLOWES AND SONS, LIMITED,
LONDON AND BECCLES.

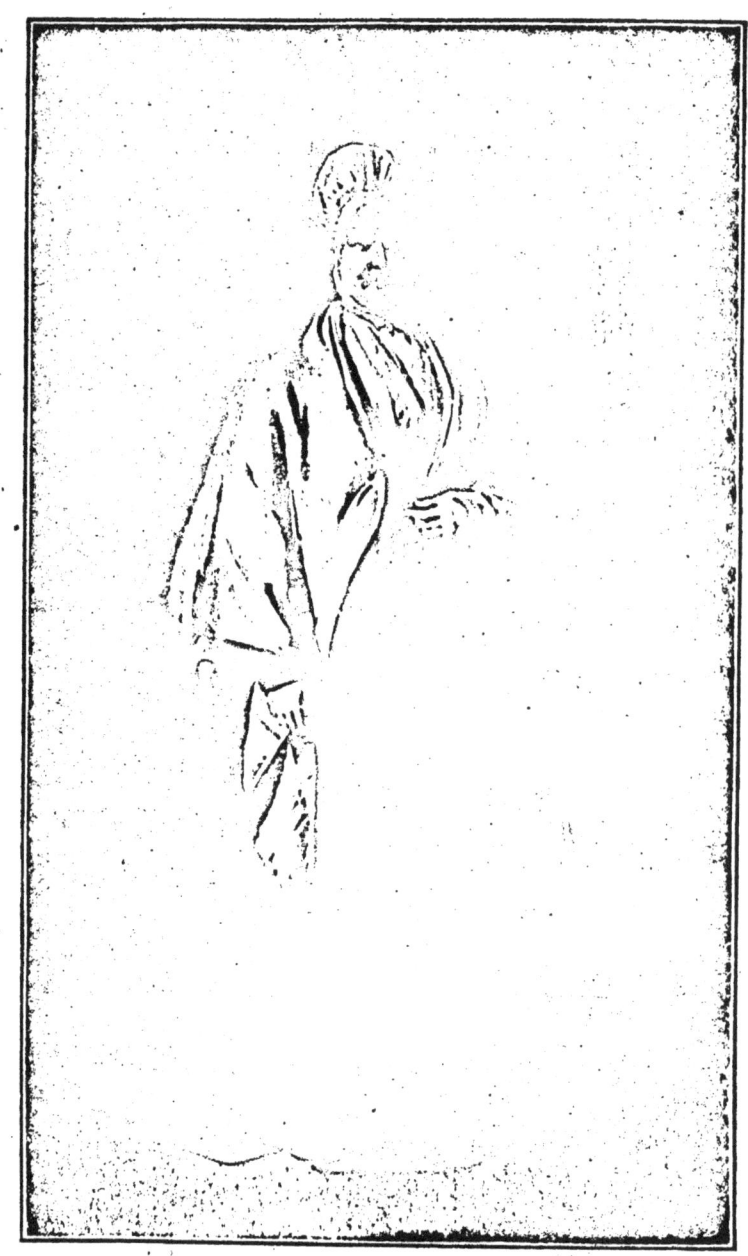

MRS. ELIZABETH FRY.
(*From the Portrait by George Richmond, R.A.*)

[*Frontispiece.*

PREFACE

THE rise and spread of trained nursing is one of the most remarkable developments of the last half of the nineteenth century, and forms an important chapter in social progress. It is a matter for national pride that Great Britain has been the cradle of this beneficent movement. No other country can show a like record, and though America has a highly organized and efficient system of nursing, it modelled its early training-schools on that of St. Thomas's Hospital. The name of Florence Nightingale had been wafted across the Atlantic, and when the brave daughters of America volunteered to go out and nurse "the boys" during the Civil War they were inspired by the example of the heroine of the Crimea.

Fifty years ago the idea of educated women training as nurses was regarded with wonder and amazement, or at best treated as a sentimental fad. Now there is a vast army of skilled and trained women engaged in this important profession throughout the British Empire, to say nothing of other lands. No place is too remote, no climate too deadly, for the nurse to ply her ministrations. Like the soldier she obeys the call of duty, and, if need be, gives her life in the cause. In field hospital in time of war; in miner's camp or settler's hut; on Canadian prairie, in the Australian bush, or the South African veldt; on the burning plains of India and in the deadly tropics the trained nurse is to be found. At home her ministrations reach the poorest attic. Every hospital, whether civil, military, or naval, is staffed by trained nurses—our largest hospital employs upwards of five hundred nurses, including the private staff—while Poor Law Infirmaries and Asylums for the Insane have trained nurses approximating to the standard of the best General Hospitals. The advance of medical and surgical science has made the skilled nurse a necessity, and the change from the past to the present system of nursing is little short of a revolution. Nursing is the first profession for women to have been recognized by a Royal Charter, and the question of the Registration of nurses by the State has engaged the attention of a Select Committee of the House of Commons, and is pending solution.

Being but a simple scribe, with no claim to belong to the profession of nursing, my endeavour has been to take a "brief" for the history of the movement, unbiassed by any school or faction, and chiefly intent on following the main stream of facts and incidents.

No History of Nursing has so far been published, and data for this volume have been obtained by original research. No pains have been spared to obtain accurate information, and in many cases the archives of the various hospitals and nursing institutions have been consulted. The writer has received valuable help and guidance from distinguished pioneers in the nursing and philanthropic world and from eminent medical men. Without holding them in any way responsible for her conclusions, she would like to thank in particular the following ladies and gentlemen who have in various ways assisted her, or whose writings have been helpful: Miss Isabella Beaver, Sister Superior the Nursing Sisters St. John the

Divine; Sir James Crichton Browne, M.R.C.S., M.D., LL.D., F.R.S.; Miss Sidney Browne, R.R.C.; Sir Henry Burdett, K.C.B.; Miss Cadenhead; Sister Caroline, Sister Superior St. John's House; The Rev. Dacre Craven, M.A.; Mrs. Dacre Craven; W. H. Cross, Esq.; Miss Mary S. Crossland; Clinton Dent, Esq., M.A., M.C., F.R.C.S.; Sir Dyce Duckworth, M.D., LL.D.; The Countess of Dufferin and Ava; Miss French; Mrs. Follows; Miss Hadden; Dr. Harvey (Perth Hospital, W. Australia); Miss M. E. Dalrymple Hay; Mrs. Julian Hill; The Honble. Sydney Holland; Miss Amy Hughes; Dr. F. Rowland Humphreys, L.R.C.P., M.R.C.S.; Dr. Theodore Hyslop, C.M., M.R.C.P., L.M.; Dr. Robert Jones, B.S., F.R.C.S., M.R.C.P.; Miss Caroline Lloyd; Miss Eva Lückes; Miss Katharine Monk; Miss Moorhouse; The Rev. Arthur Peile, M.A., Master of St. Katharine's Royal Collegiate Hospital; Sidney M. Quennell, Esq.; Miss Eleanor Rathbone; Miss Margaret Russell; Thomas Ryan, Esq.; Dr. Shuttleworth; Miss Sarah Swift; Dr. Symes-Thompson, F.R.C.P.; C. L. Todd, Esq.; Captain Tunnard; Miss Louisa Twining; Miss Wilson, President the Midwives' Institute; and Miss Catherine Wood.

My best thanks are also given to the heads of the Medical Departments of the War Office, Admiralty, and India Office; to the Agents-General for Canada, New South Wales, Queensland, New Zealand, Tasmania, Natal, and Cape Colony, for papers and reports supplied with regard to the nursing in hospitals in their respective Colonies; and to the Matrons, Lady Superintendents, and Secretaries of the various hospitals and nursing institutions visited in Great Britain and Ireland, for their kindness and courtesy in placing information at my disposal.

CONTENTS

CHAPTER I
NURSING BEFORE 1840

Pagan indifference to the sick—St. Paul institutes deaconesses—The life and work of St. Paula—Nursing an outcome of religious devotion—Rise of general hospitals—The Hospitalières—The Hôtel Dieu—Influence of the Crusades—The Abbess Hildegarde founds a school—Nursing in monastic infirmaries—Medical Brotherhoods—The Knights Hospitallers employ women—The Grey Sisters—The Béguines—Sisters of St. Elizabeth—A new era of nursing—St. Vincent de Paul—Founds the Association of Charity—Madame de Gondi—The Ladies of Charity—Remarkable influence of St. Vincent—Duchess d'Aiguillon—Madame Goussault—Madame le Gras—St. Vincent founds the Sisters of Charity—The establishment of the Sisterhood—St. Vincent's rules—Spread of the Sisterhood—They undertake every branch of nursing—Not cloistered nuns—The humanitarian spirit—First hospital nurses in London—St. Bartholomew's—St. Thomas's—Guy's Hospital—Quaint rules—Deterioration of nursing—Dr. Gooch attempts reform in 1825—Letters to Southey—" Religious female physicians "—England apathetic—Kaiserswerth founded—Its influence on nursing in this country 1

CHAPTER II
THE PIONEER WORK OF ELIZABETH FRY

Early life of Elizabeth Fry—Her marriage and settlement in London—Prison work—Friendship with Pastor Fliedner—The Deaconess Hospital at Kaiserswerth—Resolves to found a nursing sisterhood—Letter to the Bishop of London—Queen Adelaide becomes Patroness—Queen Victoria interested—Failing health and death of Mrs. Fry 23

CHAPTER III
THE INSTITUTION OF NURSING SISTERS

Institution founded, 1840—The rules and regulations—Training of the sisters—First staff of nurses enrolled—Lady Inglis becomes president—Growth of the institution—Quaint rules—Present regulations—Letter from Thackeray—Devoted service of the Committee—The lady superintendent—Contemporary nursing in America and abroad 32

CHAPTER IV
CHARLES DICKENS AND NURSING REFORM

Caricature a factor in Reform—Dickens creates Sairey Gamp—The character taken from life—Description of Mrs. Gamp—Betsey Prig of Bartlemy's—Mrs. Gamp as night nurse—They prepare their patient for a journey—Rupture of the famous partnership—No immediate reform after publication of Martin Chuzzlewit—Dickens laments state of nursing in hospitals . . . 45

CONTENTS

CHAPTER V
ST. JOHN'S HOUSE

King's College first London hospital to give facility for training school for nurses—Sir William Bowman, Dr. Todd, and Dr. Farre initiate scheme—Foundation of St. John's House, 1848—Class of inmates and their respective duties—Strict discipline—The "Master" and his office—Removal to Westminster—Miss Mary Jones appointed superintendent—Nurses for the Crimea—Removal to Norfolk Street—Expansion of work—The daily diets—Changes in the rules—Lady and nurse pupils—Crisis in 1883—Reorganization—Sister Caroline and present *régime* 56

CHAPTER VI
THE NURSING SISTERS OF ST. JOHN THE DIVINE

Descendants of St. John's House—Sister Superior, Miss Isabella Beaver—Sister Caroline Lloyd—Early activities at Drayton Gardens—Deptford District Home—The Community to-day—Its aim—Testimony by Canon Bristow—The Medals 72

CHAPTER VII
FIRST REFORMS IN HOSPITAL NURSING

Abuses under the old system—Tipping—A word for some of the old nurses—Defects in hospital arrangements—An epoch-making reform—St. John's Sisters at King's College—Old ideas regarding gentlewomen—Character *v.* Training—Putting wards in nursing order—Plan for nursing King's College—First Nurses' Home attached to a London hospital—The Nightingale Ward—Reforms at Charing Cross Hospital—A vigilant Sister Superior—Nursing under dual control a failure—Rupture between St. John's Sisterhood and King's College—Trained nursing at Guy's—All Saints' Sisters and University College Hospital—Nursing a secular professsion 76

CHAPTER VIII
THE NIGHTINGALE FUND TRAINING-SCHOOL

The Heroine of the Crimea—Inauguration of the Nightingale Fund—Influence of the Shadow story—Adverse criticism—St. Thomas's Hospital selected for the school—Mrs. Wardroper first superintendent—Rules for probationers—Temporary quarters in Surrey Gardens—Opening of the New St. Thomas's Hospital—The Nightingale Home—Miss Crossland as Home sister—A probationer's day—Severe discipline—Pathetic story—Mid-Victorian young lady—Sumptuary laws—Miss Nightingale and "her children"—Miss Nightingale's letters to probationers and nurses—Pioneer work by St. Thomas's sisters—Influence on American institutions—Retirement of Mrs. Wardroper—Her death and memorial tablet—Resignation of Miss Crossland—The school grants certificates—Mr. Henry Bonham Carter—Mrs. Wardroper's successors 91

CHAPTER IX
HOSPITAL NURSING AND TRAINING-SCHOOLS

Dearth of trained nurses in 1862—William Rathbone founds the Liverpool Training-school—Its success—London Collegiate Hospitals in the front rank of reform—King's College Hospital—University College Hospital—Charing Cross Hospital—Ormond Street Hospital for Sick Children—The Middlesex Hospital—The Royal Infirmary, Edinburgh—Lady Augusta Stanley founds the Westminster Training-school 113

CONTENTS   xi

CHAPTER X

HOSPITAL TRAINING-SCHOOLS (*continued*)

St. Bartholomew's Hospital—Guy's Hospital—Royal Infirmary, Glasgow—
Sir Patrick Dun's, Dublin—Steeven's Hospital—St. George's Hospital—
St. Mary's, Paddington—The Royal Free Hospital—Summary of Hospital
training to-day 134

CHAPTER XI

THE LARGEST TRAINING-SCHOOL

The London Hospital—Miss Eva Lückes appointed matron—Her splendid
work—Gradual reforms—Founds the London Training-school—Preliminary
training at Tredegar House—A probationers' day—Ward probationers'
examinations—Two years' certificate—Maternity wing—Scale of payment
—The nurses' quarters—The Lückes Home—The Honourable Sydney
Holland—His work for the hospital and nurses—Work of the London
Hospital—Tragedy and humour—Queen Alexandra as president—The King
honours his nurse 153

CHAPTER XII

NURSING IN MILITARY HOSPITALS

Florence Nightingale and the Crimean War—The old army nurses unsatisfactory—Evidence of the Duke of Newcastle—Mr. Russell of the *Times*
makes an appeal—Florence Nightingale responds—Letter from Mr. Sidney
Herbert—Nursing at Scutari—Value of Miss Nightingale's work—Reorganization of military hospitals after the Crimean War—Nursing sisters first
employed at Chatham—Death of Lord Herbert of Lea—Royal Victoria
Hospital, Netley—Increase of sisters in military hospitals—System extended
to India in 1888—Military hospitals lacked nursing organization—Superfluity
of nurses—Story of soldier in South African hospital—Soudan and Egyptian
campaigns—Queen Victoria institutes the Royal Red Cross—Nursing in the
South African campaign—Sir Frederick Treves' testimony—Tommy's appreci-
ation of the sisters—Queen Alexandra's Imperial Military Nursing Service—
Miss Monk's work in organization—Rules of the service—Nurses' Home,
Millbank—Miss Sidney Brown, R.R.C.; Miss C. H. Keer, R.R.C.; Miss
Annie B. Smith, R.R.C.—THE ARMY NURSING SERVICE RESERVE—THE
BRITISH RED CROSS COUNCIL 168

CHAPTER XIII

THE NURSING IN NAVAL AND SEAMEN'S HOSPITALS

Jack as a patient—The handy man—Story of Admiral Sir Harry Keppel—In
the old days—Admiral Sir Edward Parry's appeal—Naval sisters appointed,
1884-85—"Queen Alexandra's Royal Naval Nursing Service," 1902—Its
rules and regulations—Training of male attendants—Duties of the sisters—
The Seamen's Hospital, Greenwich—Nursing on the *Dreadnought*—Training-
school at Greenwich—Branch hospital at the Royal Albert Docks—The
Tropical school—Oriental patients—Amusing story—"The Hobson Jobson"
—Characteristics of seamen—A hot and a cold pipe—A land and a sea age—
Popularity of naval nursing 192

CHAPTER XIV

THE POOR LAW NURSING SERVICE

A social blot—Opinion of Lord Shaftesbury—The old Poor Law—Recreation in
1834—Neglect of the sick—Pauper nurses—Mrs. Jameson's exposures—
Dr. Joseph Rogers at the old Strand Union—Story of a nurse—Flagrant

xii   CONTENTS

PAGE

abuses—Poor houses abroad—The Irish system good for the times—First attempts at reform in England—Dr. E. Sieveking's proposal—Lord Raynham's motion, 1856—Miss Louisa Twining—Her early efforts—The Workhouse Visiting Society founded—Its work—Mr. Gathorne Hardy's Bill, 1867—Dr. Joseph Rogers at the Strand Union—*Lancet* Commission, 1866—Mr. William Rathbone's work at the Liverpool Infirmary—Miss Agnes Jones starts the training of workhouse nurses—Her death, 1868—The movement quickened in the metropolis—Mr. Ernest Hart publishes an account of investigations—Passing of the Metropolitan Poor Law Bill, 1867—Its provisions—The Highgate Infirmary makes an experiment in trained nursing—The Workhouse Nursing Association founded 1879—Mary Adelaide nurses started 1881—Dr. Joseph Rogers reviews the changes during thirty years—The Departmental Committee of Local Government Board appointed 1892—Miss Catherine Wood—Her investigations—The Meath Workhouse Nursing Association—The Countess of Pembroke's nurses started, 1897—Nursing Orders by Local Government Board, 1896-97—Report of the Departmental Committee, 1902—Royal Commission on Poor Law appointed 1904—Decision of the Workhouse Nursing Association to continue its work, 1905—Training under the Poor Law Nursing Service—Marylebone Infirmary—Kensington Infirmary—Need of trained women inspectors in country workhouses—Further action awaited **209**

CHAPTER XV

NURSING IN ASYLUMS FOR THE INSANE

The old system—Dr. Browne's description of an asylum as it was—Treatment of the insane in ancient times—St. Vincent de Paul and Madame le Gras—Pinel's system in Paris—William Tuke founds the Retreat, York—Dr. John Conolly institutes new *régime* at Hanwell—St. Luke's Asylum—Legislation, 1815-45—Affliction of George III.—Lunacy Act, 1845—Commissioners and the attendants—Mrs. Jameson on asylum nurses—The work of Dorothea Dix in United States and Scotland—The Royal Crichton Institution, Dumfries—Dr. Browne institutes lectures for nurses—Sir James Crichton Browne tries to raise the status of nurses—First systematic attempt at training—Medico-Psychological Association Examining Board—Its course for certificate—Dr. Hyslop on the asylum nurse—Bethlem Royal Hospital—A contrast, past and present—A nurse thirty-five years ago—Claybury Asylum—Dr. Robert Jones—Nursing staff at Claybury—Rules and regulations—Berry Wood Asylum, Northampton—Dr. Harding—Dr. Robertson's "Ideals" at Larbert—Organization—Dr. Shuttleworth and the Asylum Workers' Association—Increased demand for mental nurses **238**

CHAPTER XVI

PRIVATE NURSING

The best paying and most criticized branch of the profession—Dissatisfied patients—Private nurse expected to be a paragon of perfection—Some ground for complaint—Nursing plays an increasingly important part in recovery of patient—Private nurse and district nurse compared—Need of special training for private nurses—First attempts to organize private nurses—Mildmay Institution—The Royal Scottish Nursing Institution—Miss M'Alpin's Home, Glasgow—Abuses of Nursing Homes—Princess Christian's Nursing Home at Windsor—Beginning of the co-operative movement in nursing—Miss Firth formed the London Association in 1873—Her devoted life—Progress of her association—Its rules—The Nurses' Co-operation—The Registered Nurses' Society—Large proportion of nurses take up private work—Three principal classes—Daily private nursing—Marylebone Daily Visiting Nursing Association—The Ada Lewis nurses—The bitter cry of the middle classes **261**

CONTENTS

CHAPTER XVII

DISTRICT NURSING: ITS RISE AND PROGRESS

District nursing specially commends itself to public favour—Stirring of public opinion in the fifties—Mrs. Ranyard's Bible-women—She starts a nursing branch—Its position to-day—Article on deaconesses in 1860—William Rathbone, M.P., of Liverpool—Founds district nursing—Develops quickly in Liverpool—District nursing in London—The National and Metropolitan Association started 1874—Miss Florence Lees—Her tour of inspection—Report of the sub-committee on district nursing—Miss Nightingale's appeal for funds for a district nurses' home—Training of the Bloomsbury Square nurses—The "auld lichts" of the profession—Homes of the London poor—Miss Octavia Hill—The district nurses had to overcome the prejudice of the poor—Steady increase of the Metropolitan Association—Contemporary work in Scotland—The work of religious organizations—Parish nursing—The Alexandra nurses 281

CHAPTER XVIII

THE QUEEN'S NURSES

Queen Victoria devotes the women's Jubilee gift to founding an Institute for district nursing—Provisional committee formed 1888—The institute incorporated—St. Katharine's Royal Hospital—The institute removed to Victoria Street—Mr. William Rathbone's interest in the institute—Affiliation of existing homes and associations—Organization of branches—Rules for Queen's Nurses—The council of the institute—The Irish Training Homes—Lady Dudley's scheme for district nurses—The Training Home and work in Wales—Rural district nursing—The County Associations—School nursing—Present estimate of the work of the Queen's nurses—Funds of the Institute—Resignation of Miss Peter, general superintendent, and of Miss Wade, the superintendent for Scotland—A round with a Queen's Nurse—Her civilizing and refining influence—The Queen's Nurses' Journal—Council of Superintendents—Proposal for a League of Queen's Nurses—Miss Amy Hughes. THE SCOTTISH BRANCH—Its formation—Miss Guthrie Wright, honorary secretary—Pioneer work of Miss Peter in Edinburgh—Progress of the work—The Nurse's Pension Fund—Miss Wade—Miss Cowper—Success of the Scottish Branch—Jubilee Day at the Central Home 299

CHAPTER XIX

MIDWIFERY AND MONTHLY NURSING

Midwifery closely allied with nursing—Mrs. Gamp—In early times forbidden to men—After the Reformation, midwives licensed by bishops—Ignorance and cruelty—"The Woman's Booke"—The Chamberlen forceps revolutionize the practice—Warfare between midwives and the "he-practisers"—Distinguished midwives try to educate their sister practitioners—The Society of Apothecaries' action—The Female Medical Society—Miss Nightingale's scheme—Dr. Farre shows high mortality statistics—London Obstetrical Society appoints a commission—Public opinion roused—Dr. Humphrey's articles—Efforts to bring about legislation—The Midwives' Institute founded—Its incorporation—Its objects—It drafts a Midwives' Registration Bill—Various agencies at work—Passing of the Midwives' Act, 1902—Its provisions—The Association for Promoting the Training and Supply of Midwives—The Rural Midwives' Association—Enrolment of midwives under the Act—Training for midwives and monthly nurses—The Rotunda Hospital, Dublin—Rise of other lying-in hospitals—Queen Charlotte's Hospital, Marylebone 319

CONTENTS

CHAPTER XX

MASSAGE

PAGE

Definition of massage—Revival of an ancient practice—The ideal masseuse—The rise of modern massage—The Society of Trained Masseuses founded 1895—List of the Founders—Objects of the society—Conditions of membership—Fees—Examinations—Where instruction can be obtained—Fees and length of training 334

CHAPTER XXI

INDIAN AND COLONIAL NURSING

The nursing problem in India—Lady Canning's work during the Mutiny—The women of India without medical help—Pioneers in the Zenanas—Queen Victoria receives Miss Beilby, a medical missionary—Lady Dufferin founds her fund—Its objects and organization—Report of work, 1905—Lady Curzon founds the Victoria Memorial Scholarship Fund—Nurse Training-School, General Hospital, Madras—The Cama Hospital Nurse Training-School—No standard of training in Indian institutions—Recommendations of Colonel C. H. Joubert—Difficulties of nursing and training—The Up-Country Nursing Association—Lady Minto's new scheme—The Indian Military Nursing Service instituted at the suggestion of Lady Roberts—Work of Miss Katharine Loch—Miss R. A. Betty, a senior superintendent—Lady Robert's Fund—Nursing in the self-governing Colonies—Canada—Australia—New Zealand—Tasmania—Cape Colony—Natal—South African training-schools—Its military service—The Crown Colonies and Protectorates—Lady Piggott founds the Colonial Nursing Association—Its work and progress . . . 338

CHAPTER XXII

ORGANIZATION AND REGISTRATION

The nursing profession, the first profession for women incorporated by Royal Charter—Miss Catherine Wood suggests organization—A meeting in favour at the house of Sir Henry Burdett—Original plan abandoned—A meeting at the house of Dr. and Mrs. Bedford Fenwick—The British Nurses' Association inaugurated—Princess Christian consents to become president—Rules for members—Registration of its nurses—Is incorporated by Royal Charter—List of associates to whom granted—The purposes defined in the Charter—Government of the Association—Rules for membership—Its headquarters—The nurses' settlement—The Chartered Nurses' Society—The Auxiliary Nurses' Society—Membership of the Royal British Nurses' Association—THE ROYAL PENSION FUND FOR NURSES—THE STATE REGISTRATION OF NURSES—History of the movement—A Select Committee of the House of Commons appointed to consider the question.—A resolution in favour of registration by the British Medical Association—Bill introduced into the House of Commons by Mr. Munro Ferguson—Thirty-four witnesses examined by the Select Committee—Views of the advocates for State registration—Views of the opponents to State registration—Conclusions and recommendations of the Select Committee—Deputations to the lord president of the council—Reply of Lord Crewe—The British Medical Association pass a resolution in favour of the principle of State registration—Active propaganda for Parliamentary Bills 370

LIST OF ILLUSTRATIONS

	TO FACE PAGE
MRS. ELIZABETH FRY	*Frontispiece*
(*From the Portrait by George Richmond, R.A.*)	
NURSING IN THE SIXTEENTH CENTURY	22
A Ward in the Hôtel Dieu, Paris.	
(*Facsimile of a wood engraving.*)	
CHARLES DICKENS	48
(*From the painting by David Maclise.*)	
SAIREY GAMP AND BETSEY PRIG PREPARE THEIR PATIENT FOR A JOURNEY	52
SIR WILLIAM BOWMAN	56
(*From the painting in the Board Room at King's College Hospital.*)	
MISS CAROLINE LLOYD	68
Sister Superior, St. John's House, 1870-83.	
THE ORIGINAL SISTERS' CROSS OF ST. JOHN'S HOUSE	80
ORIGINAL NURSES' BADGE (MEDAL), ST. JOHN'S HOUSE	80
CHAPLAIN'S CROSS, NURSING SISTERS OF ST. JOHN THE DIVINE	80
ASSOCIATES' CROSS, NURSING SISTERS OF ST. JOHN THE DIVINE	80
MISS FLORENCE NIGHTINGALE	88
After her return from the Crimea.	
(*Photo by Keene, Derby.*)	
MRS. WARDROPER	96
Matron of St. Thomas's Hospital, 1854-87; Superintendent of the Nightingale Fund Training-School, 1860-87.	
MISS MARY S. CROSSLAND	102
Home Sister, Nightingale Fund Training-School, 1875-96.	

MEDAL WORN BY THE HEAD NURSES AT GUY'S HOSPITAL UNDER THE
OLD RÉGIME 144

RAPHAEL GOLD MEDAL FOR MASSAGE, GUY'S HOSPITAL . . . 144

CAZENOVE GOLD MEDAL, GUY'S HOSPITAL 144

MISS EVA LÜCKES 152
 Matron of the London Hospital since 1880; Founder and Superintendent of the Nurse Training-School.
   (*Photograph by C. Vandyk, London, S.W.*)

THE HON. SYDNEY HOLLAND 160
 Chairman of the London Hospital.
   (*Photo: Enid Wigram.*)

A BANDAGING CLASS AT TREDEGAR HOUSE 164
 The Preliminary Nurse Training-School of the London Hospital.

MISS FLORENCE NIGHTINGALE 168
   (*From the bust at Claydon.*)
 This bust was presented to Miss Nightingale by the soldiers after the Crimean War, and was executed by the late Sir John Steele.

BADGE OF QUEEN ALEXANDRA'S IMPERIAL MILITARY NURSING SERVICE 172

BELT CLASP OF QUEEN ALEXANDRA'S IMPERIAL NAVAL NURSING SERVICE 172

BADGE OF THE ARMY NURSING SERVICE RESERVE 172

BADGE OF QUEEN ALEXANDRA'S IMPERIAL NAVAL NURSING SERVICE 172

SIR FREDERICK TREVES 176
 (*From the painting by Luke Fildes, at the London Hospital Medical College.*)

MISS CHADWICK, R.R.C. 180
 Matron, The Curragh, Ireland.

MISS ADDAMS-WILLIAMS, R.R.C. 180
 Principal Matron, South Africa.

LIST OF ILLUSTRATIONS

	TO FACE PAGE
MISS ANNIE B. SMITH, R.R.C.	180
Matron of the Royal Victoria Hospital, Netley.	
MISS GARRIOCK, R.R.C.	180
Matron of the Royal Herbert Hospital, Woolwich.	
SIR JOHN FURLEY	184
MISS CADENHEAD	196
Head Sister, Royal Naval Hospital, Haslar.	
MISS FRENCH	196
Head Sister, Royal Naval Hospital, Plymouth.	
MISS ALICE MARY HALL	196
Lady Superintendent, Seamen's Hospital, Greenwich.	
MISS GRAHAM KNIGHT	196
Lady Superintendent, Seamen's Hospital, Albert Docks.	
MISS LOUISA TWINING	216
Pioneer of Workhouse Nursing Reform.	
(*Photo: Elliott & Fry.*)	
MISS MARIA FIRTH	272
Founder and First Superintendent of the London Association of Nurses.	
WILLIAM RATHBONE, ESQ., M.P.	288
The Originator of Trained District Nursing.	
(*By permission of Miss Eleanor Rathbone, Author of "William Rathbone—A Memoir."*)	
MRS. DACRE CRAVEN, *née* FLORENCE LEES	292
(*Photograph by Barrauds.*)	
MISS AGNES JONES	292
Founder and First Superintendent of the Workhouse Nurses' Training-School, Liverpool.	
MISS HADDEN	296
Superintendent, Metropolitan District Nurses' Home, Bloomsbury.	
MISS M. LAMONT	296
Superintendent, Queen Victoria Jubilee Institute for Nurses—Irish Branch.	
MISS PRITCHARD	296
Inspector for Wales of the Queen Victoria Jubilee Nurses.	

The Royal Red Cross 376
Badge of the Royal British Nurses' Association . . . 376
Order of the Hospital of St. John of Jerusalem . . . 376
Badge of the Colonial Nursing Service 376

THE HISTORY OF NURSING IN THE BRITISH EMPIRE

CHAPTER I

NURSING BEFORE 1840

Pagan indifference to the sick—St. Paul institutes deaconesses—The life and work of St. Paula—Nursing an outcome of religious devotion—Rise of general hospitals—The Hospitalières—The Hôtel Dieu—Influence of the Crusades—The Abbess Hildegarde founds a school—Nursing in monastic infirmaries—Medical Brotherhoods—The Knights Hospitallers employ women—The Grey Sisters—The Béguines—Sisters of St. Elizabeth—A new era of nursing—St. Vincent de Paul—Founds the Association of Charity—Madame de Gondi—The Ladies of Charity—Remarkable influence of St. Vincent—Duchess d'Aiguillon—Madame Goussault—Madame le Gras—St. Vincent founds the Sisters of Charity—The establishment of the Sisterhood—St. Vincent's rules—Spread of the Sisterhood—They undertake every branch of nursing—Not cloistered nuns—The humanitarian spirit—First hospital nurses in London—St. Bartholomew's—St. Thomas's—Guy's Hospital—Quaint rules—Deterioration of nursing—Dr. Gooch attempts reform in 1825—Letters to Southey—"Religious female physicians"—England apathetic—Kaiserswerth founded—Its influence on nursing in this country.

BEFORE the Christian Era neither doctors nor nurses were in fashion. To quote one of Florence Nightingale's terse sentences, "Christ was the Author of the nursing profession." In Pagan times, those who had knowledge of the healing art practised it under the cloak of mystery. The sick and infirm were looked at askance, as people suffering from the displeasure of the gods, and therefore removed from the plane of sympathy. The survival of the fittest was concurred in with brutal stoicism, and the unfit left to pay the penalty of nature unheeded and uncared for.

The poor little "wasters" whom one sees in the wards of our hospitals, being lovingly tended until the flickering life is nursed back to some degree of health and vigour, would have been made short work of by our Pagan forefathers. "What will be the future of this child?" I involuntarily asked, when standing by the cot of a baby-girl of fourteen months old, who had been brought into hospital in a neglected and emaciated condition, and was reported not to have a sound organ in her puny body. "We shall bring her round," said the sister, and quoted the jocose remark of the doctor, who, when a doubt was expressed as to whether baby would live, replied, "Live! Yes, she will probably live to be the mother of a criminal." Poor little mite, there was sad truth in the cynicism. Still, the claim which even the most unpromising life has for the healing treatment is a tenet of the Christian faith, which differentiates it from the Pagan.

Not that the ancients altogether ignored the claims of the sick and wounded. The army of Xerxes carried hospital tents for the wounded soldiers, and the Roman camp had its valetudinarium. Before the Christian Era, the Hindus and Buddhists had houses for the sick, but the nursing was done by men. Amongst the Druids of Gaul were wise women, who treated the sick. In early times there was a disposition to treat anything connected with the curing or relief of disease as emanating from spirits, and the wise women, skilled in the treatment of the sick, were dubbed witches or sorceresses, in the same way that a physician was held in awe as a magician practising an occult art.

St. Paul was the pioneer of the nursing movement in the first century of the Christian Era, inasmuch as, with admirable perspicacity, he called the women of the early Church to the work of caring for the sick and infirm. The order of deaconesses which the apostle instituted was the prototype of modern religious and nursing sisterhoods. St. Chrysostom, in the fourth century, mentions forty deaconesses working amongst the sick and poor at Constantinople.

In the records of these early times the personality of that noble Roman lady, St. Paula, stands out in bold relief. A descendant of the Scipios and the Gracchi, she was born in Rome in 348 A.D. Early left a widow, Paula determined to devote her time and her wealth to the cause of the sick and suffering. Rome, still in the bonds of Paganism, did not respond to her humanitarian efforts, and with the remains of her fortune she sailed in 385 for Palestine, and at Bethlehem of Judæa, fit cradle for such an enterprise, established a community of women devoted to prayer and good works, and established a hospital for the sick. The community were under no vows and made no profession, but they lived an austere life and spent their days in making clothes for the poor, tending the sick of the district and the pilgrims overtaken by disease during their sojourn in the Holy Land. The community had a spiritual superior in St. Jerome, the friend and Master of Paula, with whom she read and studied. She is said to have had the care of the Saint when he was sick, and found him a difficult patient.

Paula began her work in a poor little house at Bethlehem, assisted by her daughter, and gradually drew around her a community of women like-minded. Later she built a hospital or Hospice on the road to Jerusalem for the benefit of sick pilgrims, and also a monastery for St. Jerome. After her death she was canonized by the Roman Church. The story of her life contains this description of St. Paula— "She was marvellous debonair, and piteous to them that were sick, and comforted them and served them right humbly; and gave them largely to eat such as they asked; but to herself she was hard in her sickness and scarce, for she refused to eat flesh, how well she gave it to others and also drink and wine. She was oft by them that were sick, and she laid the pillows aright and in point; and she rubbed their feet and boiled water to wash them; and it seemed to her that the less she did to the sick in service, so much the less service did she to God, and deserved she less mercy; therefore she was to them piteous and nothing to herself." Such is the quaint and beautiful picture of the nurse fifteen hundred years ago.

Nursing was originally an outcome of religious devotion. In the fourth and fifth centuries pious ladies, following the example of St. Paula, made it their vocation to care for the sick. The pilgrims who flocked to the Holy Land often fell ill by the way or during their sojourn contracted strange Eastern diseases. Hospices were founded on the pilgrim routes, and devout women counted it a duty and a privilege to nurse those stricken while on holy pilgrimage.

Then came the rise of general hospitals, and the demand for nurses increased. The first hospital of the kind was the Hôtel Dieu, founded at Lyons in 560 A.D. A hundred years later an Hôtel Dieu was established in Paris by Landry, Bishop of Paris. Nursing sisters, known as *Hospitalières*, were attached to these institutions. They gave their services and nursed from motives of piety, but were not nuns. Pope Innocent IV., thinking it desirable that they should have a recognized standing, placed them under the Augustine rule. The noviciate or period of training was for one year. The *Sœurs Hospitalières* grew into a large body, and to them were entrusted, in conjunction with lay brothers, the nursing care of hospitals as they were established. For five hundred years they remained the only organized nursing sisterhood. An old wood engraving preserved in the Burgundy Library at Brussels shows a ward in the Hôtel Dieu, Paris, with the *Hospitalières* performing their duties. The nurses look very imposing in their ample dresses, large aprons, and dark hoods, and the ward appears to be most generously staffed. The patients are seen lying two in a bed. In one case a dying patient is receiving the last offices of the church from a priest, and it may be imagined that the situation was not exhilarating for his bed-fellow. In the foreground of the picture two nurses are seen kneeling on the floor in the act of tying up some sacks which it is not improbable contain the dead. Putting two or more patients into a bed was a common practice in hospitals nearer home. For example, at the old London Hospital of St. Mary's Spital, there were great beds made to accommodate four patients side by side, as shown in a copy of an old print on page 22.

As in modern times the Crimean War gave the impetus to the nursing movement, so in mediæval days the Crusades formed a similar incentive. In the eleventh and twelfth centuries there was a great increase in the hospices for the sick pilgrims and the wounded Crusaders who had gone to their rescue, and a consequent call for nurses.

The Abbess Hildegarde, with a view to meeting this demand, founded in the twelfth century a school for nurses at her convent of Rupertsberg, near Bingen on the Rhine. Hildegarde made a special study of the art of healing. She cultivated medicinal plants, and in the convent garden instructed her nuns in the properties of herbs. She gave lessons in the compounding of simples and in the dispensing of medicines. Her nurses ga ne practical experience amongst the sick poor who flocked to the convent infirmary.

Hildegarde, according to the custom of the time, used her knowledge of disease to impress the credulous. She was a visionary and a mystic, and claimed the gifts of a miraculous healer. She was resorted to by persons of all ranks. She died, at the age of eighty-three, in 1180, and left behind her the "Jardin de Sante," a kind of *materia medica*, which gives an interesting idea of the knowledge and principles accepted in the Middle Ages concerning plants, minerals, and poisons, and which was doubtless reverently handed down to successive bodies of nurses at her school of Rupertsberg. Hildegarde was a great personage, the correspondent of popes and emperors, and was eventually canonized.

Hildegarde was not alone in the attention she paid to the treatment of disease. Other notable abbesses in mediæval times were skilled in such matters, and nuns studied the art of nursing. Before hospitals sprang up, the early religious foundations charged themselves with the care of the poor and the sick. In the monk's refectory was supper, a bed of straw before the fire, and a breakfast in the morning for the homeless wayfarer, and for the sick there was the conventual infirmary, where the serving brethren taught medicine and surgery to the sisters who tended the patients. In those days the line of demarcation between doctor and nurse was not so clearly defined as it later became. Women were permitted to practise surgery, and Abelard, in his letters to the nuns of the Paraclete Convent, urged them to learn surgery for the benefit of the poor. The sisters also were skilled in the compounding of medicines, and had their gardens of herbs. "From conventual hospitals," writes Lacroix, "were recruited the men and women who devoted themselves entirely to tending the sick." There were also a number of matrons and elderly women who belonged to a corporation which was specially employed upon obstetric medicine, at that time forbidden to men.

The nursing sisters under religious rule gained good practical experience in the infirmary attached to their religious house, and also in the public room for the reception of the sick, which formed part of all large monastic institutions. This public room or hall for the sick poor, was the prototype of the out-patients' department of a modern hospital, for thither came the indigent sick, the halt and the lame, and the casualty cases of the countryside, to be treated by the brethren and sisters. Neither did these early nurses lack difficult and interesting cases, for the Crusaders, returning from the Holy Land, were often the victims of strange diseases, contracted in the East, which to-day would be nursed with absorbing interest in our Tropical schools of medicine. Also the holy relics preserved in priory and monastery drew patients of high and low degree, afflicted with all manner of complaints. Monarchs and great prelates sought healing at the monasteries. If they recovered it was of course a miracle, but to-day one sees in these recoveries testimony to the medical knowledge of the monks and the good nursing by the brethren and sisters.

These conventual nurses were not without instruction from the doctors of their day, who also belonged to the religious Orders. They had the benefit of the medical learning in the ancient texts, copied and handed down by the monks and ascetics and had gre latitude in their ministrations. At the beginning of the fifth century the practice of medicine and of surgery was free. No authorization was required, and a gifted sister combined doctoring, dispensing, and minor surgery along with her practical nursing. Many of the notable physicians and surgeons left their religious establishments and travelled through Europe in monastic attire to practise their skill, leaving the sick in the infirmaries at home to the care of the well-trained brethren and sisters.

Medical Brotherhoods devoted to the care of the sick and suffering also sprang up, the most notable being the Knights Hospitallers of the Order of St. John of Jerusalem or the Knights of Malta who built a hospital at Jerusalem in 1042, and afterwards removed to Malta, and the Knights Templars, or Soldiers of the Temple at Jerusalem, founded by nine Christian Knights in the year 1118. The Templars wore the mantle of Esculapius over their military attire to show that they united the art of healing with that of war. They grew into a rich and mighty Order and their establishments were church, almshouse, and fortress combined.

The Hospitallers were distinguished from the Templars by associating women in their healing work. They employed not only nursing sisters but sought the assistance of the various corporations of women in the care of the sick and wounded. At this period regular doctors were scarce, and the great ecclesiastical surgeons considered bleeding, cupping, and minor operations beneath the dignity of their attention, and left such matters to barbers and to women. The Hospitallers freely availed themselves of women attendants upon the sick, and accorded them honour and dignity. The early records do not go into the question of salary, but if Hugh of Lucca, the famous physician of Parma, received only a lump sum of six hundred livres for his services as long as he lived, one may safely assume that nurses were not paid extravagant fees. Indeed, the actuating principle in the care of the sick was religious duty, not professional gain.

The *Hospitalières*, whom we have seen were employed in the Hôtels Dieu, or first general hospitals, were succeeded by other Orders of nursing sisters. Among these were the *Sœurs Grises*, or Grey Sisters, who were under the rule of the Franciscan Order, just as the *Hospitalières* were under the Augustine rule. The Grey Sisters were not secluded in cloisters, took no vows of celibacy, but voluntarily devoted themselves to visiting the sick in hospitals, and in their own homes, and in other charitable deeds. They comprised women of all ranks, from queens to humble maidens. They underwent a period of one to three years' training for their work. Later, the Grey Sisters became a vocation apart.

Another important body of nursing sisters during the same period sprang up in Flanders under the name of the Béguines. They took no vows and might leave the community at any time. They wore black russet gowns and stiff white hoods. Their Béguinage at Ghent grew into a wonderful colony where six hundred sisters lived. They nursed, amongst other institutions, the ancient hospital of St. John, familiar to all visitors to Bruges. There one may still see the sisters tending the sick poor just as when they attracted the admiration of Howard the Philanthropist. "There are twenty of them," he writes in 1776; "they look very healthy; they rise at four, and are constantly employed about their numerous patients." He further relates, "They prepare as well as administer the medicines. The directress of the pharmacy last year celebrated her jubilee or fiftieth year of her residence in the hospital." In describing at the same period a visit to the principal hospital at Lyons, Howard refers to the sisters, " as making up as well as administering" all the medicines prescribed, "for which purpose there was a laboratory and apothecary's shop, the neatest and most elegantly fitted up that can be conceived."

While France had its *Hospitalières*, the Netherlands its *Béguines*, Germany had an order of nurses styled Sisters of St. Elizabeth, after that noble philanthropist, " Elizabeth of Hungary." They were attached to the hospitals, and dispensed in the pharmacie. When visiting their hospital in Vienna a little more than fifty years ago, Mrs. Jameson describes the Sisters of Elizabeth with their sleeves tucked up at work at the counter, weighing and compounding medicines in a most business-like manner. They had also an out-patients' department, and prescribed for the sick.

So through early and mediæval times women were organized as nursing sisterhoods. They were skilled in practical work, according to the light of the time; they treated disease, performed minor surgery, prepared and dispensed medicines, and appear to have been more or less independent of the doctors. The medical profession, as an organization, had not indeed come into being. Side by side the two branches for relieving human sickness had worked on religious lines. The first medical school was founded at the monastery of Monte Casino, and the first school for nurses by the Abbess Hildegarde at Rupertsberg. The noble art of healing had declined since the days of Hippocrates, and the men who professed it were regarded as alchymists, sorcerers, and the workers of charms. In the sixteenth century surgery and medicine first took rank as experimental science, and those who practised it were organized into the two great classes of physicians and surgeons. There appears to have followed a corresponding decline in the part which women played as healers of the sick. Irregularities, and disorders too, became rife in the monastic institutions, and the sisters under rule were, like the brothers, not free from reproach.

At the beginning of the seventeenth century a new era of nursing opened with St. Vincent de Paul, the humble shepherd lad, tending his father's flocks in the village of Pouy, who became the famous ecclesiastic and philanthropist of Paris, and founded organizations which contained the germs of most of the present-day social schemes. His Sisters of Charity were the most numerous and widespread organization of nurses ever founded.

The work began at Châtillon-des-Dombes, in the diocese of Lyons, where St. Vincent was a humble *curé*. It chanced one day that two young ladies of beauty and fortune, Madame de Chassaigne and Madame de Brie, entered the church, where St. Vincent was preaching. They were arrested by his words, and determined to quit their life of pleasure and devote themselves to the service of the poor. During an epidemic that decimated Châtillon they heroically worked amongst the stricken people. They also began to take poor families under their care. St. Vincent, however, felt that, to be effective, the work must be organized, and on December 12, 1617, in the hospital chapel, he founded the first of his schemes, the Association of Charity, the members of which pledged themselves to become the servants of the poor. Thirty similar associations quickly sprang up in the rural districts of France, and ladies of wealth and position devoted themselves to the work. Foremost amongst these was Madame de Gondi, a noble and saintly woman, in whose household St. Vincent had lived for many years as tutor to her sons. It was at her instance that he organized the Priests of the Mission, a lay brotherhood devoted to works of charity and religious missions, who had their central home at St. Lazare, Paris.

In Paris, too, St. Vincent later gathered around him influential women, who were banded into an association of Ladies of Charity. They devoted themselves to the care of the poor, to orphan and foundling children, and to the sick in the Hôtel Dieu. Four ladies together visited the hospital daily, no light undertaking, considering that at this period patients with infectious diseases were in the same ward, and sometimes put in the same bed as those suffering from non-contagious disease. The air was so offensive that the morning nurses entered the wards holding before their mouths a sponge saturated with vinegar. There is no record as to whether St. Vincent was a believer in ventilation, but, at any rate, his Ladies of Charity were instrumental in introducing various reforms into the Hôtel Dieu. Members of the Association also visited hospitals in the country districts of France, and, in modern phraseology, tried to raise the tone of nursing.

The good Saint had remarkable faculty for influencing young and beautiful widows. Indeed, the lives of many of his Ladies of Charity were as romantic as they were saintly. There was the Duchess d'Aiguillon, married at sixteen and a widow at eighteen, dowered with beauty and riches, an ornament of the Court, and destined by her uncle, Cardinal Richelieu, for the bride of a royal prince. She was a lady-in-waiting to Mary de Medicis, but left the Court to become a disciple of St. Vincent. Madame Goussault, wife of the President of the Court of Exchequer, left a widow and mother of five children when still in her prime, was President of the Ladies of Charity. She was a woman not only of piety, but of great prudence and common sense, and St. Vincent constantly sought her advice. Madame le Gras, *née* Louise de Marillac, also a young and beautiful widow, threw herself with special ardour into the work, and became the first Mother-General of the Sisters of Charity, the most famous outcome of St. Vincent's reforming crusade. The saint had also a marvellous influence over young girls. " Mademoiselle, you are not made for this world," he would sometimes say to the daughter of a house where he was calling, and the young lady not infrequently renounced the follies of fashionable life and entered the service of the poor. St. Vincent had a more effective way than merely preaching at the "smart set "; he inspired them to work.

For some time the Ladies of Charity laboured in Paris, meeting in each other's houses. Their enthusiasm was remarkable. They sold their jewels to give to the poor, and some of the noblest born dressed as servants and tended the sick in their own homes. The queen sympathized with the work, and it became a hobby of Court ladies. But, like most fashionable hobbies, it was not, in the majority of cases, very deeply rooted, and it soon became necessary to find dependable *bonâ fide* workers. Respectable young peasant girls were brought to Paris, and trained to visit the sick, under the direction of the Ladies of Charity. Next they were organized by St. Vincent, placed in a Home in Paris, under the care of Madame le Gras, and received the name of Sisters of Charity, later to be known throughout the civilized world as the Sisters of St. Vincent de Paul.

The first of the sisters to enroll was Marguerite Nazeau, a poor shepherdess, who had taught herself to read while minding her flock. Strict but simple rules were laid down by St. Vincent for the sisters, and they were governed and inspired in their duties by Madame le Gras, who was truly the Mother of the Sisters of Charity.

Thus founded in 1633, the organization spread, until in the course of twenty years two hundred houses and hospitals were established, and gradually the sisterhood spread all over Europe. In 1651, Madame le Gras, feeling that her own life and that of St. Vincent were drawing to a close, desired that the work should be perpetuated, and wrote to the Saint regarding a constitution for the sisters. A scheme was submitted to the Archbishop of Paris, and after some negotiations, a set of rules for the governance and guidance of the community was prepared, based upon those so long inculcated by Madame le Gras. When the letters of sanction were received, St. Vincent assembled the sisters on the 8th of August, 1655, and at a most solemn and impressive meeting sealed the act of their establishment. St. Vincent was Superior-General, and Madame Le Gras the Mother-General, Julienne Loret, first assistant, Mathurine Guérin, treasurer, and Jeanne Gressier, bursar. The sisters signed the document, and St. Vincent sealed it with the seal of his mission—Jesus Christ, with His arms extended to receive all who came to Him. This document of the incorporation of the Sisters of Charity, the most renowned nursing sisterhood in the world, is preserved in the National Archives in Paris. Every Wednesday until the close of his life St. Vincent came to explain to his dear sisters the rules which he had given them. "You, sisters," said he, "have given yourselves to God to assist the sick poor, not in one house only, as is done by the sisters of the Hôtel Dieu, but everywhere as our Lord did." The Saint did not wish them to be cloistered nuns. They were to leave their houses and go forth and visit the sick in every town, in every land, protected by the purity of their womanhood. They were to be in the world, though not of it. St. Vincent urged the virtues of chastity, humility, and poverty. He did not wish to have Superioresses in the houses; all the sisters were to be equal. A modest dress was designed to be worn by the sisters in all lands. When some suggested that the dress might be modified to meet different localities, St. Vincent replied, "It comes to this, that they will have as many different hats or bonnets as there are cities and countries." He permitted no deviation in costume. "You shall be known," was his constant reminder, "as

Sisters of Chàrity, servants of the sick poor. Oh, what a beautiful title!"

Madame Le Gras, the Mother-General, died March 15, 1660, and was by her own desire succeeded in that office by Sister Marguerite Chétif. A few months later, September 27, St. Vincent, now in his eighty-fifth year, also passed away. His heart was preserved in a silver case presented by the Duchess d'Aiguillon, one of the most famous of his Ladies of Charity, who had used her influence for the spread of the Sisters of Charity.

Though the sisterhood had lost its founders, it continued to go forward in the spirit which they had so nobly inculcated. From France they passed to Italy, Austria, Spain, Portugal, Ireland, and eventually to England and Scotland. They crossed the Atlantic with the French settlers in Canada, and spread to the United States, where, during the Civil War, they administered to the needs of Northerner and Confederate alike. In the East they became familiar figures in the streets of Constantinople, Smyrna, Alexandria, Jerusalem, Damascus, Algiers, and penetrated into Persia, Abyssinia, and China, winning respect and admiration even from those who differed from them in religion. In the early stages of the Crimean War our soldiers had cause to bless the good sisters of St. Vincent de Paul. It was their ministrations to the wounded of our allies which moved England to send forth its Florence Nightingale and her "angel band."

The sisters founded more than two thousand houses, and established hospitals, schools, orphanages, crèches, and workshops. There is no branch of modern nursing which they did not initiate. They nursed in the hospitals all over the continent, tended the sick poor in their own homes, ministered to the soldiers on the battlefield in the campaigns of 1652–58, took charge of military hospitals in besieged towns. They were conspicuous at the siege of Dunkirk, and in the military hospitals established by Anne of Austria at Fontainbleau. They were to be found in Naval hospitals, and nursed the galley-slaves, the most pitiful and neglected of all human beings, and also the criminals in prison. In plague-stricken Poland they went fearlessly amongst the sick. They survived the first French Revolution, when every other religious institution was condemned. After the Reign of Terror, the Consular Government established the sisterhood by a decree of the Minister of the Interior on the ground that, " the services rendered to the sick can only be properly administered by those whose vocation it is and who do it in the spirit of love." It was decreed that, " Citoyenne Duleau, formerly Superior of the Sisters of Charity is authorized to educate girls for the care of the hospitals." In 1848, when the first faint dawn of our own modern nursing movement began, there were some twelve thousand women at work in the organizations of St. Vincent de Paul. Howard had noted their work in continental hospitals, and Elizabeth Fry and Florence Nightingale each bore her tribute to the labours amongst the sick of the good Sisters of Charity.

This remarkable organization marks the transition period between nursing as a strictly religious vocation and nursing from the humanitarian point of view. The *réligieuse*, who tended the sick in her conventual infirmary was chiefly actuated by the desire to perform meritorious deeds. She nursed as a penance, in the same spirit that she mortified the flesh by doing other menial offices, or by self-inflicted torture. Her own soul, not the body of the patient, was her chief concern. A devotee who desired to emulate saints and martyrs, chose the nursing of the sick poor as the most humiliating and disagreeable thing she could do, and hoped thereby to perfect her salvation.

St. Vincent de Paul taught his sisters that nursing and the care of the poor and distressed were a duty they owed to humanity. Women who wished to live apart from the world telling their beads in cloistered cell the world and perform her duties in all humility, counting herself a servant of the sick poor. Here we have, in the early dawn of the seventeenth century, the beginning of the humanitarian spirit which to-day actuates our social philanthropy, as manifested by the hospitals, infirmaries, asylums, and district nursing organizations, supported by the public all over the land. St. Vincent lived at the period when the religious brotherhoods and sisterhoods were in a state of decadence. There was licentiousness on one hand and over-religious zeal on the other. The sisters in the hospitals were so intent on proselytizing that even the Pope found it expedient to publicly admonish them. St. Vincent's aim was to found a sisterhood whose functions were more strictly limited to the duties of nursing.

The first hospital nurses in London were the sisters attached to St. Bartholomew's, the first general hospital established in the Metropolis. It was founded by Rahere in 1102 on its present site close to the old Priory. The "staff" at the Dissolution consisted of a master, eight brethren, and four sisters, living under the Augustine rule, with three surgeons and one physician. They made up one hundred beds. It requires a stretch of the imagination to picture "Barts" in those days, when it stood in saintly isolation on the outskirts of the city, its wards tended by brethren and sisters in religious garb, and its affairs administered by the Prior. The butchers of Smithfield did not then ply their trade without its gates. The Rahere Ward of this most ancient and interesting hospital is a reminder of its early days.

St. Thomas's Hospital or almonry, founded considerably later near London Bridge in 1213, and dedicated to the martyr, St. Thomas-à-Becket, was nursed in similar manner by brethren and sisters, as also was St. Mary's Spital, which made up one hundred and eighty beds. So it will be seen that in pre-Reformation days a hospital system with physicians, wards, and nurses had sprung up, and we are inclined to think that the nursing was superior to that which prevailed later before the modern movement began.

The Dissolution of the Monasteries, 1525-40, gave the death-blow to early nursing. From conventual infirmary, monastic almonry, and hospital, the sick, the old, and the infirm were turned out to die in the streets, beg for alms and pity from door to door, or at best to drag their sick bodies to the miserable places which they called home. The sisters, like the patients, were driven forth, and many sought asylum in foreign lands. Whatever view may be held regarding the laxity of life and lapse of duty which prevailed in the great religious houses prior to the Reformation, it must be acknowledged that their dissolution told hardly on the poor and suffering, and was a great set-back to the beneficent care of the sick. For a time London was without hospitals, and the country districts without infirmaries for the sick poor. Six hundred religious establishments with their respective provision for the care of the suffering and helpless, were swept away. "No hospitals, no asylums, no almonries, no charities at all! No schools even!" writes Sir Walter Besant. "One cannot picture it, one cannot realize it."

Another chapter in early nursing opens with the reconstruction of the chief London hospitals on lay principles which later took place. St. Bartholomew's again opened its gates, and its "nursing staff" consisted of twelve sisters and a matron. There was, besides an hospitaller to receive the sick, discharge the convalescent, and administer religious comfort, a Renter clerk or secretary, a butler, and a porter. The matron, who now appears upon the scene of history, was enjoined to see that the sisters "do their duty unto the poor, as well in making of their beds and keeping their wards, as also in washing their clothes and other things." There were to be no idle hours for the new order of nurses; when not occupied in the foregoing duties they were to spin and do housework. The leading idea in these early regulations savoured of the old conventual spirit, special stress being laid on the fact that the sisters were to "charitably serve the poor in all their griefs and diseases." They were enjoined to cultivate habits of sobriety and discretion, and above all things to "avoid, abhor, and detest scolding and drunkenness, as most pestilent and filthy vices, and to shun the conversation and company of all men."

St. Thomas's Hospital, which sank into decay after the Dissolution, was repaired and enlarged for the relief of the sick and lame, by the citizens of London under the patronage of the young King Edward VI. A Charter of Corporation was granted for its foundation in 1553. A hundred years later a part of the hospital was reserved for the sick and wounded from the fleet during the war with the Low Countries. In 1732, St. Thomas's came to the front as a leading London hospital. It had been reconstructed, and now contained four hundred and eighty-five beds. There were twenty wards for the reception of patients. A sister, or "female superior," was in charge of each ward, and had under her two or three nurses. A matron controlled the domestic arrangements, and was the recognized head of the female staff. As at St. Bartholomew's, stringent rules were laid down for the conduct of the matron, sisters, and nurses, and one of the ancient regulations mentions chastisement with a birch rod as a form of correction for a refractory matron! Think of it, probationers!

In addition to the restoration of some of the hospitals originally founded under monastic rule, new institutions sprang up in London and other parts of the country as the result of private charity. The best known of these is Guy's Hospital, founded by Thomas Guy, a charitable citizen of London, in 1724. He had for many years been a generous benefactor to St. Thomas's Hospital, and was in the habit of sending there "diseased and friendless objects" to be provided for at his expense. Sixteen years before his death he built and furnished three wards at St. Thomas's Hospital for the reception of sixty-four patients, and rebuilt two large houses at the front of it. For eleven years he contributed one hundred pounds a year to St. Thomas's. Then it occurred to him that he would found a hospital himself on ground almost facing the old St. Thomas's, for the purpose of receiving the chronic and incurable cases dismissed or turned away from that institution. The eccentric old bachelor, who jilted the servant maid he had engaged to marry, because she presumed to countermand an order about a paving stone, died in 1725, before the hospital was completed, but his will contained a provision for its government and maintenance. The body of Thomas Guy rests in a stone vault amongst those of departed physicians and surgeons in the large and eerie crypt beneath the hospital chapel, which contains an elaborate monument to his memory. His statue stands in the quadrangle, and is illuminated on festive occasions. The hospital has been enlarged, and equipped far beyond the most enthusiastic dreams of its founder, and has, so far as modern exigencies permit, carried out his intention of specially benefiting the friendless poor, and those suffering from chronic disease. It was provided in his will that not only the incurable, but ordinary patients should be received into the wards of his hospital at the discretion of the authorities.

The nursing at Guy's in the old days was conducted on similar lines to that of St. Thomas's. From an examination of the old rules we find that there was a sister attached to each ward who had the care of the patients, and the superintendence of the nurses. A room for each sister was placed contiguous to her ward. The sisters attended operations, and exercised discretion in giving medicine during the night when it was not necessary "to call up the apothecary." "The sisters," we are informed, "are usually selected from a higher class of females than the nurses, and are frequently widows in reduced circumstances." Another quaint entry notifies that "the matron being advanced in years" requires an assistant. Evidently compulsory retirement on account of age was not then enforced.

A great feature at Guy's Hospital in the old days was the sister or head nurse (probably a portly widow "in reduced circumstances") sitting in state in the middle of the ward, and wearing suspended round her neck on a black ribbon, a large silver medal, bearing a representation of the hospital. Such a personage was calculated to instil the most frivolous young probationer with becoming awe. The nurse's medal is now a relic of the past, but the gold and silver nursing medals awarded at Guy's, though much less imposing in size, bear a portrait of the founder in flowing wig on one side, and on the reverse a representation of the hospital.

We cannot here attempt to trace in detail the decline and fall of nursing before the modern movement set in. The various hospitals as they sprang up all appear to have started on strict lines with regard to the conduct of their nurses, but without special provision for training. The ward sisters had learned by experience some amount of practical nursing, and they instructed the nurses within the narrow limits of their knowledge. Here came in the differentiation between the conventual and the lay nursing. The sisters of a religious community were often gentlewomen by birth, and superiorly educated for their times. They lived in an atmosphere of learning, and were instructed in the care of the sick by brethren skilled in medicine and surgery. Their conduct, too, was actuated by self-sacrifice, and a religious motive. The lay governors who succeeded the ecclesiastical rule in the old hospitals, though they started well, do not appear to have been able to maintain a respectable, to say nothing of an efficient, nursing standard. A calling which was without any standard for training naturally fell into the hands of uneducated women. Lacking knowledge, refinement, and the religious stimulus, which was a powerful factor in early times, the nurses in hospitals and kindred institutions had become, at the beginning of the nineteenth century, a social scandal, and a menace to the community.

Dr. Gooch, a distinguished physician, raised the question in 1825, in a series of letters published in the "Correspondence of Robert Southey." While touring in France and Belgium, Dr. Gooch had been much struck by the work in the hospitals of the Sisters of Charity. "Let all good Christians," he wrote, "join and found an order of women like the Sisters of Charity in Catholic countries; let them be selected for good plain sense, kindness of disposition, indefatigable industry and deep piety; let them receive—not a technical and scientific—but a practical medical education. For this purpose let them be placed as nurses and pupils in the hospitals of Edinburgh and London, or in the County Hospitals." He further suggested that they should be examined by competent physicians. He desired to see not mere nurses, but a set of "religious female physicians." Probably the good doctor went a little too far, and the faculty took fright. Southey was sympathetic with the views of Dr. Gooch, but nothing was accomplished.

While England remained apathetic, an epoch-making experiment was started in Germany by Pastor Fliedner, a humble Lutheran clergyman, and his devoted wife, which resulted in the establishment of the world-famous Kaiserswerth, near Düsseldorf on the Rhine, in 1836, for the training of Protestant deaconesses to tend the sick poor. It was the first training school for nurses on modern lines. It is not within the scope of this book to enter into a detailed history of Kaiserswerth, except so far as it influenced the pioneers of nursing in our own country. At the time of the Crimean War, Kaiserswerth had one hundred and ninety sisters and deaconesses, including sixty-two probationers. Of the sisters, eighty were stationed in different parts of Germany, five in London, three in Constantinople, five at Jerusalem, and two at Smyrna, and an important Deaconess Institution had been established at Pittsburg, United States. The starting of Kaiserswerth aroused some interest amongst the hospital authorities in this country, but did not produce any immediate result. In 1840, Elizabeth Fry visited the institution, and, inspired by what she saw, returned home to crown the efforts of her beneficent life by an attempt to raise the standard of nursing in her own land. As Kaiserswerth was the result of unprofessional and private enterprise, so also was the first institution for the training of nurses in England.

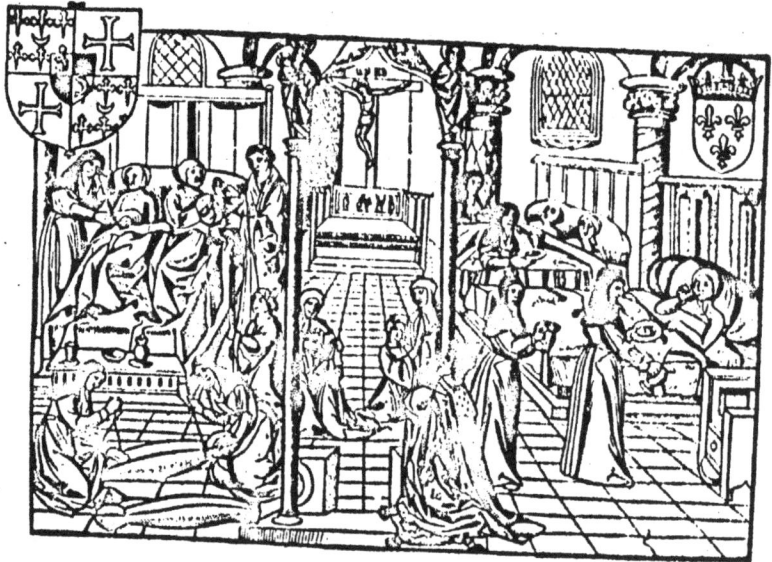

NURSING IN THE SIXTEENTH CENTURY.
A Ward in the Hôtel Dieu, Paris.
(*Facsimile of a wood engraving.*)

CHAPTER II

THE PIONEER WORK OF ELIZABETH FRY

Early life of Elizabeth Fry—Her marriage and settlement in London—Prison work—Friendship with Pastor Fliedner—The Deaconess Hospital at Kaiserswerth—Resolves to found a nursing sisterhood—Letter to the Bishop of London—Queen Adelaide becomes patroness—Queen Victoria interested—Failing health and death of Mrs. Fry.

To Elizabeth Fry belongs the honour of having founded the first known institution in this country for the training of nurses for the sick. The fact receives but little attention from her biographers, who, indeed, could hardly be expected to foresee that nursing would develop on such wide lines and attain to a position which would render its beginning a sign-post in the social history of the country.

Mrs. Fry was a woman of ideas as well as of philanthropy. Her tireless spirit was ever seeking a new outlet to benefit humanity. In her later years, when labour on behalf of prison reform had lifted her to a pinnacle of renown, the sight of a solitary coastguardsman pacing to and fro within view of her invalid's room at Brighton moved her with the desire to provide him with something to read, which resulted in the scheme for Coastguards' Libraries. In like manner, visits to the homes of the poor where sickness had no care or relief save fleeting charity, and her knowledge of the distress amongst people of limited means in time of illness, led her to devote the last years of her life to founding a nursing sisterhood. Thus the institution of trained nursing formed the coping-stone to the fabric of one of the noblest and most beneficent lives which the world has known.

The events in a life which had this important consummation may be briefly summarized. Elizabeth Fry was born May 21, 1780, in her father's town house in the city of Norwich, not at Earlham, as stated in the "Dictionary of National Biography," and was the third daughter of John Gurney, banker, a member of the Society of Friends. Her mother, Catherine Ball, was a descendant of John Barclay, the Apologist of the Quakers. The Gurneys were an old family highly esteemed in Norfolk. Elizabeth, the "dove-like Betsy" as her mother called her when a child, grew into a beautiful and attractive girl, full of spirit and somewhat self-willed. As her family did not follow the tenets of the strict Quakers, she had considerable latitude in dress and amusements. Indeed, Elizabeth was an acknowledged belle in quaint old Norwich, and considerably dazzled the provincial youths when she appeared at a county ball. In the vicinity of her father's country house of Earlham Hall, two miles from Norwich, she rode, light as a bird, in a scarlet riding-habit. She loved pleasure, and tripped about in coquettish scarlet shoes, but withal her young heart was overflowing with goodness.

A change came over the gay, buoyant girl in her eighteenth year, when she was deeply moved by William Savery, the American preacher, who was conducting services in Norwich. About the same time, too, she was impressed by a dream, in which she saw herself standing on the seashore, while the waves dashed up to engulf her. After she had resolved to devote herself to the cause of God and humanity she had a similar dream, only this time her feet were planted firmly on a rock, and the stormy waves could not disturb her. At nineteen, Elizabeth began philanthropic work by starting a class in a laundry for poor children. A year later, after some misgivings as to whether she should give up her maiden life and its freedom for work, she became the wife of Mr. Joseph Fry, a merchant in London. Mr. Fry, being a junior partner in his father's firm, had his house in St. Mildred's Court, close to his business, and there brought his bride.

The Frys were " plain ' Quakers, and the young wife conformed to the strict tenets of her husband's family. Her fair curls were tucked away beneath a plain-fitting Quaker cap, from which her pretty, girlish face looked forth with bewitching demureness. She wore a gown of Quaker grey, with a loose white handkerchief crossed over her bosom, and when she went out, a broad-brimmed beaver hat. She proved an exemplary wife and mother, and the first thirteen years of her married life were devoted chiefly to the care of her children, of whom she had nine. She saw a good deal of the misery of the London poor in the back streets near St. Mildred's Court, especially in time of sickness, and often ministered to their wants. At "meeting" she became known as a speaker of remarkable power, and the pathos of her voice gave promise of the marvellous effect which it was destined to exercise over the prisoners in Newgate. At twenty-nine years of age she was recognized as a "minister" in the Society of Friends.

When, on the death of his father, in 1809, Mr. Fry removed from St. Mildred's Court to the family mansion of Plashet, in Essex, Mrs. Fry entered upon a life of extended influence. We see her as the dignified mistress of Plashet opening her house to the philanthropists of the day, and forwarding various movements for the relief of the poor and suffering, while to her humble neighbours she was ever the friend in need. Her hours of relaxation were spent with her children out in the woods and lanes, gathering roots to stock a wild-flower garden.

Mrs. Fry believed that every woman had her individual vocation, and in following it would fulfil her mission. As a very young girl, she had, at her own urgent request, been taken over a prison, and there saw misery which for ever engraved itself on her tender heart. Her active interest in prison reform began in February, 1813, when, with some other Quaker ladies, she went to visit the female prisoners in Newgate. There she found an appalling condition of things. Three hundred women and children were crowded into four rooms, with no other attendants, day or night, than two rough men. There was no classification of the prisoners; the innocent and guilty, tried and untried, misdemeanants and the worst felons, were all huddled together. Most of them were half naked, and they slept on the bare floor without bedclothes. They cooked and washed, ate and slept in the same room. While it was difficult to get food, the prison tap was always running for those who could procure money from their friends for drink. It was a scene of hell upon earth which met the eyes of Mrs. Fry and her friends. When describing it before the Committee of the House of Commons, she relates, with characteristic restraint, "the swearing, gaming, fighting, singing, dancing, and dressing up in men's clothes were too bad to be described, so that we did not think it suitable to admit young persons with us."

It was not, however, until four years later, 1817, that Mrs. Fry was successful in organizing a scheme of amelioration. She got a matron appointed, started a school for the children of the prisoners, obtained permission to visit the condemned women, and started Bible readings in the prison. She founded the British Ladies' Society for the Relief of Female Prisoners, and upon the board sat eleven Quakeresses and one clergyman's wife. Branch societies were ultimately formed in the provinces, and machinery was set in motion which resulted in some measure of prison reform throughout the country. Mrs. Fry and her helpers roused public opinion until the House of Commons appointed a Committee to inquire into the state of the prisons, and many of her recommendations were adopted. There being no other place available, Mrs. Fry listened to the debates on what was practically her own measure through a ventilator in the House of Commons.

We cannot here follow Mrs. Fry through her years of strenuous work on behalf of prison reform, and other philanthropic work, but must pass to the period bound up in the history of nursing.

In the spring of 1840, Mrs. Fry, accompanied by her brother Samuel Gurney, his daughter Elizabeth, her friend, William Allen, and his niece, Lucy Bradshaw, visited the Continent, on a tour of prison inspection. At Berlin Mrs. Fry was entertained by and received great attention from the Prussian royal family, who were most favourable to her work. Passing on to Düsseldorf, she addressed the prisoners in jail, her words being interpreted by "a valuable man," Pastor Fliedner, who had, during a visit to London, witnessed Mrs. Fry's work for prison reform, and on his return home founded at Düsseldorf, in 1826, the first German society for improving prison discipline. At the time of Mrs. Fry's visit the "valuable man" was at the head of the Kaiserswerth Institution, which he and his devoted wife were developing. Founded in 1836, it had its beginning in 1833 in a small summer-house in the pastor's garden, where Madame Fliedner received destitute discharged female prisoners. At the time of Mrs. Fry's visit in 1840 the Deaconess Hospital at Kaiserswerth was not only training its own body of "nursing sisters," but was sending out branches which resulted in the foundation of kindred institutions throughout Germany. Kaiserswerth was the parent of all Protestant nursing institutions, and it is impossible to over-estimate its influence on the early growth of nursing. There our own Florence Nightingale, Agnes Jones, and others distinguished in the world of nursing were trained, and there Mrs. Fry received, as we have seen, the inspiration which resulted in the establishment of the first institution for training nurses in this country.

Mrs. Fry was quick to act, and two months after her return home, started, July, 1840, a "Society of Sisters of Charity," to visit and attend the sick. Mrs. Fry's daughter, writing on the subject, says: "Mrs. Fry's habitual acquaintance with the chamber of sickness, and with scenes of suffering and death, had taught her the necessity that exists for a class of women to attend upon such, altogether different and superior to the hireling nurses that are generally to be obtained. Her connection with M. Fliedner, and all she learned from him, personally and by letter, of his establishment at Kaiserswerth, stimulated her desire to attempt something of the kind in England."

Before the period at which she instituted trained nurses, Mrs. Fry had been passing through the furnace of affliction and trial. Business reverses had reduced her husband from affluence to straitened means. They had left their beautiful home of Plashet and settled in an unpretentious house in Upton Lane, within sight of Greenwich Park. It was close to the grounds of Ham House, the residence of Mrs. Fry's brother, Mr. Samuel Gurney, and in her sister-in-law Mrs. Fry found a valuable helper in her various schemes. Her own health was broken, and she had had much anxiety through severe illnesses, and several deaths in her immediate family, and these circumstances played their part in turning Mrs. Fry's attention to the need of trained nurses for families of the middle and the wealthier classes, as well as amongst the destitute poor. A mishap, by which Mrs. Fry herself nearly poisoned a sick daughter whom she was nursing, also brought vividly home to her the risks run by the amateur nurse. To quote her own account of the incident, she writes in her diary, May, 1841: "Our dearest L—— being again extremely ill, I, in my hurry, gave a wrong medicine of a poisonous nature; my fright at first was inexpressible. We sent for the doctor, who gave an emetic." Fortunately, the patient recovered. This occurred a few months after Mrs. Fry had started her nursing scheme, and doubtless tended to confirm her in the wisdom of the enterprise.

The profound respect which Mrs. Fry's character and work inspired in high places, brought helpful patronage to her venture. Amongst the archives of the institution is a letter to the Bishop of London, which we reproduce in facsimile.

"Upton, 5th Month, 1841.

"Elizth Fry presents her respects to the Bishop of London [Dr Blomfield] and if convenient to the Bishop to receive her she proposes calling upon him in St James's Sq^{re} about twelve o'clock this morning as the Queen Dowager wished the Bishop of London would inform Elizth Fry his views respecting the new institution for the Protestant Sisters of Charity. Elizth Fry would have written before had not the illness of her daughter made it so very uncertain whether she could attend to any engagement for a future day."

"To the Bishop of London."

The interview was given, and Mrs. Fry records in her diary: "June 28th, 1841. My sister Gurney [Mrs. Samuel Gurney] and my dear friend Charlotte Upcher, went with me to the Bishop of London on Sixth Day, on the subject of the Sisters of Charity. It has been a great pleasure to me, the Queen Dowager giving her name as patroness."

The letter in which Earl Howe communicated the willingness of Queen Adelaide to give her patronage to the new society, runs as follows:—

"Bushey House,
"July 8, 1841.

"My Dear Mrs. Fry,

"Queen Adelaide commands me to state with what sincere pleasure she will place her name in your Society of Sisters of Charity. Her Majesty adds that you may call upon her as an extra nurse if *short-handed*.

"Seriously, it is satisfactory to find any little objection the Archbishop had felt now removed, and Her Majesty will gladly become an annual subscriber to your excellent and, I am satisfied, most useful institution.

"Believe me, with the greatest respect,
"Very truly and faithfully,
"Howe."

Although Earl Howe did not, like his Royal mistress, facetiously offer his services as an emergency nurse, he was, on his own account, a generous subscriber to the society.

There appears to have been some objection taken by the Archbishop or the Bishop of London to the title of "Sisters of Charity," which Mrs. Fry first gave to her nurses; and Queen Adelaide later wrote to Mrs. Fry suggesting that the name should be changed to "Nursing Sisters," which was accordingly done.

Through the influence of the Queen Dowager, the young Queen, who was married in the year that the nursing institution was founded, took great interest in the scheme, and received Mrs. Fry at Buckingham Palace. One feels sure that when Queen Victoria endowed a training institute for district nurses with the women's jubilee gift her thoughts travelled back to the early efforts of Elizabeth Fry to initiate trained nursing for the sick poor. The Duchess of Gloucester was one of the first patronesses of the "Nursing Sisters," and the famous portrait of Mrs. Fry, by George Richmond, was dedicated to the Duchess of Gloucester "at the wish of Mrs. Fry's family in acknowledgment of Her Royal Highness's uniform kindness and encouragement to her in her benevolent labours." Mrs. Fry was also supported in her nursing scheme by Harriet, Duchess of Sutherland, Mistress of the Robes to the young Queen, the Marchioness of Cholmondeley, the Dowager Lady

Grey, and by the liberality of Mrs. Hoare, and various members of the Fry and Gurney families, and other philanthropic people.

Failing health prevented Mrs. Fry from taking an active part in the management of the institution which she had founded. The work was carried on by her daughter, who acted as hon. secretary, and her sister-in-law, Mrs. Samuel Gurney, the hon. treasurer, and by a committee of ladies in sympathy with her aims. Mrs. Fry remained president of the institution until her death. During her last illness she was attended by one of her own nursing sisters. She passed to rest Oct. 12, 1845, with these characteristic words upon her lips—" Love ! all love ; my heart is filled with love to every one."

CHAPTER III

THE INSTITUTION OF NURSING SISTERS

Institution founded, 1840—The rules and regulations—Training of the sisters—First staff of nurses enrolled—Lady Inglis becomes president—Growth of the institution—Quaint rules—Present regulations—Letter from Thackeray—Devoted service of the Committee—The lady superintendent—Contemporary nursing in America and abroad.

THE first institution for the training of nursing sisters was, as we have already seen, founded July, 1840, by the most famous woman philanthropist of modern times under the patronage of royal and distinguished persons. The first meeting of the ladies' committee was held in a house at White Hart Court, E.C., and there the first candidates tremblingly presented themselves for selection. The Nurses' Home was first established at Raven Row, Whitechapel, within easy distance of the London Hospital, where some of the probationers were sent for training, and also in the midst of a poor population, to whom the sisters freely ministered in sickness when not otherwise engaged.

Raven Row, which is historic as the locality of the first Nurses' Home, is to-day a squalid little turning by the Eastern Post Office, Whitechapel, and one imagines that it was not very salubrious in 1840. A dirty card in a broken and patched window, bearing a scrawl, "Here lives a good nurse," surmounted by Jewish characters, was the only reminder I recently found of the connection of Raven Row with nursing.

In the summer of 1841, the sisters and the ladies of

the Committee met at Raven Row to celebrate the first anniversary of the Institution—an historic athering viewed in its relation to the present widespread nursing movement. A year later (1842), the sisters removed to a new Home in Devonshire Street, Bishopsgate, and the venture being now on a business footing, a salaried superintendent and secretary were appointed to oversee the little household of nurses and conduct the affairs of the Institution. The first superintendent, Mrs. Kennion, was "passing rich on forty pounds a year." But, alas for human frailty, this good lady, several years later, incurred the displeasure of the Committee "by privately leaving the Home for her marriage without making a communication." This breach of conduct is severely commented on in the minute-book, and it was certainly a bad example for probationers. However, the institution survived the shock, and we may charitably suppose that the privacy of the superintendent's marriage was the result of extreme modesty on her part, or possibly a thoughtful attempt to save the nurses the expense of subscribing for a wedding present.

The Home was removed to larger premises at 16, Broad Street Buildings, E.C., in the spring of 1847, and in 1850 it made yet another removal to 4, Devonshire Square, Bishopsgate. These premises were subsequently purchased by the Committee in 1872, and still remain the Home of the Institution.

The rules and regulations for the nursing sisters were drawn up in accordance with Mrs. Fry's idea, that the care of the sick was a Christian duty to be undertaken by women who brought a religious spirit as well as aptitude and intelligence to the task. At that time the hireling nurse was, broadly speaking, a scandal to the community, and Mrs. Fry's aim was to lift nursing out of coarse and sordid conditions into the higher realm of work performed, in the first instance, for its own sake. She did not lose sight of the fact that "the workman is worthy of his hire," and provision was made for the payment, free board, lodging, and clothing of the sisters upon lines which left their minds untrammelled by too much consideration of personal profit. Still the nurses were to be something more than good earnest women desirous of tending the sick. They were to be a trained and organized body. Mrs. Fry's power of mind was equal to her goodness of heart, and she invariably made organization the pivot of her philanthropic reforms. An examination of the rules for her nurses, the first, it must be remembered, to be drawn up in this country, show that in Mrs. Fry's scheme lie the germs which have sprung into being in the numberless institutions and training homes for nurses throughout the land.

The aim and object of the Institution of Nursing Sisters is thus set forth by Mrs. Fry and her helpers. It was founded with "a view of supplying a deficiency long felt and complained of by the public, that of experienced, conscientious, and Christian nurses of the sick ; and also to raise the standard of this useful and important occupation, so as to engage the attention and enlist the services of many who may be desirous of devoting their time to the glory of God, and for the mitigation of human suffering.

"The plan on which it proceeds is simply this— conscientious, religious women are selected with great care, and their characters minutely inquired into. They are then placed in one of the public hospitals, and regularly trained for a certain period, in order to prepare them for the performance of their important duties. At the expiration of this period of probation, if their conduct and qualifications be found satisfactory, they are received as sisters, supplied with an appropriate dress, and a copy of rules for the regulation of their conduct. They are allowed an annual stipend, and maintained in a Home provided for them during the intervals of their engagements in private families or hospitals. A part of their leisure time whilst here is devoted to the gratuitous nursing of the sick poor in the densely peopled and wretched districts that immediately surround their Home."

The account goes on to explain that it is hoped " to secure an asylum for the valuable women (when past labour) the vigour of whose days shall have been thus spent." The spirit of this was later realized by the Superannuated Pension Fund.

The rate of payment to be charged to the public was a matter of anxious consideration. Mrs. Fry's great object was to provide trained nurses for a fee suited to the pockets of people of straitened and of moderate means. In the early stages of the institution, those employing the services of the nurses remunerated according to their ability, later a guinea a week became the recognized fee for a nurse, less being taken under exceptional circumstances, while it was left to the generosity of the better-off people to supplement the fee by gifts to the funds of the society.

"The sisters," runs the account, "are not permitted to receive any private remuneration, and it is requested that in no case they be informed of the amount paid for their services, as it is desired that their minds should be kept perfectly free from secular matters, to attend to their own sufficiently responsible duties."

The nurses were principally selected from the higher domestic or small farming and trading classes. No probationer was admitted who could not read and write, which meant a higher social distinction then than now. Mention is not made of a knowledge of arithmetic, and possibly this was not insisted on, lest it might lead to a worldly calculation of profits! Though the candidate was required to be of "unblemished reputation and Christian faith," she was allowed freedom as to her creed provided it was Protestant. After successfully passing the term of training (which at first was only three months), the probationer received a certificate from the matron of her particular hospital—Guy's granted the first certificates to Mrs. Fry's nurses—which was laid before the Committee, who, if they in all respects approved the candidate, bestowed a certificate printed on vellum and stamped with the stamp of the institution. On receipt of this the probationer passed to the position of a sister, and began active work under the Superintendent of the Home. On a sister ceasing her engagement she was required to return her certificate to the Board of Management, an excellent precaution to prevent the public being imposed on by a possibly untrustworthy nurse.

The regulations for dress and conduct were rigid. The sisters were to wear " a neat and becoming uniform," consisting indoors of print dresses, voluminous aprons—brown holland for the probationers—and plain muslin caps. The outdoor uniform was a quaintly cut dress of Quaker grey stuff with long black cloak, and black bonnet, having no trimming save a long black veil. In no case were " gold ornaments or jewellery, lace, embroidery, feathers, or artificial flowers " to be worn. There is, however, a shocking tradition that some of Mrs. Fry's nurses smuggled pink roses into their bonnets! The flesh was weak even in " the good old times!" Judging from some of the minute-book entries there appears at first to have been some trouble in satisfactorily arranging the sumptuary laws. Some objection about dress having been raised on the part of the sisters, the Committee promptly enacted that the sisters should *always* appear in the dress of the institution. Another item refers to shawls for the sisters, which were to be " of black silk, the lining to be selected by Mrs. Bradshaw."

In regard to the age of a candidate, no hard-and-fast rule was laid down. She must give promise of steadiness and maturity of judgment, but must not be so far advanced in life as to be unfit for active exertion. The engagement was for three or five years, subject to three months' notice by the sister if for good and sufficient reasons she wished to retire.

There were strict rules to prevent unseemly levity of

conduct. Male visitors were not admitted to the Home ; neither was a sister allowed to enter a place where spirits were sold, or to bring spirits into the house.

The early records of the institution are not absolutely stainless. We find occasionally a sister dismissed for breach of the rules, and one for " haughty and imperious conduct." It is further set down that " some of the sisters have been seen entering places where spirits are sold, and inviting each other to partake of the same ! " How the Sairey Gamps and Betsey Prigs of that day must have chuckled over these little lapses on the part of the " new-fangled nurses."

The training given to these pioneer nurses could not be other than very elementary, but if they did not get lectures on anatomy, physiology, and hygiene, they at least obtained some practical experience in the hospital wards. I have heard the training of these early days described "as much cleaning, scrubbing, and polishing, varied by sitting at the bedside or standing in the out-patients' department." It greatly depended on the good-will of the head ward nurses as to how much knowledge the probationers were allowed to obtain, and some were not well-disposed towards the new invasion, and promptly hurried the probationers away when the doctors came round, and there was anything likely to be learned. Even the old-fashioned ward nurse or sister could be cryptic and dragon-like, and more intent on magnifying her office than on imparting information. At first the training period was for three months, then six months, rising later to one year, at which it remained stationary for a long time. The institution paid a training fee of a guinea a week to the hospital for each probationer.

The first probationers were sent to Guy's Hospital, an institution likely to commend itself to Mrs. Fry on account of the charitable aim of its founder to give special consideration to the poor in chronic illness, and the medical staff would be wishful to further the efforts of a philanthropist of Mrs. Fry's reputation. Others were sent to the London Hospital, but in 1842 such " was the uncleanly state of that establishment," a minute records, " that the secretary is desired by the Committee to inform the Committee of the London Hospital that unless an improvement be made the nursing sisters cannot be allowed to continue on duty there." The remonstrance had some effect, as the sisters did continue in the service of the " London." The simple circumstance is, however, noteworthy as instancing the good influence of the better class of nurse on the sanitary arrangements of the hospitals. The Augean stable must perforce be cleaned if decent women were to enter, and, small as was their number, Mrs. Fry's nurses did make their influence felt on the metropolitan institutions.

The work of the nursing sisters was threefold. They went as paid nurses into private families; they did district nursing gratuitously for the poor, and they joined the nursing staff of several of the London hospitals as well as receiving their probationary training in those institutions. We find in 1845 that some of the sisters were placed at Hanwell to become acquainted with mental nursing, others were sent to the Orthopædic Hospital, and to the newly founded German Hospital at Dalston. Their services became in demand by the clergy, and one finds now and again a sister engaged to take charge of the sick poor in a parish. When, in 1854, the Crimean War was raging, several of the sisters volunteered for service, and joined the ever-memorable band of nurses who went out with Florence Nightingale to Scutari. It will thus be seen that this pioneer institution supplied workers in all branches of nursing, civil and military, so far as the scant opportunity of the time afforded.

The first twelve sisters who passed the Committee may not be known to fame, and their knowledge and experience was limited; but it is of interest to record their names, as representing the first trained and certificated staff of nurses in this country. They were—

Sister Jane Wade	Sister Elizabeth Smith
„ Jane Frances	„ Ann Clift
„ Maria Godfrey	„ Elizabeth Barwick
„ Mary Tarling	„ Hannah Cornish
„ Mary West	„ Mary Cordingly
„ Mary Taylor	„ Sarah Holland

Points to be noted in this early organization are the application of the terms "sister" and "probationer" to the nurses, the adoption of a nurses' uniform, provision of a nurses' home, training at a hospital, the granting of certificates, government by a code of rules, and the careful selection of candidates, as to character, health, and age, at a time when the hireling nurse was often a woman of no character, and her age and health were not specially considered.

After the death of Mrs. Fry, Lady Inglis, who had been a prominent supporter, became president of the institution. Progress was, however, very slow. After it had been in existence for nearly seven years, Mrs. Fry's daughter wrote: "The exertions of this little society have been hitherto greatly circumscribed, and it may be looked upon more as an experiment than as an object attained. The help of the nursing sisters has been sought and greatly valued by persons of all classes, from royalty to the poorest and most destitute."

The real growth of the Institution began in 1872, after its removal to 4, Devonshire Square, and it is interesting to find it still flourishing in this secluded bit of old-world London, in the heart of the city, and close to the Meeting House, where Mrs. Fry's voice was often heard. The Quaker element is no longer represented in its management. The last of the grey-gowned ladies have long since disappeared from the Committee; but it remains a tradition of the institution that application for a nurse from a member of the Society of Friends receives priority of attention. The outdoor uniform of the sisters from your institution, and beg it to accept the other five pounds. With the thanks and good wishes of your obliged serv^t·

"W. M. THACKERAY.

"To Mrs. Robinson,
　"Lady Superintendent."

The Institution of Nursing Sisters continues its quiet course of prosperity, favoured by the patronage of Queen Alexandra and a list of influential ladies, and under the management of a singularly devoted committee. The hon. treasurer, Mrs. Julian Hill, niece by marriage of Rowland Hill, has discharged her duties since 1865, without a break, a truly noble record of honorary service. Mrs. Hill retains her early enthusiasm for the work, and allows no private considerations to interfere with her attendance at committee meetings. The excellent state of the finances attest her good business management. It is an interesting circumstance, taken in conjunction with his wife's long service to the institution, that Mr. Julian Hill was taken when a small boy to hear Mrs. Fry read to the prisoners in Newgate, a memory which to-day he reverently cherishes, although, at the time, he was bitterly disappointed at not hearing a criminal trial instead, a more exciting event from a boy's point of view. Mrs. Hill is ably assisted by Lady Mackenzie, the co-hon. treasurer, who has been on the committee for some years. Mrs. Rashdall, the hon. secretary, has been upon the committee since 1880, and the co-hon. secretary, Mrs. Main Walrond, has given her valuable services to the institution since 1875. Seldom has it fallen to the lot of a society to have had its honorary officers for such long periods. The Committee sit in the order of their length of service, and that spirit of old-time dignity which distinguished the early founders still prevails at Devonshire Square.

Miss Margaret Russell, the lady superintendent, was trained at Edinburgh Royal Infirmary and at University

College Hospital. She was matron at Stroud General Hospital before becoming superintendent at Devonshire Square. Miss Russell unites to her skill as a nurse excellent business faculty, and a deeply sympathetic interest in the traditions of the institution. Her assistant, Miss Martindale, it is interesting to find, comes of Quaker stock, and thus supplies a link with the past. The undeviating course of prosperity which has attended the institution seems like the continual benediction of its saintly founder.

In concluding this sketch of the pioneer nursing society in England, it is interesting to co-relate it to early efforts in other countries. Some attempt at trained nursing was made at the New York Hospital by Dr. Valentine Seaman, at the close of the eighteenth century. His course of lectures to nurses were chiefly on midwifery, but included anatomy, physiology, and the care of children. They were published in New York in 1800.

The first organized training school for nurses in America was the Lying-in Charity, of the Quaker city of Philadelphia, founded in 1828 by Joseph Warrington, M.D., a member of the Society of Friends. He belonged to the Medical Department of the University of Pennsylvania, and for many years was obstetric physician to the Philadelphia Dispensary. While performing the duties of that position he realized the need of trained maternity nurses for the poor. His institution was incorporated by an Act, dated May 7, 1832. The original title was "The Philadelphia Lying-in Charity for attending indigent females at their own homes," which was changed to its present title, "The Philadelphia Lying-in Charity," by special Act, dated May 12, 1888. The nurses are housed in a special home connected with the hospital during the intervals of their active work in the six districts of the city. Ellwood Wilson, M.D., assisted Dr. Warrington for many years in the medical service of the institution, and afterwards became president of the society, and collected funds for the erection of the present building, the cost of which was fifty thousand dollars. It is interesting to note that the first effort to establish systematic training for nurses in the United States was, as in England, due to the Quakers. Later, in 1838, the Quakers of Philadelphia started a Nurse Society to improve the standard of nursing and to share the work of tending the sick, then almost wholly in the hands of Roman Catholic Societies.

In Europe, the Deaconess Institution at Kaiserswerth, founded by Pastor and Madame Fliedner in 1836, was the first Protestant institution to train a nursing sisterhood. The influence of this organization on Mrs. Fry has been already referred to. It also supplied a trained matron and nursing staff to the German Hospital at Dalston, founded in 1845, a time when trained matrons were unknown in the London hospitals. That institution was founded under the auspices of Queen Victoria and King Frederick William IV. of Prussia, for the benefit of German residents in this country. A new building with a hundred beds was opened in 1864. The nursing staff, now largely obtained from the Sarepta Deaconess Institution at Bielfeld, consists of twenty sisters, including the head, and of five male attendants.

CHAPTER IV

CHARLES DICKENS AND NURSING REFORM

Caricature a factor in reform—Dickens creates Sairey Gamp—The character taken from life—Description of Mrs. Gamp—Betsey Prig of Bartlemy's—Mrs. Gamp as night nurse—They prepare their patient for a journey—Rupture of the famous partnership—No immediate reform after publication of Martin Chuzzlewit—Dickens laments state of nursing in hospitals.

THE next important event which followed the efforts of Elizabeth Fry in nursing reform, was the publication of "Martin Chuzzlewit," which struck a blow at the hireling nurse in the characters of Mrs. Gamp and Betsey Prig. Fiction and caricature have played an important part in social history by focussing abuses in so strong a light that men and women were compelled to look and condemn. Cruikshank gave the death-blow to hanging as a punishment for counterfeiting the old one-pound note by his ghastly caricatures, and Dickens combined with a skill never surpassed the art of the novelist with the aim of a social reformer. Poor Miss Flight, grown crazy with the hopelessness of prolonged litigation, aroused public indignation against the Court of Chancery, which ended in some measure of reform. Oliver Twist, the pauper lad, hungry-eyed and ever craving for "more," revealed the abuses of workhouse management and dealt a blow at "Bumbledom," which continues to this day. In like manner Sairey Gamp and Betsey Prig, the immortal examples of the private and hospital nurse of fifty to sixty years ago, have played an incalculable part in revealing the low status of nursing in the good old times, and to their creator belongs an honoured place in the roll of early nursing reformers. What "Uncle Tom's Cabin" was to the abolition movement, "Martin Chuzzlewit" was to nursing reform.

"In all my writings," says Dickens, "I hope I have taken every available opportunity of showing the want of sanitary improvements in the neglected dwellings of the poor. Mrs. Sarah Gamp was, four and twenty years ago, a fair representation of the hired attendant on the poor in sickness. The hospitals of London were, in many respects, noble institutions, in others very defective; I think it not the least among the instances of their mismanagement, that Mrs. Betsey Prig was a fair specimen of a hospital nurse, and that the hospitals, with their means and funds, should have left it to private humanity and enterprise to enter on an attempt to improve that class of person—since greatly improved through the agency of good women."

It was during the summer of 1842, while walking in the green lanes around the cottage he had hired at Finchley, that Dickens thought out the character of Mrs. Gamp. The original was an old nurse hired by a lady friend of the novelist's to take charge of a patient very dear to her, and the habits of this person as told to Dickens were faithfully portrayed; among them that peculiarity which Mrs. Gamp had of rubbing her nose along the top of the tall fender in her patient's room as she soliloquized and enjoyed the heat of the fire. Although Dickens called Mrs. Gamp a fair representation of the hireling nurse for the sick poor, it may be noted that he drew her from one attending in the house of wealthy people.

"Martin Chuzzlewit" began to appear in parts, January, 1843, and ran until 1844, when it was published in book form, and dedicated to the great heiress, Miss Coutts, subsequently to become the Baroness Burdett Coutts. Doubtless the revelations which it contained regarding the ways and characters of women entrusted with the care of the sick was an incentive to the philanthropic efforts of Miss Coutts in hospital reform, and has borne fruit in the many benefactions of the baroness to nursing institutions. It is clear from the preface to one of the later editions of "Martin Chuzzlewit," that Dickens had been accused of exaggeration in the portrayal of the characters. "I have never touched a character precisely from the life," he writes, "but some counterpart of that character has incredulously asked me, 'Now, really, did I ever really see one like it?' . . . Though Mrs. Gamp considers her portrait to be quite unlike, and altogether out of drawing, she recompenses me for the severity of her criticism on that failure by awarding unbounded praise to the picture of Mrs. Prig." Dickens admits, however, that "in writing fiction he never had any disposition to soften what is ridiculous or wrong," so we may take it that the characters of Mrs. Gamp and Mrs. Prig, though drawn from the life of his time, lost nothing in the telling.

A distinguished literary man and woman, whiling away time at a tedious reception, undertook to confess their mutual ignorance regarding literary masterpieces.

"I have never read 'Pilgrim's Progress,'" said he, with the air of a man who had let fall a bombshell. "And I," said she, after gasping with pious horror at her companion's confession, "have never read 'Pickwick.'" After that one would not be surprised to find that there are some people who have not read "Martin Chuzzlewit," and to whom "Sairey Gamp" is only a name mysteriously connected with umbrellas and nursing. In any case we make no apology for reviving her personality as an example of the old-time nurse. "She was a fat old woman, this Mrs. Gamp, with a husky voice, and a moist eye, which she had a remarkable power of turning up, and only showing the white of it. Having very little neck, it cost her some trouble to look over herself, if one may say so, at those to whom she talked. She wore a very rusty black gown, rather the worse for snuff, and a

shawl and bonnet to correspond. The face of Mrs.
Gamp—the nose in particular—was somewhat red and
swollen, and it was difficult to enjoy her society without
becoming conscious of a smell of spirits." She lodged
at a bird fancier's in Kingsgate Street, High Holborn, in
the first-floor front, her window being "easily assailable
at night by pebbles, walking-sticks, and fragments of
tobacco-pipe," thrown by panting husbands with faces as
white as muffins. She was a widow, the lamented Mr.
Gamp having ended his days at Guy's Hospital, where
he was last seen by his spouse "a-lying with a penny-
piece on each eye, and his wooden leg under his arm."

Mrs. Gamp was, in her highest walk of art, a monthly
nurse, but she did on occasions condescend to nursing of
a less interesting character, and also undertook the laying
out of the dead. It is with her "funeral face," and
carrying a large bundle, a pair of pattens, and a species
of gig umbrella, "the latter article in colour like a faded
leaf, except where a circular patch of a lively blue had
been dexterously let in at the top," that we first encounter
Mrs. Gamp proceeding under the escort of Mr. Pecksniff
to lay out the departed Mr. Chuzzlewit. Arrived at the
house, she lets it be known that "if it wasn't for the
nerve a little sip of liquor gives me I never could go
through with what I sometimes has to do. I says to Mrs.
Harris" (this lady being Mrs. Gamp's familiar), "'Leave
the bottle on the chimley-piece, and don't ask me to take
none, but let me put my lips to it when I am so dispoged,
and then I will do what I am engaged to do, according to
the best of my ability.' 'Mrs. Gamp,' she says, 'if ever
there was a sober creetur to be got at eighteen-pence a
day for working people, and three and six for gentle
folks—night watching being a extra charge—you are that
inwallable person.' 'Mrs. Harris,' I says to her, 'don't
name the charge, for if I could afford to lay all my fellow-
creeturs out for nothink, I would gladly do it, sich is the
love I bears 'em.'"

Having performed the last offices for the departed

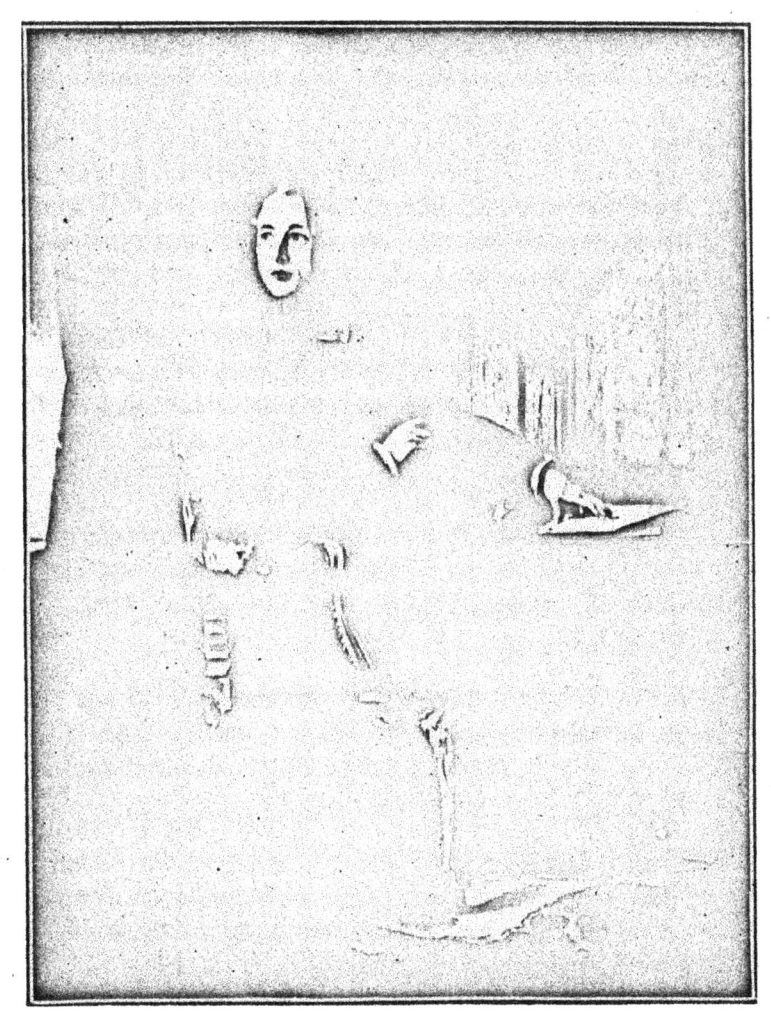

CHARLES DICKENS.

(*From the painting by David Maclise.*)

[*To face p.* 48.

Mr. Chuzzlewit, and enjoyed the funeral as it was only possible to do when long mourning cloaks, hat-bands, mutes, many plumes, and unlimited feasting and drinking were the fashion, Mrs. Gamp returned home with her new mourning to await the next job, come birth, come death.

We next see Mrs. Gamp in the capacity of a night nurse, taking turn about with Betsey Prig, " the best of creeturs." Mrs. Prig was a hospital nurse recommended by Bartlemy's, otherwise known as St. Bartholomew's, engaged at the present time in nursing a gentleman stricken with fever in the Bull, at Holborn. Thither sped Mrs. Gamp when the clock struck eight, carrying her night wrappings, and mounted the stairs of the Bull to that attic room where the fever patient tossed and moaned in his wanderings. Mrs. Prig, the day nurse, stood bonneted and shawled waiting with impatience to be gone. "Mrs. Prig was of the Gamp build, but not so fat; and her voice was deeper and more like a man's. She had also a beard."

"' He's quiet, but his wits is gone. It an't no matter wot you say,' confided the day to the night nurse.

"' Anythin' to tell afore you goes, my dear?' asked Mrs. Gamp, settling her bundle down inside the door, and looking affectionately at her partner.

"' The pickled salmon,' Mrs. Prig replied, ' is quite delicious. I can partick'ler recommend it. Don't have nothink to say to the cold meat, for it tastes of the stable. The drinks is all good.'

" Mrs. Gamp expressed herself much gratified.

"' The pbysic and them things is on the drawers and mankleshelf,' said Mrs. Prig, cursorily. 'He took his last slime draught at seven. The easy-chair an't soft enough. You'll want his piller.'"

No sooner had Mrs. Gamp entered upon her occupation of the sick chamber than, bending over her patient— a young man, dark with long black hair showing against the whiteness of the bed-clothes—she proceeded to professional examination. Not with a view to the comfort or relief of her patient, the last thing which would be likely to occur to a nurse of Sarah Gamp's class, but moved by a ghoulish delight in the horrible, she pinned the delirious man's arms against his sides, and exclaimed, "He'd make a lovely corpse."

After this cheerful diagnosis, Mrs. Gamp began preparations for passing a comfortable night, and turned her attention towards supper. One sometimes hears of ructions between the modern private nurse and the household servants, but the immortal "Sairey" was equal to a regiment of unwilling housemaids. She rang her bell with authority, and on the appearance of the maid said, with a tone expressive of weakness—

"'I think, young woman, that I could pick a little bit of pickled salmon, with a nice little sprig of fennel, and a sprinkling of white pepper. I takes new bread, my dear, with jest a little pat of fresh butter, and a mossel of cheese. In case there should be such a thing as a cowcumber in the 'ouse, will you be so kind as bring it, for I'm rather partial to 'em, and they does a world of good in a sick-room. If they draws the Brighton Old Tipper here, I takes *that* ale at night, my love, it being considered wakeful by the doctors. And whatever you do, young woman, don't bring more than a shilling's-worth of gin-and-water warm when I rings the bell a second time: for that is always my allowance, and I never takes a drop beyond!'" The references to the cucumber being good in the sick-room and the opinion of the doctors in favour of Mrs. Gamp's favourite tipple are ingeniously thrown in.

After supping to her satisfaction, Mrs. Gamp makes the soothing reflection, "'What a blessed thing it is to make sick people happy in their beds, and never mind one's self as long as one can do a service!'" Then, draining her glass, she bethought herself of the patient's medicine, and by the simple process of clutching his

windpipe to make him gasp, poured it down his throat.
Remembering Betsey Prig's parting injunction, Mrs. Gamp
next took the pillow from under his head to add to the
comfort of the couch which she improvised for herself out
of two easy-chairs. This was no imaginary touch on the
part of the novelist, for even in a much later period than
the one he described, hospital nurses were often discovered
serenely sleeping before the ward fire on the appropriated
pillows and blankets of the patients whom they were
supposed to be night-watching.

Having arranged a comfortable couch, Mrs. Gamp
divested herself of her false curls, put on a prodigious
nightcap, grimy and yellow, a night jacket, and over that
a watchman's old coat, the sleeves of which, tied round
her neck, made her look as though she were in the
embrace of one of those worthy guardians of the streets.
Soon she slept heavily, did this exemplary night nurse,
while her fever-tossed patient moaned the night away in
high delirium. At length his ravings roused her, and
coarsely mocking his wild speech, Mrs. Gamp got up,
not to soothe the fevered brow or moisten the parched
lips, no nonsensical sentiment of that kind for her, but to
"bile the kettle" and get herself a cup of tea. Awaiting
this desirable consummation "she sat down so close to
the fender (which was a high one) that her nose rested
upon it; and for some time she drowsily amused herself
by sliding that feature backwards and forwards along
the brass top, as far as she could, without changing
her position to do it." She maintained all the time
a running and scornful commentary on the patient's
wandering speech. Mrs. Gamp's attitude before the
high fender, sliding her nose backwards and forwards
along the top, was, as we have already seen, taken from
the life.

At length morning broke, and at eight o'clock Mrs.
Prig, the day nurse, promptly relieved duty. The doctor
also came, and appears to have shown little concern about
the nursing of his patient.

We next encounter the sisterhood when their patient has struggled to the first stage of convalescence, and they are preparing him for a journey into the country. "He was so wasted, that it seemed as if his bones would rattle when they moved him. His cheeks were sunken, and his eyes unnaturally large. He lay back in the easy-chair like one more dead than living, and rolled his languid eyes towards the door when Mrs. Gamp appeared as painfully as if their weight alone were burdensome to move.

"'And how are we by this time?' Mrs. Gamp observed. 'We looks charming.'

"'We looks a deal charminger than we are, then,' returned Mrs. Prig, a little chafed in her temper. 'We got out of bed back'ards, I think, for we're as cross as two sticks. I never see sich a man. He wouldn't have been washed, if he'd had his own way.'

"'She put the soap in my mouth,' said the unfortunate patient, feebly.

"'Couldn't you keep it shut, then?' retorted Mrs. Prig. 'Who do you think's to wash one feater, and miss another, and wear one's eyes out with all manner of fine work of that description, for half-a-crown a day! If you wants to be tittivated, you must pay accordin'.'

"'Oh dear me!' cried the patient, 'oh dear, dear!'

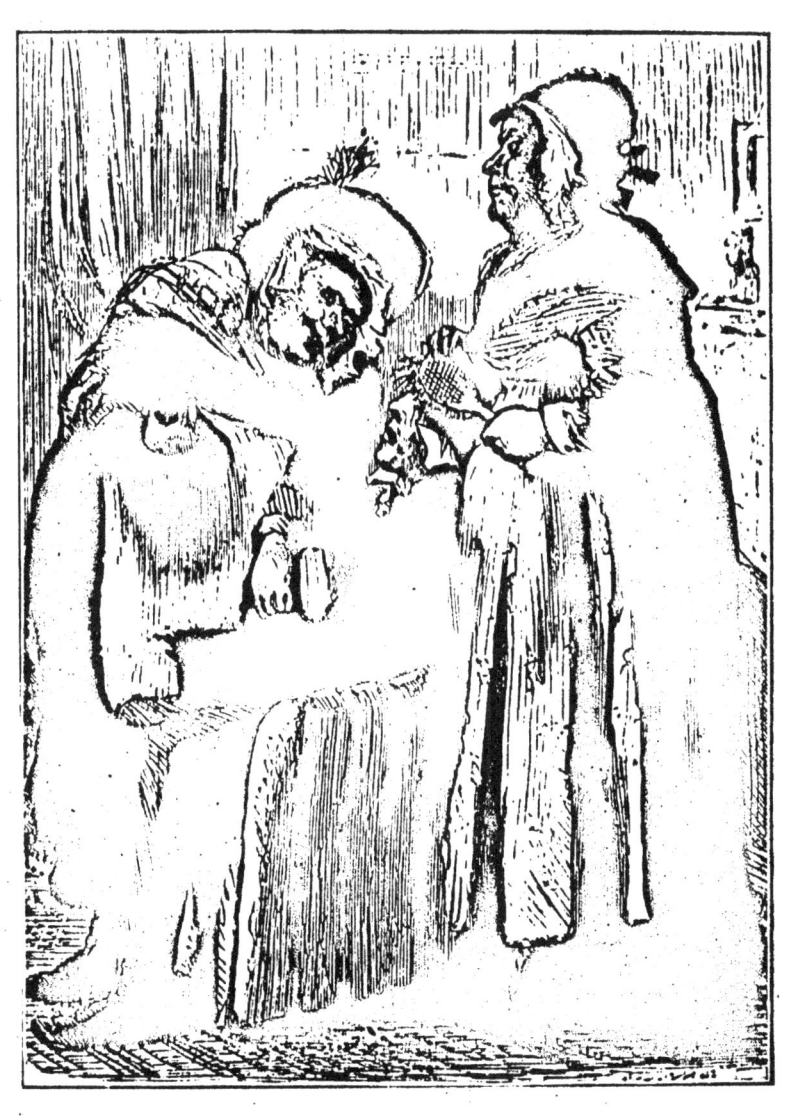

SAIREY GAMP AND BETSEY PRIG PREPARE THEIR PATIENT FOR A JOURNEY.

[*To face p.* 52.

"'There!' said Mrs. Prig, 'that's the way he's been a-conducting of himself, Sarah, ever since I got him out of bed, if you'll believe it.'

"'Instead of being grateful,' Mrs. Gamp observed, 'for all our little ways. Oh, fie for shame, sir, fie for shame!'"

Here Mrs. Prig seized the patient by the chin, and began to rasp his unhappy head with a hair-brush, one of the hardest kind of instruments producible by modern art, and the patient's eyelids became red with the friction. It is at this juncture that the artist has depicted the famous sisterhood and their patient.

When his toilet was at length completed, Mrs. Gamp gathered her bundle, pattens, and umbrella together, and thus took leave of Betsey Prig—

"'Wishin' you lots of sickness, my darling creetur',' Mrs. Gamp observed, 'and good places. It won't be long, I hope, afore we works together, off and on, again, Betsey; and may our next meetin' be at a large family's, where they all takes it reg'lar, one from another, turn and turn about, and has it business-like.'"

Such a desired climax to their professional partnership was, fortunately for the patients, not destined to come to Sairey Gamp and Betsey Prig. They later parted in wrath, amid bitter recriminations at the memorable feast in Mrs. Gamp's lodgings, enlivened by something stronger than tea, though for appearance sake, kept in an old tea-pot.

"'Betsey,' said Mrs. Gamp, filling her own glass, and passing the tea-pot, 'I; will now propoge a toast. My frequent pardner, Betsey Prig!'

"'Which, altering the name to Sairah Gamp, I drink,' said Mrs. Prig, 'with love and tenderness.'

"'Now, Sairah,' said Mrs. Prig, 'joining business with pleasure, wot is this case in which you wants me? *Is* it Mrs. Harris?'"

Mrs. Gamp replied with dignity that there could be no question of partnership with such a patient as Mrs.

Harris, whose constant words "'in sickness is and will be,' "Send for Sairey!"'" Whereat Betsey Prig, shutting one eye and folding her arms, exclaimed, "'Bother Mrs. Harris!'" adding the memorable and tremendous words, "'I don't believe there's no sich a person.'"

The thunderbolt had fallen, the identity of Mrs. Harris was questioned, and Mrs. Gamp rose in her wrath and denounced her "pardner." As Mrs. Gamp pathetically said, "'the words she spoke of Mrs. Harris lambs could not forgive, nor worms forget!'"

And so we leave the famous sisterhood, with their dram-drinking, snuff-taking, and coarse brutal habits, to whom human sympathy, the first requisite for a nurse, was unknown.

Few characters, even of the laughter-provoking Dickens, have caused such perennial amusement as Sairey Gamp and Betsey Prig; but it was not for the sake of comicality that they were introduced into the story of "Martin Chuzzlewit;" Dickens wrote of them with a set purpose. Ever the friend of the distressed, his heart bled for the poor in time of sickness, when they suffered neglect and torture at the hands of the untrained hireling nurse. Betsey Prig, of St. Bartholomew's, was typical of a class all too prevalent in the great London hospitals. Dickens wrote at a period when the poor in sickness and misfortune were treated as though they were criminals. The prisoners in jail, thanks to John Howard and Elizabeth Fry, had received some mitigation of their hard conditions, but the public conscience had not yet been aroused by the sad state of the sick poor in hospitals and workhouse infirmaries.

No immediate result in the betterment of the condition of the sick poor followed the publication of "Martin Chuzzlewit," still the leaven was working and people who shook with laughter over the sayings and doings of Sairey and Betsey were unconsciously having their eyes opened to the abuses exposed. The evils did not, however, glare so vividly then as they do now in retrospect.

The coarse unskilled nurse was put up with as a necessary evil which no one knew how to get rid of. Sanitary matters were viewed differently in those days by all classes. The old hospitals, reeking with infection and filth, were not places in which gently nurtured women could nurse; therefore, with a few exceptions, the Gamps and Prigs had the field to themselves. Even in private homes sick-nursing was more or less loathsome by reason of the lack of knowledge of hygiene to keep the patient sweet and the sick-room habitable. In time of illness people sought nurses whose sensibilities were not too fine, if there were no relatives to perform the task for love.

Six years after the publication of "Martin Chuzzlewit" we find Dickens lamenting that "hospitals with their means and funds should have left it to a private enterprise in this year 1849 to enter on an attempt to improve that class of patient," who was confided to the care of such examples of the hospital nurse as he had drawn in Betsey Prig. The private enterprise to which Dickens refers was the foundation of St. John's House, the next step to be recorded in the history of nursing.

CHAPTER V

ST. JOHN'S HOUSE

King's College first London hospital to give facility for training school for nurses—Sir William Bowman, Dr. Todd, and Dr. Farre initiate scheme—Foundation of St. John's House, 1848—Class of inmates and their respective duties—Strict discipline—The "Master" and his office—Removal to Westminster—Miss Mary Jones appointed superintendent—Nurses for the Crimea—Removal to Norfolk Street—Expansion of work—The daily diets—Changes in the rules—Lady and nurse pupils—Crisis in 1883—Reorganization—Sister Caroline and present *régime*.

Up to the year 1847 little real advance had been made in nursing reform. The institution of nursing sisters, though a noteworthy beginning, made slow progress, and the trenchant and humorous pen of Dickens had not roused hospital boards of management to introduce a better order of things. To King's College Hospital belongs the honour of having made the first attempt to introduce a higher class of nursing. The minute-books of the hospital record that King's " was the first hospital in London in which the superior nursing of patients, and the use of the wards as a training school were extended to a voluntary nursing sisterhood ; " a fact which is of special interest now that the famous college hospital is soon [1906] to be removed from its historic site in Lincoln's Inn Fields to meet a more extended field of usefulness in South London. The three eminent physicians of King's, Mr. (afterwards Sir) William Bowman, Dr. Todd, and Dr. Arthur Farre, were the leading spirits in initiating the scheme which resulted first in the foundation of the famous St. John's House, and later in the

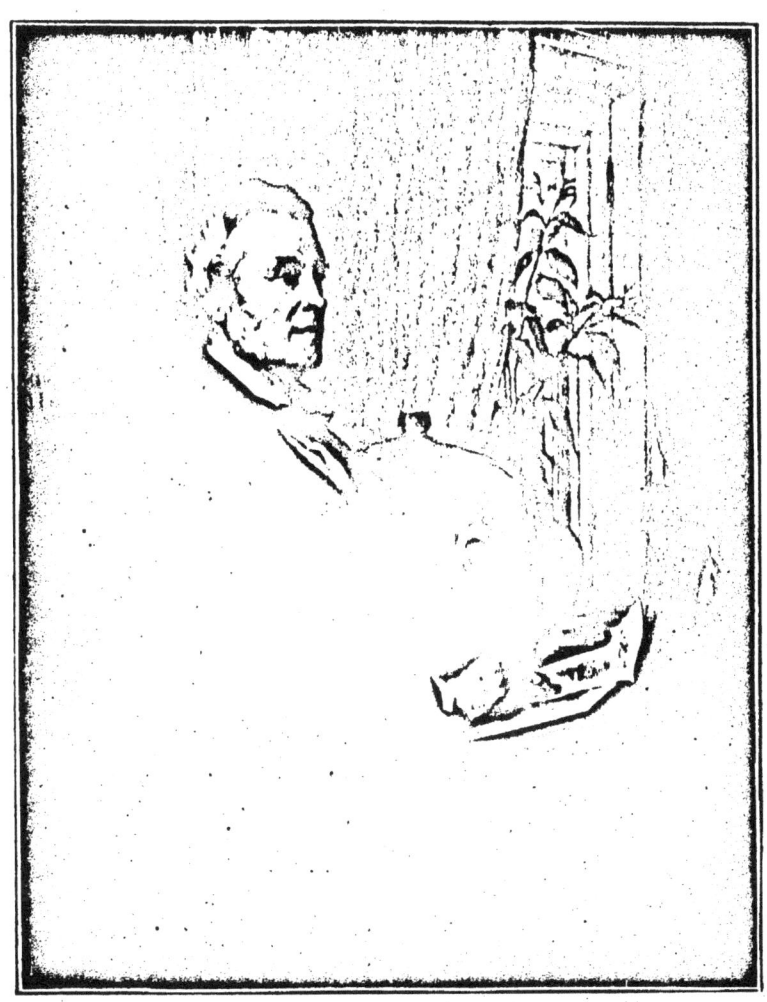

SIR WILLIAM BOWMAN.
(*From the painting in the Board Room at King's College Hospital.*)

nursing charge of the hospital being undertaken by its sisterhood.

In the autumn of 1847 Mr. William Bowman, then recently appointed joint Professor of Physiology at King's College Hospital with Dr. Todd, addressed a circular letter to eminent medical men and others interested in philanthropy, seeking co-operation in an attempt to improve the status of nursing by the establishment of a training institute for nurses. The result was an inaugural meeting at the Hanover Square Rooms, July 13, 1848, under the presidency of the then Duke of Cambridge, supported by Dr. Blomfield, Bishop of London, and many other eminent persons. The Queen Dowager Adelaide gave her patronage to the scheme, and it was supported by the Archbishop of York, the Bishops of Lichfield, Salisbury, Gloucester and Bristol, Ripon, Norwich, Oxford, Chichester, Llandaff, and Manchester, Canon Wordsworth and Canon Jelf, and Earl Nelson and Earl Harrowby.

Although the scheme primarily issued from the medical faculty at King's, it was from the first taken under the wing of the Church, as instanced by the imposing array of bishops who were among the promoters. In these early stages of reform, there was a disposition to return to the actuating principle of pre-Reformation days, and to regard nursing as a religious vocation. Possibly the public mind had been so disgusted by the conduct of the worldly hireling that it was convinced that nothing but a religious motive would keep a nurse in the straight path. This idea was to some extent evident in Mrs. Fry's institution, and became most pronounced in the new Sisterhood of St. John's. At the inaugural meeting, the aim of the institution was thus set forth : "It is proposed to establish a corporate or collegiate institution, the objects of which would be to maintain in a community women who are members of the Church of England, who should receive such instruction and undergo such training as might best fit them to act as nurses and visitors to the sick and poor. It is either upon the council or committee of an institution founded for the training of women in an avocation peculiarly feminine. In this it forms a marked contrast to that founded by Mrs. Fry, in which a committee composed entirely of ladies managed the affairs of the society.

Dr. Blomfield became president of St. John's House, and to the end of his life took an active interest in promoting its progress, and was attended in his last illness by one of its nurses. The office has since been filled by successive Bishops of London. The rules of the institution received the approval of the archbishops; appeals were sent to the clergy to promote funds for the undertaking. A chaplain or master was appointed, the nurses and sisters were admitted at a religious service conducted either by the Bishop of London or one of his episcopal colleagues, and there are traditions at St. John's House of even three bishops taking part in the admission service of some of the sisters. No person not a member of the Established Church of England and Ireland was admissible to fill any office in the institution. It was founded at a time when the wave of Anglicanism which had its origin in Dr. Pusey's movement at Oxford was sweeping over the country. A revival of mediævalism was in fashion, and became apparent in the rules of the sisterhood founded under the auspices of the Protestant Church. The time was ripe to sympathize with its efforts, and the institution most forcibly appealed to women eager for a vocation at once religious and philanthropic. In a word, St. John's House became the religious enthusiasm of the day.

In less than a year after the inaugural meeting the organization was started as the "Training Institution for nurses in hospitals, families, and the poor," and began its work with a small staff of sisters and nurses at 36, Fitzroy Square, in the St. Pancras district of St. John the Evangelist, from which it took its name of St. John's House.

The inmates to be received into the institution were divided into three classes, probationers, nurses, sisters. No probationer was admissible without the written recommendation of a governor or subscriber. She must be at least eighteen years of age, able to read well, and to write, and to produce certificates of baptism and of character. If at the end of six months she appeared in every way satisfactory, she remained, under ordinary circumstances, at the institution for a probationary period of two years, and paid fifteen pounds, or in special cases less, towards the cost of her maintenance. She was trained in the particular duties of a nurse, performed domestic duties in the house, and attended upon the sick in hospital or private residences as the authorities directed. At the end of her probation she received a medical certificate of competency, and was, if duly approved, placed upon the list of nurses of the institution.

The nurses received board, lodging, medical assistance, washing, and clothing, and one pound per month for their services. In some cases the fee was higher. They nursed in hospitals and private families, and when required attended the sick poor. If at the end of five years they had proved themselves worthy, they received from the council a certificate, and were entered upon the house list of certified nurses. Women who had not been probationers of St. John's House were received as nurses if they were able to bring medical certificates of health and competency, and guarantees as to character.

The sisters, women of superior birth and education, were divided into resident and non-resident. They must have attained the age of twenty-five, and had to furnish the same kind of certificates as the probationers. In cases of applicants under the age of thirty, and not widows, the council required the sanction of parents. The resident sisters lived in the house, and received board, lodging, washing, medical assistance, and certain fixed articles of dress, towards which they paid fifty pounds per annum in quarterly instalments. The institution did not, however, accept the property of a sister beyond her annual income, so long as she continued a member of it.

The non-resident sisters had to bring the usual certificates required by the institution, and were permitted to live at home with their families or in private houses approved by the authorities. They were allowed to join the common table of the institution on specially arranged terms, no other payment being required from non-resident sisters.

The duties of both classes of sisters were defined as—

1. *Within the House.*—To assist the master and lady superintendent in the instruction and general training of the probationers, and in the domestic management.

2. *Out-of-doors.*—To assist the lady superintendent in visiting the sick poor at their dwellings, subject to the directions of the clergyman of the parish, accompanied by one or more probationers, to superintend any of the probationers assigned to their care out of the institution, and to aid in attendance upon the sick at hospitals.

The usual fee charged to private families by the institution for the services of a nurse was one guinea per week for full duty, and ten shillings and sixpence for occasional duty. The fees belonged to the funds of the institution, and nurses were forbidden to receive gratuities on pain of dismissal. The rules as to dress were severe. The wearing of jewellery and fashionable hair-dressing were forbidden. The gowns and bonnets provided for the nurses were of a quaint style calculated to chasten the spirit of the most frivolous-minded young woman. The cap was similar to that worn by the Deaconesses at Kaiserswerth.

The probationers were sent for six months' training to a hospital, but lived at and remained under the control of St. John's House. If the technical training did not amount to much in these early years, the probationers were well drilled in matters of conduct. The sisters marshalled them two and two, like a string of school-girls, when they went to the hospitals or attended divine service. They were not allowed to talk at meals, and scarcely to enter a room unless summoned. A humble " proby " would scarcely presume to sit in an easy-chair, certainly not if one of her superiors was present. Scoldings were a part of the day's discipline in keeping with the spirit of that time, which pinned its faith to the axiom that young people, and especially those in training, were generally in need of scoldings. A refractory probationer was handed over to the stern admonitions of the " master," who chastened a wild spirit with religious exercises. The peculiar position of young women training in public hospitals, where they were brought into contact with medical students and others not of their own sex —a departure over which Mrs. Grundy shook her head nearly to decapitation—engendered a rigid discipline on the part of those responsible for the innovation. The question of nursing as an avocation for ladies and respectable young women was on its trial, and measures to save the venture from reproach could not be too strict. Though the old St. John's Sisters were undoubtedly martinets, they were splendid disciplinarians.

The first lady superintendent of St. John's house was Miss Elizabeth Frere, a sister of Mr. George Frere, a member of the council of the institution. Another member of the family was Sir Bartle Frere, Governor of the Cape. Miss Frere laboured assiduously for the first six months in organizing the institution, and to her initial work the first success of the enterprise was due. It may be noted, as an interesting coincidence, that Miss Frere bore the name of Elizabeth, and her initials were the same as those of the pioneer in nursing reform—Elizabeth Fry. Having put the house into working order, Miss Frere was succeeded by an officially appointed superintendent, Mrs. Elspeth Morrice.

In keeping with the fact that St. John's House was a religious foundation, the head of the institution was the chaplain, quaintly termed in mediæval style the "Master." He must have taken Priest's Orders in the Established Church, and be a married man or a widower. One fails to understand why a widower would be a less dangerous person in the house of a sisterhood than a bachelor. The first Master of St. John's was the Rev. F. Twist, and his wife gave some assistance in the household management.

Not only did the master direct the religious instruction of inmates, prepare the probationers for confirmation when necessary, and perform the morning and evening service, but he exercised control over the nurses and the household matters. He interviewed candidates and judged their suitability for nursing; gave orders to the tradespeople; and with him the lady superintendent discussed the domestic conduct of the establishment. In the early years he instructed the nurses on their district work and received their reports. It appears, from the records, that when the master found himself involved in subjects beyond his knowledge, he consulted Dr. Todd or some other medical man; more particularly with regard to the qualifications of probationers.

We find him pronouncing one candidate "too diminutive in person to discharge the duties of nurse efficiently;" and another "self-conceited and ill-tempered." It was also his painful duty to admonish a nurse after service in chapel for not joining audibly in the responses. The timetable of the master's day in 1849 affords an interesting peep into the routine of St. John's House—

- 7.30 Prayers in chapel; or
- 8.0 Service in St. John's Church.
- 10.0 Interview with the lady superintendent, when all details about the house, nurses, etc., were discussed and settled. Instruction to individual nurses.
- 12.0 Instruction for "Sisters," Tuesdays, Thursdays, and Saturdays, on the parables of our Lord.
- 1.0 Dine with inmates, at least three times a week. Show house to visitors.

3.0 Instruction for probationers, Tuesdays, Thursdays, Saturdays, on "The Book of Common Prayer," or private interviews with nurses, etc.

4.0 House committee (Mondays). Office hours—10 to 1; 3 to 5.

No doubt the master had his trials under the item of "interviews," not only with the nurses, but with ladies who came to engage them; however, he possessed his soul in silence, or at least abstained from relieving his feelings after the manner of an entry in an old diary at the Devonshire Square Institution, where a much-tried superintendent records : "Another lady called to hum and ha and fiddle-faddle, for she did not know what she wanted. I promised to help her when I knew what she really did require, and I did not lose my temper ; but very nearly !" One feels sure the diarist practised abnormal self-restraint.

Difficulties early beset St. John's House from the outside. The inhabitants of Fitzroy Square were aghast at having in their midst a colony of nurses. Even the brass plate on the door of the house was an offence in the nostrils of the "genteel" neighbourhood, and there was a genuine terror of contagion. It must be admitted that in the unsanitary conditions of many of the old London hospitals, a nurse fresh from the wards was the last person one would care to encounter. So strong was the antagonistic feeling that, in 1853, the institution, with the approval of the Bishop of London, removed to 5, Queen's Square, Westminster, and found sanctuary under the wing of the venerable Abbey. The Westminster Hospital became the chief training-place for the probationers, and in the district around the sisters and nurses tended the sick poor. They also did useful work in London and country hospitals, and occasionally took nursing charge of some village stricken with an epidemic. The private nursing was successfully continued.

Soon after the removal to Westminster, Miss Mary

Jones, a friend of Miss Florence Nightingale, was appointed lady superintendent of St. John's House, and under her able management it made good progress. The outbreak of the Crimean War in the following year roused public attention to the need of trained nurses as it had never been roused before, and St. John's House was brought more prominently into view, while its inmates were inspired with enthusiasm to render service to the wounded soldiers. Six of its nurses, Rebecca Lawfield, Emma Fagg, Ann Higgins, Elizabeth Drake, Mary Ann Coyle, and Mary Ann Burnett proceeded, October 23, 1854, under charge of the master, to Paris to join Miss Nightingale's first contingent for the East. A few months later followed a second detachment of twenty nurses, prepared and selected by the superintendent, Miss Jones. Four of the first party returned from Scutari, unable to face the discipline and privations of the work, and Nurse Elizabeth Drake died of fever at Balaclava. Of her the lady-in-chief wrote, August 16, 1855: "I have lost in her the best of all the women here. . . . I feel like a criminal in having robbed you of one so truly to be loved and honoured. It seemed as if it pleased God to remove from the work those who have been most useful to it. His Will be done!" In the cemetery at Balaclava, Miss Nightingale erected a small marble cross to the memory of Nurse Elizabeth Drake.

The Crimean period quickened the activities of St. John's House, and a great expansion of the work followed, the most important being an arrangement entered into in 1856 to undertake the nursing of King's College Hospital. This was followed in 1865 by a similar arrangement with the newly founded Galignani English Hospital in Paris, and in 1866 with Charing Cross Hospital, and in 1871 with the Children's Hospital at Nottingham; but this important work, which raises the whole question of the reform of nursing in hospitals, will be more fittingly dealt with in a separate chapter, and we will here briefly conclude the story of St. John's House in other particulars.

Soon after undertaking the nursing of King's College Hospital, the institution removed to commodious premises in Norfolk Street, Strand, to be near the scene of the new field of labour. St. John's House, Norfolk Street, became widely known as a centre, not only of nursing, but of beneficence and religious life. The sisters, at their own expense, built a chapel to their house, and decorated it in a most artistic manner. The Fra Angelico pictures above the altar were copied from the originals in Rome by an artist engaged by Captain Lloyd, the brother of Sister Caroline Lloyd. Daily services were held in the chapel by the master, and there the special admission services for sisters and nurses took place, under the auspices of bishops and distinguished clergy. The sisters, on admission, received a silver cross, with the badge of the institution, and the nurses a medal with a similar device. The Rev. H. A. Giraud succeeded the Rev. C. P. Shepherd as chaplain in 1857, and held the position for many years. Mr. Giraud was also chaplain to King's College Hospital. At various times Churchmen of distinction, like the Bishop of Bedford and Dr. Vaughan, Master of the Temple, were honorary chaplains of St. John's House. As years went by, the duties of the chaplain were confined to religious work, and the household and nursing arrangements, in which the master had at first co-operated, were left in the hands of the superintendent, who was now known as lady, and eventually as sister superior.

A most interesting feature of St. John's House was the daily "diets," established in 1867 by an arrangement of the Knights Hospitallers of the Order of St. John of Jerusalem, with the Council of St. John's House, that a midday meal should be given to six convalescent patients from King's College Hospital, and a similar number from Charing Cross Hospital. These diets were prepared under the superintendence of the sisters, and dispensed to the needy convalescents in the quaint old wainscoted hall of St. John's House, an unspeakable boon to the deserving poor, who frequently came out of hospital to face the struggle of life all over again. To guard against abuse a sister and nurse visited the patients who received the diets. Independently of this, a sisters' fund was started, for providing food and clothing for the sick poor whom the nurses of the institution found in distressing circumstances. A visitor to the hall of St. John's House, when the diets were being dispensed, would have been reminded of the hospitality to the sick and poor which distinguished the conventual infirmary in olden days. It was a revival of mediæval England in the heart of the Strand.

As the years went by changes took place in the rules and regulations of St. John's House. Eighteen was soon found too young to admit a probationer, and the age for a time stood at from twenty-five to forty. A gradual increase took place in nurses' wages, which rose from a maximum of £20 per year to £28. A pension fund was started for disabled nurses, also a pension scheme for those past work. A convalescent home for sick nurses was started at Ashstead, and received kindly support from the late Mrs. Gladstone. Mr. Gladstone was also deeply interested in the work of St. John's House.

The introduction of "lady pupils" and "nurse pupils" was another development of the work, started with a view to training superintendents and nurses for other institutions. The lady pupils were received at St. John's House for a period of six or twelve months, and gratuitously trained to take positions at the head of public or private nursing institutions, cottage hospitals, etc. They paid a sum for maintenance while in residence at St. John's House. No one was now received as a sister who had not been first a lady pupil. The nurse pupils were trained for a similar period for other institutions. In this way important pioneer work was done to provide lady superintendents and nurses for institutions in the provinces, and so spread some of the leaven of nursing reform over the country.

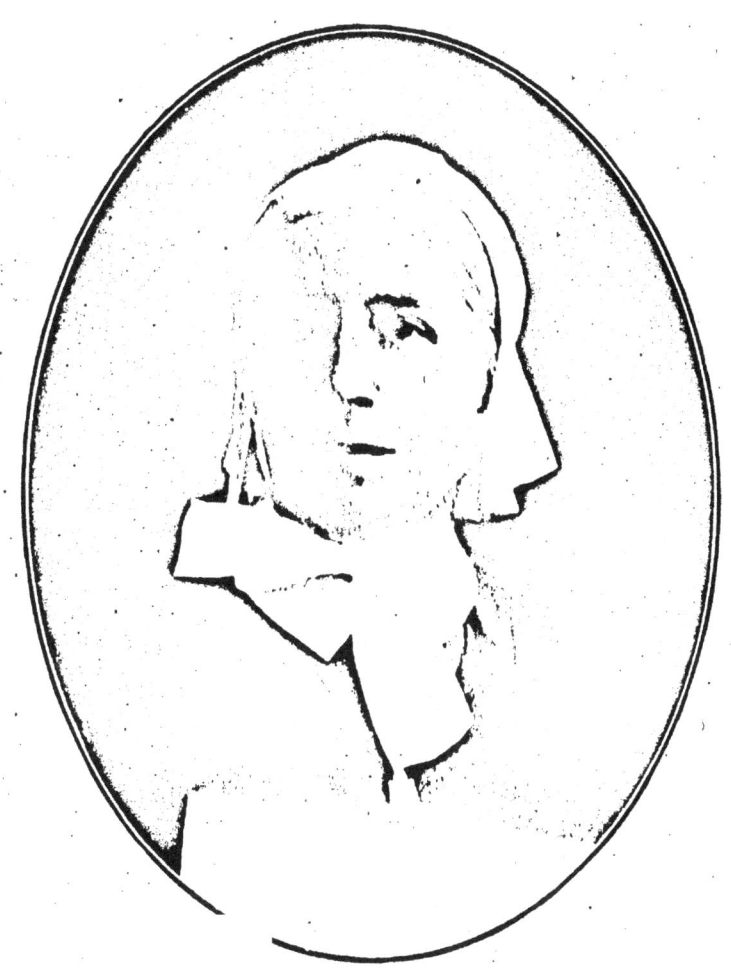

Miss CAROLINE LLOYD,
Sister Superior, St. John's House, 1870-83.

[*To face p.* 68.

During the cholera epidemic of 1866, the sisters and nurses of St. John's rendered valuable service in London. They also nursed St. George's Workhouse through an epidemic. In 1879 a staff of sisters and nurses were sent to Woolwich and Netley, to relieve the nurses going from those establishments to the British Army in South Africa. The list of cottage and smaller country hospitals where the St. John's nurses have at various times rendered service is a long one, and the demand for them in private families was for many years in excess of the supply. The sisters did most beneficent work in the slums of the old Clare Market. Protected by the uniform which the most abandoned had learned to respect, they passed unmolested down alleys where a policeman dare not go. On one occasion a sister was robbed of her purse, but the thief, finding to whom it belonged, secretly restored it to St. John's House. The presence of these devoted women did much to quell the drunken brawls and obscene behaviour in one of the worst of London slums, at a time when "slumming" had not become the fashion.

In 1867 Miss Mary Jones resigned the position of lady superior, which she had held for thirteen years, and was succeeded by Mrs. Hodson, who had been for many years a sister of St. John's House. In 1870, Miss Caroline Lloyd, who had also long been a sister, became superior, and was the last sister to hold the office under the original *régime*. She left in 1883, and with the sisterhood and many of the nurses, founded the community of the Nursing Sisters of St. John the Divine at Drayton Gardens, South Kensington. The crisis which led to this secession arose in connection with the authorities of King's College Hospital, and is dealt with more particularly in the next chapter. The council of St. John's House remained, though the sisterhood had departed, and in time the nursing was reorganized, under the charge of the All Saints' Sisterhood, a religious community which had its home in the adjoining parish to that where St. John's House had its birth. In 1893 another change took place, when the council placed its nursing under the care of the Sisterhood of St. Peter's, Mortimer Road, Kilburn, and a new *régime* was inaugurated by Sister Caroline, the present superior, under whose beneficent and tactful rule the institution has pursued a course of peace and prosperity in the historic house in Norfolk Street. The demolition of the premises is imminent, and ere long the Strand will lose the institution which has lived and worked in its midst for upwards of forty-five years. Other premises have been secured in Queen's Square, Bloomsbury, and there a new St. John's House will begin its career.

The activities of the institution comprise private and hospital nursing and work amongst the sick poor. All nursing candidates must be members of the Church of England, single women or widows, between the ages of twenty-five and thirty-five. Good, strong, active women of fair education are eligible. The salary for private nurses is from twenty-eight pounds to thirty pounds a year, which is augmented by a weekly commission of two shillings whilst at a case, and at the end of each year a cash bonus based upon the surplus shown in the accounts of the preceding year. A comfortable home, board, lodging, uniform, laundry, etc., are provided for the nurses, with no extra expense, when they are not at work. They receive medical care and attention when ill. A pension or bonus is awarded to any nurse leaving the institution after serving it efficiently for a certain number of years. There are now some twenty nurses on the pension list, one having drawn her pension for twenty years. There is an alternative scheme of payment, in which a higher rate of salary, beginning at £30, with an annual rise of £1 until £40 is reached, is given, but with this there is no pension. All nurses receive a three years' training in a general hospital, and are kept in touch with the advancing knowledge of their profession by nursing in hospitals from time to time. The institution supplies nurses at from two to three guineas per week. It has also a convenient arrangement for sending out daily nurses at two and sixpence an hour, five shillings for half a day, and ten and sixpence per day or night. Monthly nurses are supplied at ten to fifteen guineas per month, and certificated masseuses attend at the rate of seven shillings an hour, and less by the week. All money for the services of nurses belongs to St. John's House.

The aim of the sister superior is to make the institution as much like a home as possible. There are practically no rules except punctuality to meals. The superior governs her household on the principle that nurses need refreshment of mind. Four to six weeks' holiday is given to each nurse during the ear.

In 1901 the superior started the League of St John's House Nurses, which has for one of its objects the State registration of nurses. Pleasant little At Homes take place during winter, at which present and former nurses meet for talk and relaxation, and tea, music, and recitation beguile the time. *The St. John's House News* is the organ of the league, and an interesting feature in it is the "History of St. John's House," to the early chapters of which I am much indebted.

The president and visitor of the institution is, as in former days, the reigning Bishop of London. The Rev. E. F. Russell is chaplain, and takes a constant interest in the work and in the social gatherings, and is, we feel sure, a less feared personage than were the old "masters" of St. John's. The Council is composed of nineteen gentlemen, chiefly belonging to the Church and to the medical profession. The treasurer is the Rev. Prebendary Arthur J. Ingram, M.A., the physician Sir Hugh Beevor, Bart., the trustees the Rt. Hon. John G. Talbot, M.P., Prebendary Ingram, and Laurie Frere, Esq., and the secretary is Ernest R. Frere, Esq.; the latter two names recall the interest taken by the Frere family in St. John's House from its foundation nearly sixty years ago.

CHAPTER VI

THE NURSING SISTERS OF ST. JOHN THE DIVINE

Descendants of St. John's House—Sister superior, Miss Isabella Beaver—Sister Caroline Lloyd—Early activities at Drayton Gardens—Deptford District Home—The Community to-day—Its aim—Testimony by Canon Bristow—The medals.

CLOSELY allied with the history of St. John's House, of which indeed they are the lineal descendants, are the nursing sisters of St. John the Divine, of Drayton Gardens, South Kensington. Though separated from the old foundation, the sisterhood has a heritage in the earlier history of St. John's, and several of its present members are representatives of the noble band of pioneer women who laboured in the cause of the reform of nursing at King's College and Charing Cross Hospitals.

Miss Isabella Beaver, the sister superior at Drayton Gardens, did good work in the old days at King's, in helping to bring about the cleanliness and improved sanitary conditions of the wards. She was sister in charge of the surgical ward at King's College, in which Lord Lister made his experiments after his appointment as professor in clinical surgery in 1877. In her own personality Miss Beaver affords an example of the religious enthusiasm and the devotion to principle and duty which distinguished the old St. John's Sisterhood.

The institution at Drayton Gardens was established in 1883, after the rupture which took place between the medical staff and the St. John's sisters at King's College Hospital. The first sister superior at Drayton Gardens was Miss Caroline Lloyd, who since 1870 had been superior at St. John's House, Norfolk Street, and had carried out drastic measures of reform at Charing Cross Hospital. She resigned her position as superior shortly after removal to Drayton Gardens, but continued her valuable services in connection with that institution until her retirement in 1894. Now in vigorous old age, Sister Caroline fights her nursing battles o'er again, and has an entertaining fund of reminiscence.

Although after their settlement in 1883 at Drayton Gardens, the connection of the sisters with King's and Charing Cross Hospitals ceased, they were active in new ventures. They started a little hospital at Lewisham, which has since been enlarged, and where their probationers are now trained. It has a pleasant Nurse's Home attached. In the following year, 1884, they opened a new hospital for women and children at Poplar, and a Crèche for poor children in the same district. These charities are no longer continued, but the sisters have now a district Nurses' Home at Poplar, from which nurses work amongst the riverside population. In 1884 they founded a hospital for women and children at Morden Hill, Lewisham, now known as St. John's Hospital, which is nursed and administered at great sacrifice by the Community. The work at the Deptford District Home is a great boon to that poor and populous neighbourhood. The waiting-room is much appreciated by the children on their way to school, who turn in to have burns and scalds, cuts, broken chilblains, and other injuries to which the little ones are prone, attended to by "nurse," and some get leave to come again during the dinner hour to have a dressing changed. This surgery presents a motley throng of juvenile patients.

The community associated with Drayton Gardens to-day numbers about twenty sisters and between seventy and eighty nurses. Both district and private nursing is undertaken. The probationers are trained at St. John's Hospital under the resident house surgeon, and attend lectures by the sisters. The midwives take the usual course at the Midwifery Institution. The good work amongst the poor is continued in Lewisham, Poplar, and Deptford, and a Convalescent Home is supported at Littlehampton, and is a great boon to weary and enfeebled women. At the mother house in Drayton Gardens the Sister Superior is assisted in the management by her old friend and fellow-worker, Sister Grace Hurt, whose family were neighbouring proprietors to the Nightingales of Lea Hurst—a district where nursing enthusiasm must have been catching. The venerable Earl Nelson, who took an active part in the founding of St. John's House, subsequently gave his support to the sisterhood at Drayton Gardens, and still remains amongst its patrons, which include Princess Christian of Schleswig-Holstein, the Countess of Winchelsea, Lord and Lady Mountgarret, Lady Foley, Sir Edmund Hay Currie, and John E. Linklater, Esq. The hon. chaplain is Canon Bristow, and the services for the admission of sisters and nurses are held at Southwark Cathedral. Hector F. Monro, Esq., is the hon. treasurer, and Sir John Dickson-Poynder the hon. secretary. Dr. Talbot, the Lord Bishop of Southwark, is the visitor.

The aim of the Community of St. John the Divine is to ensure a high standard of character and skill in nursing the sick, whether rich or poor, in their own homes and in hospitals, by giving ladies and respectable women sound training under a superior and sisters, with a comfortable and well-ordered home when unemployed. There is a pension fund for nurses,* and it is of interest to find that one of the latest put upon the pension list is Nurse Cole, the oldest of the Charge Sisters who accompanied the community when they separated from St. John's House, and had worked with them in the old days at King's College Hospital. She has a record of thirty-eight years of conscientious and devoted service in her profession.

* They are affiliated through the institution to the Royal Pension Fund for Nurses.

Canon Bristow thus records his testimony to the self-
sacrificing services of the sisterhood amongst the sick
poor : " In times of increased facilities for pleasure, and
increased softness of living, it is a happiness to think of
lives thus spent for the commonwealth, and to realize
that by their means many a mother has been restored to
her family ; many a breadwinner enabled to return to his
labour ; and many a sufferer strengthened and comforted
in times of extreme sickness, and aided in 'crossing the
bar' by the reverent devotion of those who, like their
Master, care for body and soul."

The badges worn by the community differ from those
of the old St. John's Sisterhood. The sisters wear a perfectly plain Latin cross in silver, the associate sisters a
Maltese cross in silver, with an eagle in the centre, and
the nurses a similar medal in bronze. A highly cherished
insignia is the large bronze Maltese cross containing in
the centre a representation of the St. John's House nurses'
medal, which was struck for those nurses who came away
from Norfolk Street with the sisterhood in 1883. It is
worn by the chaplain, Canon Bristow, and by the visiting
bishop for all services. Specimens of these various medals
were buried under the foundation-stone of the St. John's
Hospital when it was laid by the Duchess of Albany.

CHAPTER VII

FIRST REFORMS IN HOSPITAL NURSING

Abuses under the old system—Tipping—A word for some of the old nurses—Defects in hospital arrangements—An epoch-making reform—St. John's Sisters at King's College—Old ideas regarding gentlewomen—Character *v.* Training—Putting wards in nursing order—Plan for nursing King's College—First Nurses' Home attached to a London hospital—The Nightingale Ward—Reforms at Charing Cross Hospital—A vigilant Sister Superior—Nursing under dual control a failure—Rupture between St. John's Sisterhood and King's College—Trained nursing at Guy's—All Saints' Sisters and University College Hospital—Nursing a lay profession.

In order to appreciate the reform in hospital nursing started in 1856 by St. John's House, one may instance the abuses which then existed. Drunkenness, callousness, and immorality were the chief sins of the old hospital nurse, as the records of various institutions prove. One hospital still preserves the black-list book in which the causes for the dismissal of members of the "female nursing staff" are set down. It is an illuminating document on the character of the old-fashioned nurse. One is dismissed for drinking the patients' brandy, another for gross immorality, others for returning to the hospital in the middle of the night in a drunk and disorderly manner, for thefts from the patients, and for turning them out into the cold so that they might use their beds. Another was dismissed for impertinence to the chaplain. Such conduct, when discovered, was of course punished by dismissal, as this particular record proves. Hospital authorities did not condone such offences even in the good old times. A corrupt system had, however, grown up through engaging nurses without demanding a character. Women cut off from respectable occupation were in those days to be seen standing outside the big London hospitals, like dock labourers waiting for a job. They were summoned to the wards as exigency demanded, and combined scrubbing and nursing as required. This class of woman was in demand for night nursing, the chief care of the sick at night being then covered by the phrase "a woman to sit up." This the nurse often proceeded to do by taking the patients' pillows and blankets, and making herself comfortable before the ward fire. The brandy she administered in strictly homeopathic doses to the patient, and in lesser dilution to herself. Wine was a luxury not to be wasted on the sick. A low state of morality was engendered by the presence of male convalescents, who assisted the nurses in the wards. In these days they would be sent out of hospital to a convalescent home.

The system of tipping was an abuse which widely prevailed in the hospitals under the old nursing *régime*. If a patient was to have good attention, either he or his friends must tip the nurse. An old St. John's sister relates that when first she took charge of a ward vacated by the old staff, she was offered tips ranging from one shilling to five pounds, sometimes accompanied by the remark—"Look here, young woman, just you see after my wife, and there's that for you," attempting to slip a coin into her hand. It is further related that doctors were sometimes driven to tip, and would say to a night nurse in charge of an anxious case, "If I find this patient alive in the morning, there will be five shillings for you." This might have been intended as increased wages for extra attention, but the principle remained the same. Rarely could the old hireling be trusted to give the frequent nourishment and constant watching which meant life or death to the patient without some such stimulus.

As a contrast between the old and new style, the

case may be instanced of a sister who a few years ago was dismissed from a London hospital for having thoughtlessly accepted a box of pocket-handkerchiefs from a grateful lady patient. She was an excellent nurse, highly valued by her hospital, but the breach of discipline could not be overlooked. Patients, it appears, cannot be cured of sending presents to nurses, but the recipient promptly returns such gifts to the donor, or, if sent anonymously, the articles are handed over to the hospital authorities. Little romances are not infrequent in connection with such gifts. At one hospital a valuable ring sent by a gentleman patient to the ward sister waits in the secretary's drawer to be claimed.

While there is no question that the low esteem in which the occupation of nursing was held in the first half of last century, and even later, brought women of undesirable character into the work, it must be acknowledged that there were some good nurses even in the old days. A doctor relates that he remembers one of these "untrained" nurses in his hospital who was so clever in accident cases that she would tell the house surgeon what to do. Other gentlemen who have long held positions in connection with hospitals give strong testimony in favour of the general good behaviour and skill of many of the old nurses. And I have met a few survivals of the old *régime* still occupying minor positions on the staff of hospitals, who impress one by their long years of splendid devotion to the sick and the dignity of their characters, though they are without skilled training or much education. The old hospital nurses, who prided themselves on being able to take the initiative, were a little contemptuous of the routine obedience of the trained staff. "Trained nurses, indeed!" said one. "Why, if a trained nurse were told to put poultices on a man, she would go on poulticing his body while it was being carried down to the mortuary!"

The old surgical nurse must have been a woman of iron nerve, and one almost questions whether her modern successor could have faced the work in the days when operations were performed without anæsthetics. However, though instances of skilled and devoted women stand out amongst the old nurses, there were not enough of these geniuses in the rough to go round.

The hospital arrangements of that time were insanitary and generally defective. Wooden bedsteads, often draped with old and dirty curtains, were in use, and vermin abounded. A sister who had charge of a surgical ward at "King's" relates that the nurses kept an old pair of forceps to nip up from the bed-curtains the insect which should not have been there. Patients often kept the old clothes in which they were brought to the hospital beneath their mattresses, thus adding to the insanitary and infectious state of the wards. Sometimes two patients were put in one bed in a crowded hospital, and a visitor going the round of the Edinburgh Royal Infirmary, before the nursing in that now admirable institution was reformed, saw three male patients in one bed. When the doctors were expected, the least ill of the patients in an overcrowded bed were hustled into clothes or a blanket, and put to sit by the ward fire, returning to bed when the doctor had finished his rounds for the night. At other times a partially convalescent patient in a crowded ward would be roused from his slumbers and given a shilling to sit up in his blanket by the fire while an emergency case was put into his bed, the latter being *unchanged* for the reception of the new patient.

In many of the hospitals patients died like flies from preventible causes. Hospital fever was a recognized complaint. A healthy man came in, perhaps with a broken leg, and remained to die of fever, brought on by the infectious and insanitary condition of the wards. This state of things must be viewed comparatively, for in the earlier part of last century hygiene was not practised even in respectable families. The daily bath and the open window at night were at best regarded as fads, and people drew their curtains closely around their four-post beds with righteous complacency. People lived in happy disregard of germs and microbes, and a holy horror of ventilation. The Lister school had not arisen, and the surgeon at an operation did not consider his dress in relation to the patient, but strictly as regarded himself. He kept his oldest coat hanging in the hospital to wear at an operation. Now his newest coat would not be considered suitable, and he must be covered in a sterilized garment, and ply sterilized instruments, with sterilized hands covered with sterilized gloves, and even have his feet encased in rubber goloshes. In the old days a surgeon received a new gown on his appointment to the house staff of a hospital, and it served him for operations probably as long as he remained. There is, I believe, a tradition that the surgeon's gowns were occasionally cleaned.

The dieting in hospitals was as defective as the sanitary arrangements. Little attention was paid to special cookery for the sick. An allowance of bread and other articles of food was dealt out each day to the patients, who kept the supply in a locker by the side of the bed. Discipline was lax, and patients obtained from their friends salt fish or other dainties according to fancy, and it was no unusual thing to see a patient wrapped in his blanket cooking a herring at the ward fire during the absence of the head nurse, who probably was discussing a pint of porter with her cronies downstairs.

If the preparation of food was often promiscuous, so also was the administration of medicine. It was frequently left in the hands of the patient, who had, probably side by side on the top of his locker, a bottle of medicine and a bottle of lotion, scarcely distinguishable from each other, and sometimes he took the poisonous lotion, with lamentable results. The tending and feeding of patients at night were no part of hospital routine. In a general way the patients after eight o'clock in the evening were left without attention until breakfast next morning. Many cases proved fatal for want of timely care and nourishment.

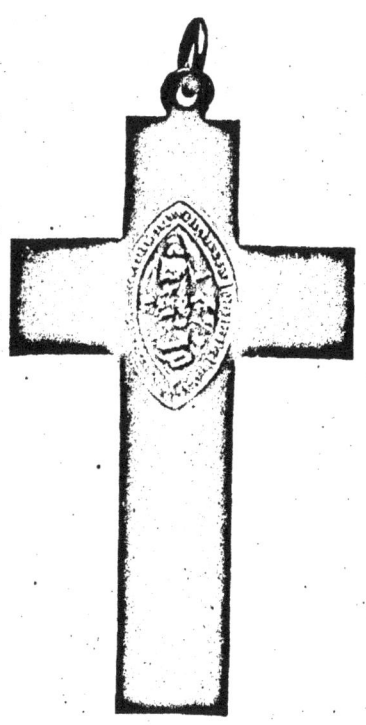

THE ORIGINAL SISTERS' CROSS OF
ST. JOHN'S HOUSE.

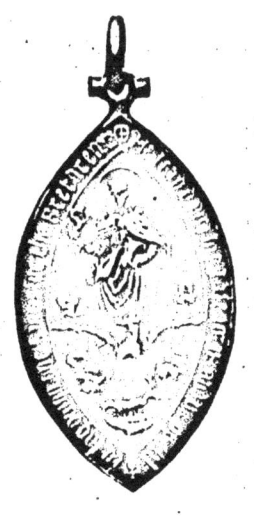

ORIGINAL NURSES' BADGE
(MEDAL).
St. John's House.

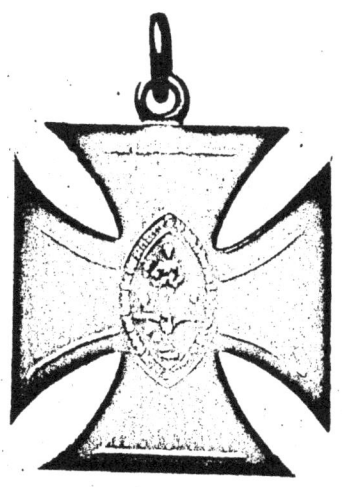

CHAPLAIN'S CROSS,
Nursing Sisters of St. John the Divine.

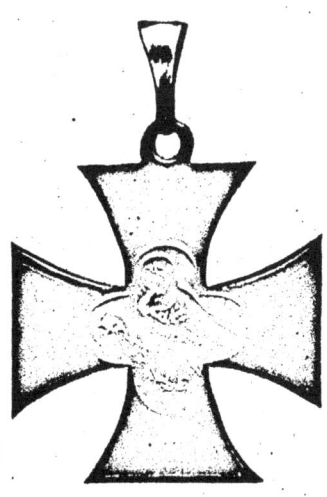

ASSOCIATES' CROSS,
Nursing Sisters of St. John the Divine.

There appears also to have been great lack of delicacy and refinement in the wards. Patients were washed in public, and they died in public. Screens round the beds, now a feature in every hospital, to insure privacy to the patient when being washed or examined, and freedom from disturbance when dying, were rarely, if ever used. The following story is told by a modern nurse of her first experience as a ward sister in a Midland hospital. Screens and the new style of nursing were being gradually introduced. Some of the doctors were a little impatient about screens, or perhaps careless in their use. During the absence of the sister in question to fetch a screen, the medical man began to strip the patient—a woman—preparatory to examination. When the sister returned she burst into tears from a sense of outraged delicacy. The doctor, a gentleman of the olden school, who took the common hospital usage as a matter of course, was quite taken back at the distress he had innocently caused. The sequel is entirely to his credit. After leaving the ward he sought the matron and made an apology for the incident, expressing pleasure at the introduction of a refined woman as a ward sister, and undertaking to support her efforts in every way. This may be taken as a fair example of the sympathetic attitude of experienced medical men towards the superior class of nurses.

An epoch in the history of reform in hospital nursing occurred in 1856, when the committees of King's College Hospital and St. John's House entered into a term of agreement that the sisters and nurses should take over the work, "in order to introduce a higher class of nurses and a better system of nursing into the wards of the hospital, and to carry out more fully than hitherto one main object of St. John's Institution—that of training and providing nurses for the sick in hospitals, as well as for private families and the poor." The agreement was dated March 31, 1856, and was to hold good for two years. The scheme received some assistance from an anonymous donation of one hundred pounds sent the previous year to Miss Mary Jones, Lady Superior of St. John's House, by "a sister of an officer fallen in the Crimea," who desired that the money should be devoted to a fund for building a suitable residence for St. John's House, and to enable the House to make arrangements for taking charge of the sick in King's College Hospital.

The day on which the sisters and nurses of St. John's took formal possession of the wards of the hospital was a dramatic occasion. The old staff, with looks of scorn and derision, stood bonneted and cloaked in the hall, and departed in high dudgeon when the new nurses arrived. With the true spirit of Sairey Gamp and Betsey Prig, these hirelings of the old *régime* declined any assistance to the new-comers, who were left to find out the "bad cases" for themselves, and to put in order wards purposely left in dirt and disorder. By night the sisters and nurses who had arrived in dainty uniforms are described as having "looked like a set of sweeps or charwomen."

It cannot, of course, be claimed that the early St. John's sisters who entered upon the work of hospital reform were trained nurses according to the modern idea. With the exception of the Deaconess's Institution at Kaiserswerth, no training school for nurses existed. Moreover, in those days it was *infra dig.* to suggest training from a professional standpoint to a gentlewoman. Given the Christian desire to serve the sick, it was assumed that by birth, breeding, and education she was qualified to take a position of authority and responsibility in hospitals and kindred institutions, and her services were always gratuitous.

At that period it was not so much a question of "trained nursing," as of introducing methods of order, discipline, and cleanliness into the wards. To-day, when a poor patient is received in a hospital he is stripped of his old clothes, bathed or washed, combed and brushed, put into clean attire in a clean bed, and then is described as being "in nursing order." In like manner the pioneer work of the St. John's sisters primarily consisted in getting hospital wards as well as the patients into nursing order. Character went for more than training, and a refined and educated woman with a homely knowledge of nursing was with confidence, and indeed gratitude, placed in charge of the sick by medical men.

One of the old pioneer sisters, asked where she got her training, replied : "There was no training to be had. I wanted to do something for the sick poor, and, putting on a cap and apron, I went to the hospital. A sister whom I knew had just been called away, and asked me to take charge. I was introduced to the doctor as 'a new sister,' and the only question he asked to test my capabilities was, 'Can you make egg-flip?' Fortunately I was able to answer 'Yes,' at which he smiled approval, waved his hand, and said, 'This is your ward ; I leave you in charge.'"

We may in imagination follow the summarily inducted sister. She made her egg-flip with care and attention, we feel sure ; we know also that she administered the prescribed wine and brandy to the patient and not to herself. If she attempted night duty, she did not take the patients' pillows and make herself comfortable before the ward fire. She gave medicine and food according to medical orders. She looked under beds, routed out the patients' lockers, and allowed the underlings no peace until floors were scrubbed and dust removed, and endeavoured to obtain from the house steward or matron a more plentiful supply of clean bed-linen. We know, too, that her voice was low and sympathetic to the sufferers, and her hand soft and soothing to the weary brow. In a word, she brought into the ward, so far as in her power lay, a refined woman's sense of order and cleanliness, the inherent power of a gentlewoman to compel decency of act and word in her presence, and the ability to control subordinates. If she could not furnish the doctor with a report of a patient's case in technical terms, her observation was guided by intelligence, sympathy, and a cultivated conscience.

The nursing sister of those days was usually a p e woman. Nothing but the highest motives would idavd induced a gentlewoman to break through the prejudices of her class. Oldfashioned training, too, stood her in good stead. She had known the Spartan discipline then meted out to youth in all well-regulated families, and had acquired habits of endurance, and of obedience to authority. She had far less need of a course of sick-room cookery than has the modern probationer, for in country home or parsonage she had followed the example of mother and grandmother in cooking special dishes with her own hands, while she would likewise be versed in the compounding of simple remedies. Such things were a part of a gentlewoman's education when curls and spencers were in fashion. One can imagine a sister embarking on her nursing career with neatly copied recipes from the cherished manuscript of her grandmother's "Cookery and Household Book." Probably at home she had been the right hand of the family doctor, for people could not then telephone for a nurse when illness broke out, and the want was supplied by some "dear girl" or maiden aunt. An interest in nursing purely for the work's sake made the sister quick to acquire knowledge, to be obtained through the kindness of the medical staff and the study of such books as existed. She watched and observed the patients, and so, through the school of experience, surmounted in some degree the lack of systematic training.

The arrangement of King's College Hospital with St. John's House worked so satisfactorily for the first two years, 1856–58, that a renewal of the contract was entered into with mutual satisfaction. The experiment, which was the first made in a London hospital to give the patients superior nursing, and the use of the wards as a training school for nurses, was watched with curiosity, and some anxiety. Miss Nightingale visited the hospital, and expressed great satisfaction at the improvement effected, specially remarking upon the cleanly and homely look of the wards.

The plan upon which St. John's House nursed the hospital was as follows: The lady superior placed one of the sisterhood in the hospital as "sister-in-charge" of the nursing establishment there, and associated with her, and subordinate to her control, were other sisters who took charge of wards, superintended the work of the nurses, the training of probationers, and assisted in the general domestic management of the hospital. At first the latter was in the hands of the house steward, and the dual arrangement retarded the progress of efficient nursing, as the steward did not always see eye to eye with the sister-in-charge in regard to the supply of linen for the wards and the dieting of the patients. A great advance was made when some years later the nursing and domestic arrangements were combined under one head. All the members of St. John's House engaged in the hospital remained under the sole authority of the sister superior and the sister-in-charge, but in nursing matters the sisters and nurses acted in strict obedience to the medical staff.

In 1860 a gift of one thousand pounds to the hospital by Mr. S. F. Wood, of Hockleton, Yorkshire, and the Inner Temple, London, enabled the committee to add another story to the hospital to provide nursing quarters for the sisters and their staff. There, high up above the chimney-pots, with an outlook across to St. Clement Danes, over the congested district of the Strand, and the courts and crowded alleys of the old Clare Market, the St. John's sisterhood arranged a comfortable nurses' home, the first to be attached to a London hospital. There was a little oratory connected with the quarters, as the nursing staff did not then use the College Chapel. This funny old top story has remained the nurses' home at King's up to the present time. When the hospital is removed to the new site in Camberwell, a nurses' home will be provided worthy of an institution which was in the vanguard of hospital nursing reform.

Two years after the building of the old nurses' home, the ward below it, named after Miss Nightingale, was opened January, 1862, for the reception of poor married women during their confinement, and for the training of midwifery nurses for country districts under the sisterhood of St. John's House. This was the first attempt to found a midwifery school for nurses in this country. The scheme owed its origin to Miss Nightingale, who allocated a portion of the fund raised as a testimonial for her services in the Crimea to that purpose. The ward was under the charge of Dr. Arthur Farre. However, the experiment did not succeed. The juxtaposition of the lying-in and surgical wards in days when antiseptic precautions were unknown, resulted in a terrible mortality amongst the women from puerperal fever, and the ward was closed December, 1867. Since then it has been used as a children's medical ward, and bears the name of the Pantia Ralli Ward. Subsequently, a maternity home was established at Ashburnham Road, Chelsea, where the midwifery work begun in the Nightingale Ward was carried on under improved conditions. The home was supported by public subscriptions, and nursed for some years by St. John's House.

In 1865, St. John's House extended its work by taking over the nursing of the Galignani English Hospital at Paris, an admirably appointed little institution, containing twenty-five beds, and situated in the beautiful suburb of Neuilly. It was founded by the liberality of the brothers W. and J. A. Galignani, and its nursing was from the first placed under the Superior of St. John's House.

A year later, 1866, the institution undertook an important piece of new work by taking over the nursing of Charing Cross Hospital on similar lines to those followed at King's College. The sisters and nurses who went to the new scene of labour had a hard task to face in "regenerating" this hospital. Owing to the difficulty which still existed in procuring respectable women as nurses, it was necessary to have some of the old type of nurses at work in the hospital, and the presence of these called for strict discipline. Often in the middle of a stormy night did Miss Caroline Lloyd, who was sister superior at St. John's 1870–83, don her bonnet and cloak, and cross the Strand from Norfolk Street to Charing Cross Hospital to see that there was nothing improper going on in the wards or dormitories. At last it became a saying in the hospital, " It is a stormy night; we shall have the sister here." This vigilance gave rise to the nickname of "ward prowlers," which the medical students, some of whom then lived in the hospital, gave to the St. John's sisters.

The Superior's midnight visits were justified, for occasionally she surprised a party of students and nurses regaling themselves with an oyster and porter supper downstairs, or an after-theatre tea-party before a ward fire. The hilarious conduct of the revellers was scarcely conducive to the rest of sick people. Sometimes the sister discovered more serious breaches of conduct. Raising the moral tone of a hospital, to say nothing of the nursing, must have been an exciting experience in these early days of reform. In 1871, a further branch of work was added by taking over the nursing of the Children's Hospital, Nottingham.

The arrangement for the nursing of the two important London hospitals, by St. John's House, proceeded for many years in comparative harmony, and much good was effected, as the appreciative entries in the minute-books of King's College prove.

It was inevitable that sooner or later nursing under the dual control of St. John's House and the hospital authorities of King's College and Charing Cross would induce friction. The sisters in their zeal were occasionally given to magnify their office, and sometimes to intrude the religious teaching of their particular tenets upon the patients. The medical staff resented the appearance of criticism on the part of the sisters, and were desirous of having the nursing staff absolutely under the control of the hospital. An arrangement which had been admirable as an experiment in reform, became impracticable as years went by.

The first serious break in the cordial relations which had so long existed between St. John's House and King's College occurred in 1874. It fills many pages in the minute-book of that period, and need not be dealt with in detail. Friction had arisen between the sister matron and the hospital authorities regarding the control and dismissal of nurses and matters of domestic management. On January 2, 1874, the council of King's College passed a resolution that "if the sister matron did not care to reconsider her relations from their point of view they should have to call for her removal." On February 9, the hospital, in a letter, sent its ultimatum that "the sisters and nurses must owe obedience to the hospital authorities." This eventually brought about a new arrangement under Miss Parry, known as Sister Aimée, who, as sister matron, reorganized the domestic arrangements on workable lines, and was able to introduce many needed reforms with regard to mealing, the supplies of linen to the wards, and other matters which had formerly been controlled by the house steward. Miss Parry had been sister-in-charge of the nursing staff of King's College since 1868.

The new arrangement continued for nine years until 1883, when a more serious rupture occurred. It is unnecessary to go into detail regarding a circumstance which created much sensational criticism at the time, and called forth a lengthy leader in the *Times* for August 8, 1883. The facts in brief are that, Miss Parry, the sister matron, complained to the chairman of the hospital of the unbefitting manner in which a patient in the obstetric department had been treated

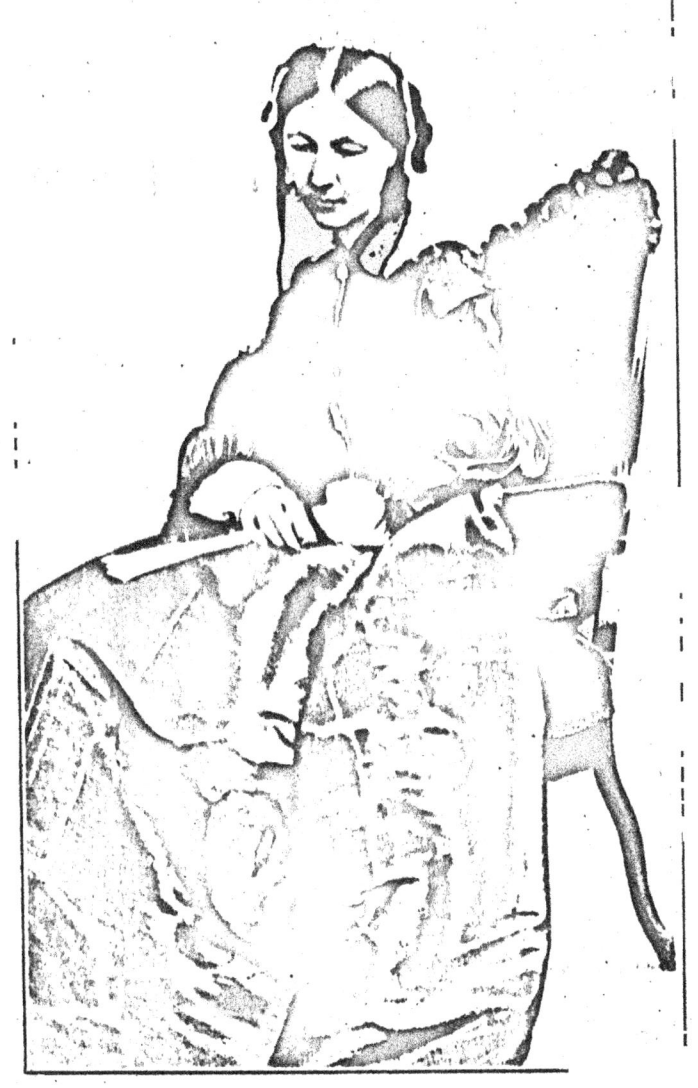

MISS FLORENCE NIGHTINGALE.
After her return from the Crimea.
(*Photo by Keene, Derby.*)

by one of the medical officers. The complaint was investigated, and the committee exonerated the medical officer. Thereupon the Medical Board of the hospital urged for the dismissal of the sister matron, and the committee of St. John's House consented to her retirement. The sister superior of St. John's, Miss Caroline Lloyd, her colleagues in the sisterhood, and many of the nurses, resenting the treatment of the sister matron, withdrew their connection with St. John's House, and formed themselves into the sisterhood of St. John the Divine at Drayton Gardens, South Kensington, an institution already dealt with.

The nursing both of Charing Cross and King's College Hospital by St. John's House ceased in 1883, and this first important and long-continued experiment in hospital nursing reform came to an end.

Among the pleasant reminders of the care and taste bestowed upon the wards at King's College by the St. John's Sisterhood, are the prettily designed and artistically decorated wooden fireplaces at either end of the different wards, which were the work of Sister Aimée and her friends.

The early reforms at University College Hospital were initiated by the All Saints' Sisterhood, a religious community founded by Miss Brownlow Byron and the Rev. Upton Richards, the first vicar of the parish of All Saints, for work amongst the poor and sick. It began its work when Dr. Tait was Bishop of London. The sisterhood had a Nursing Home in Fitzroy Street, and for many years, until 1899, had charge of the nursing at University College. The sisters, in their nun-like garb, with long black stuff dresses and hanging sleeves, were a striking feature in the wards; but it was an anachronism which could not exist side by side with modern dress and methods. University College followed suit with the other hospitals, and organized its own nursing staff under a trained head—Miss Hamilton, now matron of St. Thomas's.

While paying all honour to the important pioneer work in hospital nursing accomplished by the devoted members of the sisterhoods dealt with in this chapter, the time had come when nursing was no longer to be regarded as a religious and philanthropic vocation, but as a profession. The first step in this direction was the founding of the training-school at St. Thomas's Hospital by Miss Florence Nightingale and Mrs. Wardroper.

CHAPTER VIII

THE NIGHTINGALE FUND TRAINING-SCHOOL

The Heroine of the Crimea—Inauguration of the Nightingale Fund—Influence of the Shadow story—Adverse criticism—St. Thomas's Hospital selected for the school—Mrs. Wardroper first superintendent—Rules for probationers—Temporary quarters in Surrey Gardens—Opening of the new St. Thomas's Hospital—The Nightingale Home—Miss Crossland as Home sister—A probationer's day—Severe discipline—Pathetic story—Mid-Victorian young lady—Sumptuary laws—Miss Nightingale and "her children"—Miss Nightingale's letters to probationers and nurses—Pioneer work by St. Thomas's sisters—Influence on American institutions—Retirement of Mrs. Wardroper—Her death and memorial tablet—Resignation of Miss Crossland—The school grants certificates—Mr. Henry Bonham-Carter—Mrs. Wardroper's successors.

THE year 1860 is a memorable one in connection with the history of nursing, for it saw the establishment of the first training-school for probationers as an integral part of a hospital. The training of nurses had, as we have seen, been in progress for some years at King's College, but under the control of the separate organization of St. John's House. The new school was placed under the control of the St. Thomas's Hospital; its object was to train nurses for work in hospitals, and it bore the honoured name of "Nightingale." It came into existence as a direct outcome of Florence Nightingale's heroic work in the Crimean campaign. In the summer of 1855, when the country rang with plaudits for the work which she and her noble band of nurses had accomplished for the wounded soldiers, people were anxious to offer Florence Nightingale some tangible proof of the nation's gratitude. Mr. and Mrs. S. C. Hall approached Mr.

Sidney Herbert (afterwards Lord Herbert of Lea), the famous War minister, under whose auspices Miss Nightingale had undertaken her task, to inquire what form of testimonial would be most acceptable to the lady whom England delighted to honour. Mrs. Sidney Herbert answered the query in the following letter to Mrs. Hall :—

"49, Belgrave Square, July, 1855.

"MADAM,

"There is but one testimonial which would be accepted by Miss Nightingale.

"The one wish of her heart has long been to found a hospital in London, and to work it on her own system of unpaid nursing, and I have suggested to all who have asked for my advice in this matter, to pay any sums that they may feel disposed to give, or that they may be able to collect, into Messrs. Coutts' Bank, where a subscription-list for the purpose is about to be opened, to be called the 'Nightingale Hospital Fund,' the sum subscribed to be presented to her on her return home, which will enable her to carry out her object regarding the reform of the nursing system in England."

A meeting was held at Willis's Rooms, November 29, 1855, presided over by the late Duke of Cambridge, who, during his service in the Crimean campaign, had witnessed Miss Nightingale's heroic work in the hospital at Scutari. Many distinguished people addressed the gathering, but the most telling speech was made by Mr. Sidney Herbert, who read the following extract from a friend's letter : " I have just heard a pretty account from a soldier describing the comfort it was even to see Florence pass. 'She would speak to one and another,' he said, 'and nod and smile to many more, but she could not do it to all, you know, for we lay there by hundreds ; but we *could kiss her shadow as it fell*, and lay our heads on the pillow again content.'" This "shadow story" is known wherever the English language is spoken; it inspired the muse of Longfellow, has been pictured and sung in every clime, and remains the most eloquent tribute ever paid to a woman's influence; but it is not as generally known that it was estimated to have brought at least ten thousand pounds to the Nightingale Fund, and thus to the cause of nursing. It was repeated at meetings all over the kingdom throughout the winter of 1855-56, and never failed to bring "down the house" and unloose the purse-strings. The Nightingale Fund quickly reached forty-four thousand pounds, and was subscribed to by every class of the community. The men of the services throughout the British Dominions were well represented in the list. The soldiers also subscribed for a bust of Miss Nightingale, which was executed by Sir John Steele, and presented to her after her return home.

However, although popular enthusiasm was great concerning the beneficent work for the suffering soldiery during the recent war, it did not extend in the same degree towards Miss Nightingale's scheme for establishing trained nursing. People still shook their heads over the idea of making nursing a calling for women of gentle birth, and of the exclusion from it of the uneducated, unskilled, and unfit woman. It is surprising to find that even less than fifty years ago women of good position mocked at the notion of elevating the sick nurse, and a large proportion of the public calmly acquiesced in evils which they persuaded themselves could not be remedied. Lady Palmerston's view on the subject is thus recorded in the "Life of Lord Granville": "Lady Pam thinks the Nightingale Fund great humbug. The nurses [in hospitals] are very good now; perhaps they do drink a little, but so do the ladies' monthly nurses, and nothing can be better than them; poor people! it must be so tiresome sitting up all night, and if they do drink a little too much they are turned away and others got." The sentiments are characteristic of old "Lady Pam," who called china "chiney" to the day of her death, and hated new-fangled notions.

Society at this period reeked with such thoughtless, narrow-minded opinions, and in its defence of the foibles of the "poor women" condemned to such "tiresome work" as sick-nursing were singularly forgetful of the patient. Florence Nightingale walking the Scutari hospitals and initiating nursing reforms in the distant East was a heroine, but Florence Nightingale putting her finger on the plague-spots at home was by no means so popular. "Let the 'Gamps' and the 'Betsey Prigs' take their drops of comfort; if they fall into excess, well, so do their betters! The sick have got to be nursed, and who is going to do it? Not refined women! Preposterous idea!" And so Mrs. Grundy talked and threw cold water on the Nightingale Fund scheme as soon as Crimean enthusiasm had died down.

The application of the fund lay dormant until 1859, when, it having become apparent that Miss Nightingale's health would not permit her to undertake the arduous task of organizing and managing a hospital for nursing on a special plan, as indicated in the letter from Lady Herbert, already quoted, she placed the fund in the hands of trustees, and a council was named to administer it. Her friends, Lord and Lady Herbert of Lea, were the guiding spirits of the scheme. The object was to devote a portion of the interest of the £48,000, at which the fund now stood, in providing a training-school for hospital nurses. Miss Nightingale reserved to herself the power to advise, and her opinion was taken by the council on details of the scheme.

The hospital selected for the training-school was St. Thomas's, which then stood near London Bridge. It had, as we have seen, played its part in nursing as a monastic institution, and was reopened after the dissolution by the citizens of London, under the patronage of Edward VI. Since then it had been nursed by ward sisters and nurses, on a plan which was a forerunner of the modern system. Miss Nightingale was too practical a reformer to be influenced by mere sentiment, and if St. Thomas's had not offered something more to the purpose than an "apostolic succession" of nursing sisters from mediæval times, it would not have been honoured as the home of the Nightingale School. Its claim to the distinction lay in the fact that it had in Mrs. Wardroper a matron of singular ability, fully alive to the need of nursing reform, who had already been doing pioneer work.

At a time when the hospital matron was generally a nonentity, or worse, the personality of Mrs. Wardroper stands out in luminous contrast. The widow of a medical man, she brought superior education and refinement to the position, and a genius for supervision and organization. For thirty-four years Mrs. Wardroper was matron of St. Thomas's, and had been seven years in that position when chosen to be the superintendent of the newly formed Nightingale Training School. Matrons who to-day are accustomed to see the probationer enter their presence with awe, seem themselves to pale at mention of the name of their old chief, Mrs. Wardroper. She was a strict disciplinarian, a person not to be trifled with, and had a quick discernment of character. Official dignity masked a kind and sympathetic heart, and none knew better how to stimulate and encourage a promising pupil than Mrs. Wardroper; but to the erring, idle, or desultory nurse she was as the voice of Jove. One of her old probationers recalls the wonderment with which, when she first came to St. Thomas's, she listened to her father conversing in terms of equality with Mrs. Wardroper! Possibly she feared that the earth would open and swallow him up for his temerity. Moved by a spirit of mischief, I once suggested to an old probationer of St. Thomas's that Mrs. Wardroper was not, according to modern ideas, a "trained nurse." Eyes flashed at me over the tops of the spectacles, and the almost speechless lady coldly remarked, "Mrs. Wardroper was a fine woman!" All the nursing world will concur in that verdict.

When Mrs. Wardroper became matron of St. Thomas's there was not a sober woman on the staff. She blamed the conditions of work, and at once set about remedying those conditions by a partial division of labour. She employed some of the women for the rougher cleaning work, and kept others more at the bedside of the patients. Mrs. Wardroper improved the nurses' dietary and shortened the hours of labour. She appealed for some ladies to help her, and a few came forward. These she placed over certain sections of the work, and gave them the title of "sister," as the word "nurse" had become so degraded. Such were the conditions which Miss Nightingale found at St. Thomas's, and which led her to select that hospital for her training-school. An upper floor in a new wing of old St. Thomas's was arranged as quarters for the Nightingale probationers. Each had a small separate bedroom, and there was a common sitting-room, and two rooms for the sister-in-charge. In May, 1860, candidates were advertised for, and on June 15th the first fifteen probationers went into residence. They were under the authority of Mrs. Wardroper, the matron, and subject to the rules of the hospital. The training was for one year, and comprised practical instruction in the wards by the matron and sisters, and courses of lectures by the medical staff of the hospital. At the completion of her first year, the probationer passed on to the nursing staff of the hospital. Each probationer was required, at the end of her trial month, to sign a paper promising to remain under the authorities of St. Thomas's for three years, except under special conditions, so that though the training period, so-called, was only a year, the probationer, after going on to the staff, had a further experience of two years' work in the hospital, which was in itself a continuation of training.

Miss Nightingale's object was twofold. She wished to train ladies for superior positions as matrons and

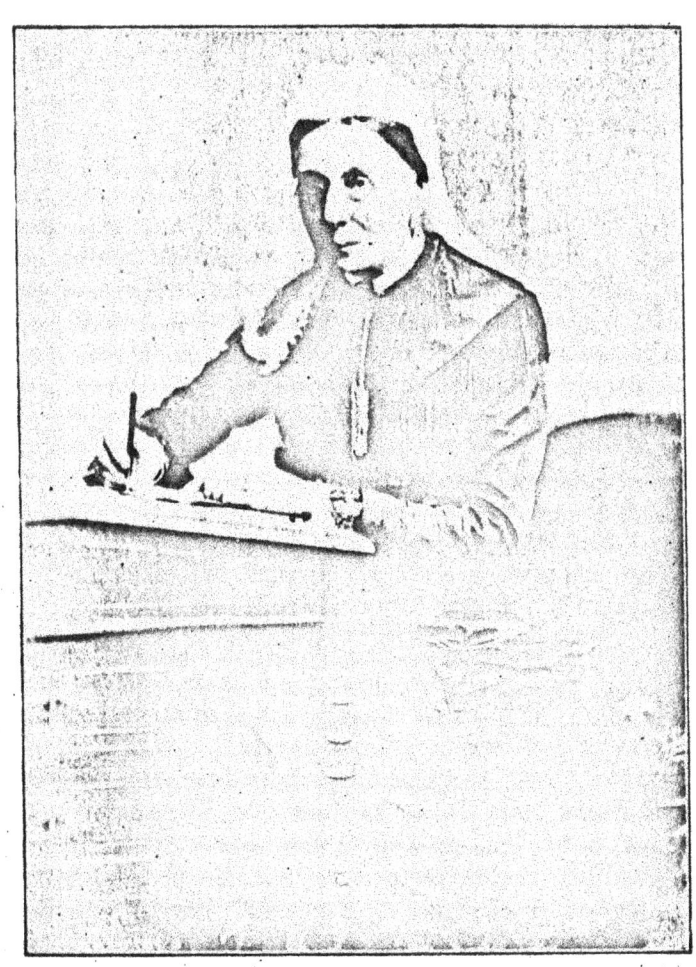

MRS. WARDROPER.

Matron of St. Thomas's Hospital, 1854-87; Superintendent of the Nightingale Fund Training School, 1860-87.

[*To face p.* 96.

superintendents, and respectable young women to serve as nurses; and the probationers were divided into special or lady probationers and nurse probationers. The lady probationers paid thirty pounds towards the cost of maintenance during the year of training, and promised, after leaving the Nightingale Home, to undertake service for *two* years on the nursing staff of the hospital at the current salary, in order to complete their training ; the period to be limited to one year in the case of those paying at a higher rate. After leaving the hospital, and having passed through the course of instruction and training satisfactorily, a lady probationer was expected to become matron or superintendent in some hospital or institution. In the old days the lady probationers were addressed as " miss."

The nurse probationer, after satisfactorily completing her year of training in the Nightingale Home, passed to the hospital staff, and was required to continue in that service for a period of three years, at the current salary. The nurse probationers received free board, lodging, uniform, allowance of two shillings per week for laundry, and the yearly sum of ten pounds, in quarterly payments.

The first year was an anxious one for the promotors of the experiment. The discipline proved too severe for some aspirants, and four probationers were dismissed during the first term. Out of those who successfully passed through probationary training and were put on the register as nurses, six were appointed on the staff of St. Thomas's, and two entered workhouse infirmaries. Miss Nightingale steadily fought opposition and criticism, and from her sick-room came stirring appeals to the young womanhood of the country to devote themselves to the noble vocation of nursing the sick. Mrs. Wardroper laboured with her raw material as only Mrs. Wardroper could, and the training-school grew and prospered, though slowly.

When the old St. Thomas's Hospital was pulled down it found temporary quarters in the Music Hall of the old Surrey Gardens, which had been Mr. Spurgeon's Tabernacle. The quaint beds with the red check curtains were brought from the old hospital.

The year 1871 saw the opening of the new palatial St. Thomas's on the Embankment, and Miss Nightingale and Mrs. Wardroper had the satisfaction of seeing the Nightingale Training School, an integral portion of the finest and most up-to-date hospital in Europe. The magnificent frontage to the river facing the Houses of Parliament, the eight imposing blocks or pavilions in which it was built, the open corridors which formed a promenade overlooking the river the whole length of the building, its magnificent operating theatres and laboratories, made St. Thomas's one of the wonders of London.

The Nightingale Home formed a special wing adjoining the matron's house, and provided accommodation for forty probationers and the home sister. There was a small separate room for each probationer, and a common sitting-room. The chief apartment was the dining-hall, usually termed the Nightingale Hall, which was decorated by mottoes specially selected by its founder. The home was refined and comfortable, but not in the least luxurious. Queen Victoria opened the hospital, June 21, 1871, and the *Times* reporter seems to have been lost in admiration of the sisters and nurses in their dainty uniforms flitting about the wards and corridors. His accounts of their attractive appearance possibly helped to make nursing popular; at any rate, the connection of the school with the much-talked-of St. Thomas's hospital gave it a *cachet* which attracted increased numbers to enroll themselves as probationers. The rules remained practically the same, but the nurses had extended facilities for studying their work in the larger hospital with its modern appliances.

The appointment in June, 1875, of Miss Crossland as home sister, marks an epoch in the history of the training-school. She became Mrs. Wardroper's right hand, and exercised an influence over the probationers which has never been surpassed. Her entry upon the work was dramatic. She arrived at St. Thomas's as a probationer, May 1, 1874, and the same evening made such a favourable impression that Mrs. Wardroper said to the then home sister, "That probationer will do for the future home sister." A year later, June 25, 1875, Miss Crossland was called to the post of honour, which she continued to hold for twenty-one years. For the first thirteen years she worked under and with Mrs. Wardroper, and played an important part in the training of the probationers. She was a strict disciplinarian, and jealous for the prestige of the first training-school. "For a nurse to succeed in her work," said Miss Crossland on one occasion, "she must not mind what she has to do; but *she must mind very much how she does it.* She must be thorough, she must be willing to learn, willing to be taught, she must be loyal to her school and teachers. It must be her aim to keep up the standard of her school, not to bring the slightest speck upon it to sully the name of 'Nightingale.'"

The following table, supplied by an old probationer of the Nightingale Training-School, gives interesting details of a typical day's work. This lady recalls that Mrs. Wardroper often used to say to the probationers, "Nursing is a hard, self-sacrificing life, and this is why our training is so very severe. Few can go on with it; it requires great strength and endurance." The table certainly confirms Mrs. Wardroper's sentiments.

PROBATIONER'S DAY AT ST. THOMAS'S

"Rose at 6 a.m.

"Breakfast, 6.30; the meal rather indifferent, but I never complained, thinking it *infra dig.* to mind about food; home sister read the morning Collect.

"Wards, 7 o'clock.—Made all the beds my side of the ward with a staff or a night nurse, for, as many helpless patients had to be moved, a skilled hand was required to help a probationer. The patients who were well enough got out of bed, and, wrapped in blankets, sat on the locker while the bed was made. The number of beds made was about fourteen, and thirty-five minutes was allowed for doing it. After this each patient was thoroughly washed—night-shirt or night-dress being taken off. The very bad cases were left until a staff nurse could assist. The patient's towel and soap were kept in his locker. The washing had to be completed in rather less than half an hour.

"8 o'clock.—The ward sister came on duty. She read short prayers from the Collects, then put out the brandies and took the temperatures of the patients. After the washings and numerous small duties for patients were over, the probationer either dusted the ward or retired to the bath-room to wash all utensils—dressing-bowls, basins, spittoons, and lavatory utensils, which had to be washed with soap, and dried. It took about an hour. In winter it was bitterly cold," adds the narrator, "and one's hands got terribly chapped. I remember grieving very much at the unsightly condition of my once pretty hands.

"9.30.—Went to the Nightingale Home. If in Edward Ward, it took five minutes out of the precious time to reach my bedroom. There I had to wash, change my dress, make my bed, and dust, and empty basins. After that I got some much-needed food—tea or cocoa, and bread and butter. We were allowed to take a piece from breakfast. We boiled water at a tiny stove in our room.

10 o'clock.—Back to the ward; gave out lunch to the patients; assisted with dressings or waited on medical patients. The house doctors came round and gave numerous orders and changes in treatment. We never had a chance to sit down, but were kept busy until dinner-time.

"12.45.—Dinner.

"1.30.—Back to the ward. The three-quarters of an hour was a precious little rest. Dinner only took quarter of an hour, afterwards we used to make tea in our rooms or go to sleep.

"2 o'clock.—The honorary doctors came round the wards. The great man was followed by a small crowd of students. The sister attended, carrying the ink pot. A probationer carried a basin of water for the "honorary" to wash his hands after touching the patient. Another probationer brought up the screens, turned down the bed-clothes, etc. Clinical lectures were often given, and after we had become acquainted with the intricate medical vocabulary *and* the terribly indistinct medical graphology we learned a good deal from these lectures. In the surgical wards wounds had to be redressed after the surgeon had finished. This often curtailed the probationer's time off, as with the extra press of work we could not leave the wards.

"3.30.—Time off until five o'clock.

"5 o'clock.—Tea, for which an hour was allowed. Once a week we might have the tea hour out, which gave two and a half hours clear off duty. Once a week at 5.30 there was choir practice with the home sister. Sometimes I played the organ in chapel; but as I could not snatch even half an hour for practice, I was very nervous and frightened.

"6 o'clock.—Wards; short prayers by the sister; washing patients and putting them comfortable for the night; medicines, poultices, dressings, liniments, rubbings all to be gone through, which occupied the time until eight o'clock. The house doctors came round to see the patients. The arrival of a fresh admission case kept a probationer extra busy and late.

"When a probationer was on special duty, the hours were: on at 7 p.m., off duty at 8 a.m.; or on at 10 a.m. and off at ten p.m., with half an hour for meals. Once I had a patient for 'special'; he was a man in delirium tremens, and I had to hold his jaw to aid the breathing. This for twelve hours in the day was very hard work.

"8.30. We left the wards and returned to the Home. Supper. Prayers at nine o'clock. Once a week home sister gave us an address.

"We had two hours off duty four days a week. The other two days we attended lectures in our off-duty time. All study was done in off-duty hours. Every other Sunday we had from four till ten o'clock, and once a month a half-day. No holiday was allowed during the probationary year, with the exception of a few days. Afterwards each nurse had a clear fortnight in the year."

Discipline was so severe that a probationer was not permitted to leave her ward even to see her nearest relatives. "On one occasion," says the writer of the foregoing diary, "my mother came up from the country to see me. She seldom could do this, and I asked the ward sister to let me leave at 12.30 instead of 1.45, all the work being finished; but she refused for no other reason except to enforce discipline."

One has to consider, in dealing with a pioneer training-school like St. Thomas's, that the girl of that period was considerably given to sentiment. High schools and athletic exercises had not accustomed her to a little of the rough and tumble of life. She was prompted to take up

nursing because the romantic side of her nature had been
stirred by the story of "Florence Nightingale, the heroine
of the Crimea," or by the pathetic career of Agnes Jones,
the Una who had lost her life in battling with the lion of
disease. Young ladies viewed nursing as a career in
which they could do all manner of kind, gracious, and
heroic actions—smooth pillows, comfort the distressed,
face contagion, court martyrdom, and be interesting at
any price. The authorities of the Nightingale School
had, plainly speaking, "to knock this out" of the heads
of their pupils, and make them realize that nursing was a
serious work, not a mere outlet for sentiment, and, like
Kipling's raw recruit, the probationer did not like the
training process.

A clergyman once made the criticism that "the training at St. Thomas's was calculated to crush all enthusiasm
and spirit in order to force the character to its idea
without making any allowance for natural bent, and was
calculated to turn young women into automatic machines
—discipline was too severely directed against natural
affection."

A pathetic story of a probationer and a suffering child
may be quoted as illustrating the kind of discipline which
shocked many excellent parents and turned some promising probationers from the work. In the Edward
Ward of St. Thomas's lay a poor boy, Harry, officially
known as No. 10. He was a bright, affectionate little
fellow, and took a particular liking to one of the probationers. It was agony to the child to be lifted, and his
cries disturbed the other patients in the ward. "I will
try and not cry out," said little Harry, "if she lifts me,"
meaning the probationer to whom he had taken a fancy.
But the ward sister was obdurate, another nurse was
directed to lift the boy, who called out piteously, and the
young probationer was reprimanded for having spoiled
No. 10. When the printed report of this particular
probationer was filled up by the ward sister to send in to
the matron, Mrs. Wardroper, against the item "Lifting

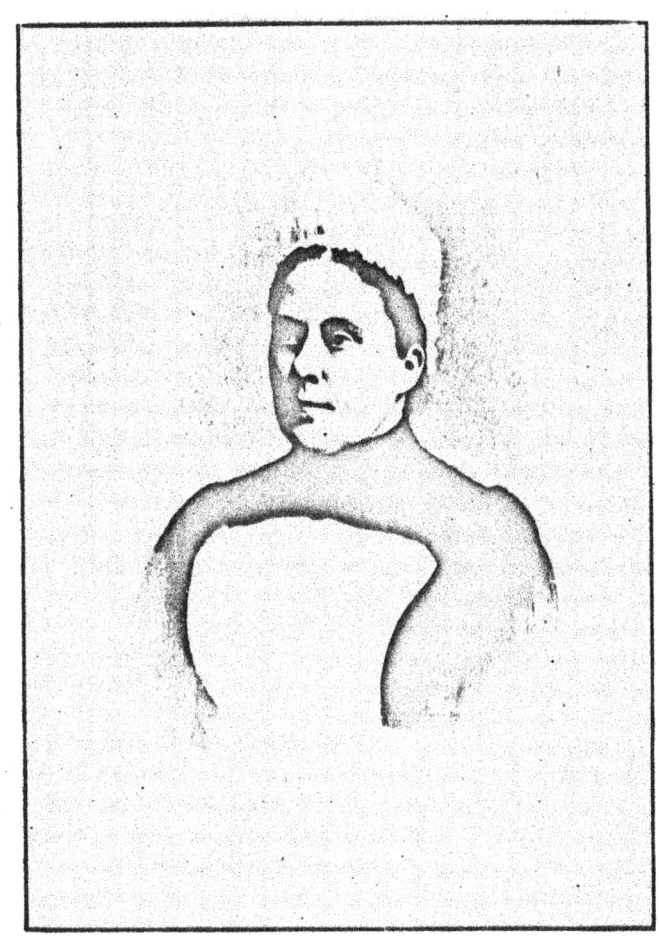

Miss MARY S. CROSSLAND,
Home Sister, Nightingale Fund Training School, 1875-96.

[*To face p.* 102.

helpless patients" was written "Bad." One can understand the sense of injustice felt by a tender-hearted girl at being disgraced for what she thought was an act of human kindness to a suffering child. On the other hand, it is equally clear that discipline could not be maintained in a ward, if patients were allowed to choose who should lift them. The nurses were not allowed to make friends with the patients, and were constantly changed from side to side in the ward. The individuality of nurse and patient was rigidly kept under, and some of the early sisters are said to have carried this to the extent of turning probationers into machines.

Thirty and forty years ago the lady probationers, prompted by enthusiasm for the new calling, went straight from sheltered homes and a life of refined ease to face the routine of a hospital training-school with less preparation than does the modern girl. One can imagine the bewilderment of the mid-Victorian young lady, brought up at home in seclusion and refined ignorance, when her hospital studies suddenly plunged her into the heart of life's mysteries, and it was not surprising that some succumbed and returned home in a state of chaotic frenzy, mind upset and body enfeebled.

The sumptuary laws also told hardly on many girls. When not in uniform, the probationers were expected to wear black or very dark plain dresses and black bonnets. A probationer who attempted to walk out in a hat was sent back to her room, and that useful compromise, the toque, had not then come into fashion. One old probationer recalls that she was severely reprimanded for having on a white straw bonnet trimmed with cream lace and black velvet, which "mother," in the rectory home had thought the pink of propriety and good taste. One adventurous spirit found a more daring outlet. She issued forth from St. Thomas's in decorous garb, but when she gained Westminster Bridge the black dress was lifted to display, O vanity of vanities! a pair of red stockings! Brilliant hose was then the fashion.

When the St. Thomas's Sisters went to do pioneer work in other hospitals and institutions, many relaxed somewhat the very strict rules of conduct and the rigid attempts at "character building" to which they had been subjected, but not St. Thomas's splendid care of its patients. "No hospital comes up to the actual nursing which St. Thomas's taught," writes an old probationer who did not altogether appreciate the strictness of her training; "every small detail with the utmost thought for the patients' comfort was considered. The nursing was technically perfect." There were, too, examples of women imbued with the tenderest human feeling. A sister in charge of the Magdalen Ward is described as "a true saint," who brought her loving influence to bear on the girls and redeemed many from their terrible life. The public little knew how much trained and educated women were needed for nursing these poor outcasts.

I have dwelt on the strict discipline of the first training-school, but there is another side to the picture. Every probationer knew that in Miss Nightingale she had a sympathetic friend. Each probationer was required once a month to write out "A Day's Work in the Ward," and the papers were sent to Miss Nightingale, who criticized and commented on their contents. From her sick-couch came the word of loving encouragement or the criticism administered with characteristic point and often humour. "Her children," she called the probationers, and her words were tender as those of a mother. Some extracts from letters written by Miss Nightingale to the probationers collectively, may be quoted in illustration.

"To the Probationers of the Nightingale Home.
"Easter Eve, 1879.

"MY DEAR FRIENDS,

"I am always thinking of you, and as my Easter greeting I could not help copying for you part of a letter which one of my brother's family had from

Col. Degacher (commanding one battalion of the 24th Regiment in Natal), giving the names of men whom he recommended for the Victoria Cross when defending the commissariat stores at Rorke's Drift. . . . He says: 'Private John Williams was posted, together with Private Joseph Williams and Private William Harrison, in a further ward of the Hospital. They held it for more than an hour, as long as they had a round of ammunition left. When the Zulus burst open the door, a hand-to-hand conflict ensued, during which Private Joseph Williams and two of the patients were dragged out and assegaied. . . . A lull took place, which enabled Private John Williams, who with two of the patients were by this time *the only men left alive* in the ward, to succeed in knocking a hole in the partition and taking the two patients with him into the next ward, where he found Private Henry Hook. These two men together, one man working whilst the other fought and held the enemy at bay with his bayonet, broke through three more partitions, and were thus enabled to bring eight patients through a small window into the inner line of defence.'"

The letter goes on to relate how similar brave deeds on behalf of the patients in another ward were enacted by Privates W. and Robert Jones, and Corporals W. Allen and F. Hitch during that terrible night at Rorke's Drift, January 22nd and 23rd, until all the patients were withdrawn from the hospital.

"*There* is a night-nurses' night's work for you!" continues Miss Nightingale. "When shall such nerves live again? In every nurse of us all. Every nurse may, at all costs, serve her patients as these brave heroic men did at the cost of their own lives. Do you see what a high feeling of comradeship does for these men? . . . Oh, let us nurses all be *comrades*, and stick to the honour of our flag and corps! . . . These great tasks are not to be accomplished suddenly; it is when discipline and training have become a kind of second nature to us that they can be accomplished every day and every night. Every feeling, every thought we have stamps character upon us, especially in our year of training. Prompt obedience is the question. We are not in control, but under control ; . . . so God teaches each one of us in time to go His way and not our own.

"Pray for me, my dear friends, that I may learn it, even now in my old age. .
"Florence Nightingale."

In another of these delightful epistles, written in response to birthday congratulations, May, 1900, Miss Nightingale writes to the nurses—

"My dear Children,
"You have called me your mother-chief; it is an honour to me—and a great honour to call you my children.

"Always keep up the honour of this honourable profession. I thank you—nay, I say our Heavenly Father thanks you, for what you do.

"'Lift high the royal banner,
It shall not suffer loss,'

—the royal banner of nursing. It should gain through every one of you. It *has* gained through you immensely.

"The old Romans were in some respects, I think, superior to us. But they had no idea of being good to the sick and weak. That came in with Christianity. Christ was the Author of our profession."

The Queen of Nurses never omits to be practical, and several pages of the letter are given up to methods in the treatment of disease—particularly consumption.

"A very remarkable doctor, a great friend of mine, now dead," she writes, "introduced new ideas about consumption, which might then be called the curse of England. His own wife was what is called 'consumptive' *i.e.* she had tuberculosis disease in her lungs. He said to her: 'Now, you have to choose; either you must spend the next six months in your room, or you must garden every day [they had a wretched little garden at the end of a street]; you must dig; get your feet wet every day.' She chose the latter, became the hardiest of women, and lived to be old.

"The change in the treatment of pneumonia—disease of the lungs—is complete. I myself saw a doctor take up a child sufferer, which seemed as if it could hardly breathe, carry it to the window, open the window at the top, and held it up there. The nurse positively yelled with horror. He only said, 'When my patient can breathe but little air, I like that little good.' The child recovered, and lived to old age . . .

"Nursing is become a profession; trained nursing no longer an object, but a fact. But, oh, if *home* nursing could become an everyday fact here in this big city of London! . . . If you ask a mother who has perhaps brought you a sick child to 'look at,' 'What have you given it to eat?' she answers triumphantly, 'Oh, it has the same as we have' (!) Yes, often including the gin. And a city where milk, and good milk, is now easier to get than in the country! . . . Now let me try to thank you, tho' words cannot express my thankfulness for all your kind thoughts, for your beautiful book and basket of flowers, and kind wishes.

"God bless you all and me, your mother-chief, as you are good enough to call me.

"My dear children,
"FLORENCE NIGHTINGALE.

"To all our Nurses."

In such way, by loving thought, apt illustration, and words of noble inspiration, has Florence Nightingale sought all through these forty-six years, since the training-school bearing her honoured name was founded, to stimulate the probationers and nurses to noble endeavour in their calling. Her heart has been ever with them, and her regard constantly demonstrated by gifts of flowers in summer, and holly and evergreens at Christmas, from the dear old home at Lea Hurst to deck the rooms of the Nightingale Home. There are cards and mottoes at Christmas, and good wishes at special festive gatherings for her "dear children" at St. Thomas's, and in days gone by parties of the nurses were invited to spend the day with their chief in the beautiful grounds of Claydon, the old home of her sister, Lady Verney.

It has been the great satisfaction of Miss Nightingale's life to see one after another of the St. Thomas's sisters passing to fields of pioneer work in hospitals and institutions in many parts of the empire, and thus carrying forward the work of trained nursing. The school was for many years the model for the various training-schools which sprang up. Dr. W. G. Thompson of New York calls the Nightingale School "the parent of the American system." The outbreak of the Civil War in America turned the attention of that country to the need of a system of training institutions for nurses, and the New York State Charities Aid Association studied its organization through the reports of Dr. Wylie, who came from New York to London to investigate the St. Thomas's School with a view to making it the model for the Bellevue Hospital, New York, and other schools throughout the United States. The children have now in some cases wrested the supremacy from the parent school. The development of trained nursing in the United States is most striking, and Japan has astonished the world by the efficiency of its nursing organization during the late war.

The St. Thomas's School has, however, a noble prestige of pioneer work. Year after year its sisters went forth to organize hospitals and institutions on the modern plan, not only in Great Britain, but in the far distant colonies and America, and even in Continental cities. And to-day France is reorganizing her nursing on the Florence Nightingale system, and with this object a nursing journal, *La Garde-Malade Hospitalière*, has been started.

Mrs. Wardroper retired in 1887, after accomplishing a remarkable record of work. She was the pioneer hospital matron of modern times. Before her advent at St. Thomas's the office of matron could scarcely be said to have been created. "Mrs. Wardroper never lectured to probationers," writes one of her old pupils, "but she trained them more thoroughly, I think, than the highly trained matron of the present day, and certainly maintained a far higher state of discipline in the hospital and wards. In her time, if a probationer had been found 'chatting' to a young medical student or surgeon, she would have been dismissed at once!" In Mrs. Wardroper's letter of farewell to "Past and Present Probationers of the Nightingale Training School," January 12, 1888, she says, "A nurse is not a good nurse who does not humbly learn something every day, who does not practise something better and better every day. Give me the joy of knowing that you all do so, remembering that we care more and more for the work, that God has given us to do for Him, for our bodies as the active willing handmaids of trained minds and loyal hearts, never forgetting that body, mind, and heart are all free gifts, to be given again freely to God, and the work which is His and ours." Mrs. Wardroper died at East Grinstead in December, 1892, in her eightieth year, deeply regretted and revered. In May, 1894, a carved stone memorial was placed to her memory in the chapel of St. Thomas's Hospital. It was the work of Mr. Tinworth. The unveiling ceremony was performed by the Archbishop of Canterbury, and a long line of nurses, together with many lay friends and hospital chaplains, formed an impressive procession. As the commemorative tablet states, Mrs. Wardroper, selected by Miss Nightingale as the first superintendent of the school of nurses in this hospital, "was eminently successful during the last twenty-seven years of her career in training and sending out, not only into Great Britain and her dependencies, but also into other lands, women capable and worthy to carry on a good work."

Miss Crossland, the able lieutenant of Mrs. Wardroper, who may be said to have created the office of home sister, retired in 1896, after occupying the post for twenty-one years. At the annual meeting, June 25, for nurses and probationers, a presentation was made to Miss Crossland. Mr. John Croft, F.R.C.S., one of the consulting surgeons of St. Thomas's Hospital and for many years medical instructor to the Nightingale School, acted as spokesman for the subscribers. The presentation consisted of an album inscribed by two hundred and eighty nurses, and a cheque for eighty pounds. Miss Crossland thanked her friends in a speech of interesting reminiscences. The secretary, Mr. Bonham Carter, read the resolution passed by the council, which was as follows :—

" Resolved that, in accepting Miss Crossland's resignation as home sister, the council desire to convey to her their very sincere regret at losing services which they so greatly value, and they wish to place on record the high appreciation of the benefits which the Nightingale School has derived from her single-minded devotion to her duties, and from her great power, not only of teaching, but also of inspiring her pupils with her own high sense of duty. They indeed feel that she may be said to have created the post of 'Sister of the Nightingale Home,' which she has for twenty-one years so wisely and so ably filled. And as some acknowledgment of the value of her work to the school and to the cause of nursing generally, they resolve to grant her a retiring allowance of fifty pounds a year, during the pleasure of the council."

Next followed the presentation of a bouquet from Miss Nightingale, to which was attached the following characteristic message :—

"To Miss Crossland, Home Sister of the Nightingale Home for twenty-one years, who has given a new life and calling to so many, in nursing the poor, body and soul, by absolute self-devotion, by training in wise discipline, loyalty, and love, as well as in technical and intellectual skill and knowledge. A grateful Florence Nightingale."

The dining-hall and corridors were beautifully decorated for the occasion with flowers sent by Miss Nightingale.

The rules of the school practically remain the same as when it was founded. The number of probationers received for training has increased, and now averages fifty. They have outgrown the limits of the Nightingale Home, and when the new home for staff nurses at St. Thomas's is completed, some additional accommodation in their former quarters will be available for probationers. An important change to be noted is the granting of certificates in lieu of gratuities, which came into force in 1904. Hitherto St. Thomas's had not granted certificates to its nurses. They are now awarded to nurses who have satisfactorily completed three years' training and service in the hospital.

A name long connected with the school is that of Mr. Henry Bonham Carter, a relative of Miss Nightingale's, and her trusted friend and adviser. As secretary for many years of the Nightingale Fund, Mr. Bonham Carter has exercised great influence at St. Thomas's, and he and Mrs. Bonham Carter have long been familiar figures at the nurses' reunions, and are deeply interested in the various branches of the nursing movement. The late Mr. William Rathbone was for many years chairman of the Council of the Nightingale Fund.

In concluding this account of the pioneer training-school a tribute should be paid to the work of Miss Pringle, who, after reorganizing the nursing at the Royal Infirmary, Edinburgh, returned to her *alma mater* to succeed Mrs. Wardroper as matron. Miss Pringle has recently published a little volume on nursing, which is of much practical interest for those entering the profession. Her successor, Miss Gordon, had a long and distinguished career as matron at St. Thomas's, and that important post is now filled by Miss Hamilton, who, like her predecessors, is an old Nightingale probationer. Eight nurses from the Nightingale School received appointments as matrons during last year, and seven entered the Army Nursing Service. There is not, I believe, any portion of the empire where pupils of this School have not gone forth to do pioneer work.

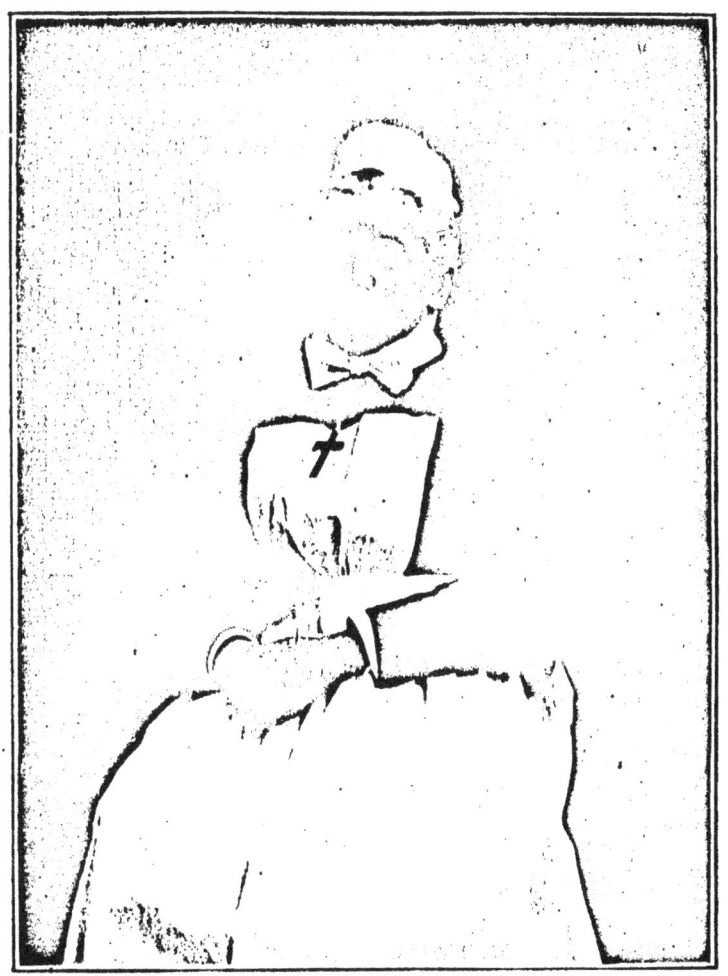

Miss Monk.

Sister and Matron of King's College Hospital, 1883-1906; Founder and Superintendent of the Nurse Training School.

[*To face p.* 112.

CHAPTER IX

HOSPITAL NURSING AND TRAINING-SCHOOLS

Dearth of trained nurses in 1862—William Rathbone founds the Liverpool Training-School—Its success—London Collegiate Hospitals in the front rank of reform—King's College Hospital—University College Hospital—Charing Cross Hospital—Ormond Street Hospital for Sick Children—The Middlesex Hospital—The Royal Infirmary, Edinburgh—Lady Augusta Stanley founds the Westminster Training-School.

THE system of trained nursing begun in the Nightingale School of St. Thomas's was by no means quickly propagated. The other large hospitals seemed disposed to cautiously watch the experiment before following suit. It was still thought that the "fancy" of educated women for becoming nurses was a passing enthusiasm which would die away as Crimean days receded, and hospital authorities probably felt that they had better not disturb the existing order of things before being sure that a supply of the new could be found to replace the old order of nurses. Reformers, too, were beset by the difficulty of procuring trained women to train others. St. Thomas's and King's College could not meet the demand for sisters to take in hand pioneer work at other institutions. This dearth had the result of calling into being the Liverpool Training-School and Home for Nurses, founded in 1862, which carried the training system into the provinces and formed an important event in the nursing movement. It was the generous gift to Liverpool of the late William Rathbone, one of its most distinguished citizens, under the following circumstances, as related by Miss Eleanor Rathbone in the most interesting memoir of her father.

extend it, but could not obtain trained women to carry out the scheme. In his dilemma he did what most people did in those days when planning nursing ventures, he asked the advice of Miss Nightingale. Her answer was brief and to the point—" Liverpool had better form a school to train nurses in its own hospital."

The Royal Infirmary, the chief general hospital of Liverpool, had, however, no facilities for training nurses. Its then staff were of the usual rough, intemperate, and untrustworthy class, and when a rise of wages had been offered to attract a more reliable kind of nurse, all save four celebrated the rise in their fortunes by getting drunk on the first quarter-day. This was scarcely the material out of which trained nurses could be fashioned. It was necessary to begin anew and form a school. Mr. Rathbone talked matters over with Mr. Edward Gibbon, Chairman of the Infirmary. This gentleman was conservative in his ideas. He, however, visited London, and inspected the nursing organization at King's College and St. Thomas's, and on his return to Liverpool told his friends that until he saw the system in these two hospitals he did not know what nursing was. He supported Mr. Rathbone's generous offer to build a Training-School and Home for Nurses and present it to the Liverpool Infirmary. It was to be managed by a committee of the infirmary, who pledged themselves to carry it on until it had had a fair trial.

It was started in 1862 in temporary premises, and was opened May 1, 1863, as "The Training-School and Home for Nurses," in Ashton Street, where it is still located. The nurses were to be trained in the wards of the Royal Infirmary, first, for work in that institution, secondly, for nursing the poor in their own homes, and thirdly, for well-to-do private patients. The school was placed under the charge of Miss Merryweather, who had been through a short training at St. Thomas's, and for many years she rendered admirable service as superintendent. The founder himself acted as honorary secretary, and Miss Nightingale was in the early years chief adviser. So this first provincial training-school grew and prospered, and in turn sent out its pupils to do pioneer work in other towns. It has now eighty-two nurses employed in the Liverpool Infirmary; twenty-one district nurses, and forty-five private nurses. Probationers are trained on the three years' system, and are required to remain a fourth year in the service of the institution, at the expiration of which time a certificate is granted. A register of nurses is kept, and a nurse's certificate may be rescinded for subsequent misconduct or inefficiency.

In London the Collegiate Hospitals were in the front rank of the reform movement. King's, as already narrated, placed its nursing under the charge of St. John's House so early as 1856, and later established a home and school for trained nurses at the hospital under the superintendence of St. John's sisters. When that arrangement came to an end in 1883, and the hospital resolved to have a nursing staff entirely under its own control, Miss Monk was appointed sister matron, and entrusted with the task of organizing the new system. Miss Monk had trained at St. Bartholomew's, and had been an associate sister at St. John's House, so that her appointment was interesting as forming a link between the old *régime* at King's and the new nursing school.

Miss Monk was a very young woman for a matron when appointed to the important post which she was destined to fill with success and distinction for a period of twenty-three years. Although she reaped the advantages of the cleanliness, order, and good routine which had been established in the wards by the St. John's sisters, Miss Monk did arduous pioneer work in training a new staff. She managed the departure of the temporary staff, which in 1883 took the place of the St. John's sisters, with consummate tact. One set of nurses departed by one door, and the fresh staff entered by another. They saw nothing of each other, and friction and unpleasantness were avoided.

The new sister matron also showed her skilful generalship in the training of her nurses. She was at first assisted by sisters from St. Thomas's. The nurses' old quarters in the top floor of the hospital were re-arranged on a better plan. The cubicles, hitherto divided by curtains, were partitioned off into separate rooms; the oratory of the St. John's sisters was devoted to other uses, and the nurses attended service in the College chapel. By Miss Monk's efforts, a sum of twelve hundred pounds was raised for the building of a new wing on to the old quarters, to provide space for a nurses' sitting-room. A special classroom was arranged for probationers, and there the assistant matron and home sister, Miss Little, gives demonstrations in practical nursing and holds classes to assist the pupils in assimilating the instruction given by the medical and surgical lecturers. The late Miss Clara Peddie (Sister Sibbald) was for many years home sister, and rendered valuable assistance to Miss Monk in bringing the nursing school of the old Collegiate Hospital to a high state of efficiency. The training is for three years, and certificates are granted for varying grades, so as to embrace nurses who show to greater advantage in the practical work of the wards than in examinations—a fair and important distinction. Miss Monk arranged a generous scheme for recreation, and worked out her plan in the form of a clock dial. By it each nurse is secured four hours off duty daily without involving the hospital in much extra nursing outlay. Probationers have also one day a month. Sisters have five hours on alternate days, two days a month, and six weeks' holiday in the year.

One wonders whether it was the fame of the medical or of the nursing staff which brought the famous canine patients to King's! The incident occurred July 31, 1887, and is treasured in the hospital archives. Early on the morning of that day two terriers came to the door of the out-patients' department, bringing with them a retriever with an injured paw bleeding copiously. They barked loudly, were admitted, and had the satisfaction of seeing their suffering friend successfully treated. One of the terriers was recognized as a dog who had been himself treated at the hospital a few days before, and now he had returned to introduce an injured acquaintance. In the Board room is a picture, after the original by Mr. Yates Carrington, representing the three dogs on the hospital steps.

It was a matter of universal regret that Miss Monk was, in the spring of 1906, compelled through ill-health to resign the position of sister matron at King's College Hospital. Her beautiful personality endeared her to every one in the hospital, and her work in the founding and development of the nursing school is a noble record of work performed with rare zeal and modest self-effacement. To Miss Monk herself it was a matter of keen disappointment and regret that she was unable to continue at her post until the completion of the removal of the hospital to Camberwell. It was also a great sorrow to her to be compelled to sever her connection with Queen Alexandra's Imperial Military Nursing Service, more especially as Her Majesty had recently placed her on the council of the British Red Cross Society, in both of which works she took the warmest interest. It will be remembered that Miss Monk rendered great service in helping to organize Queen Alexandra's Imperial Military Nursing Service in 1902-3.

It is an interesting point connecting two honoured names in the nursing profession that Agnes Jones, the pioneer of trained workhouse nursing, was the dear friend of Miss Monk's mother. Colonel Jones, the father of Agnes Jones, was a brother officer of Miss Monks' grandfather, and became her mother's guardian.

On July 30, 1906, a presentation was made to Miss Monk by Lord Methuen, Chairman of the Committee of Management of King's College Hospital, on behalf of the committee and of the meical and nursing staff of the hospital (past and present), and a number of her personal friends. Dearer still to Katharine Henrietta Monk must be the knowledge that she will ever live in the annals of the hospital as the beloved "Sister Katharine."

Miss Monk has been succeeded by Miss M. E. Ray, who comes with a great reputation from the Lincoln County Hospital. Miss Ray was trained under Miss Monk at King's College, was ward sister there for four years, after which she went as assistant superintendent to Leeds General Infirmary, and then as matron to the Lincoln County Hospital. She has now returned to her *alma mater* as head, after an absence of ten years.

University, the sister collegiate hospital, early adopted a system of trained nursing by the All Saints' Sisterhood, who undertook it by contract with the hospital. The plan worked well for many years, but when in 1899 an enlargement and reconstruction of the hospital was started, the system of nursing was changed, and a new staff organized under a trained matron. Miss Hamilton, who later became matron of St. Thomas's, filled the post for three years, and under her superintendence the University College School of Nursing was established on lines adopted by the committee in 1899. The training is for three, and the engagement to the hospital for four years.

Miss Dora Finch, who became matron in 1902, has successfully carried on the work during the period of change through which the hospital has been passing. Most of the old building has been pulled down and new erected. It must have been no light task to be matron during this transition period, involving much changing about of patients and nurses. Miss Finch was trained at St. Bartholomew's, and for eleven years worked there as "day," "night," and ward sister successively. She was matron of the Women's Hospital in the Euston

Road before coming to University College. Miss Finch has in contemplation the organization of a private nursing staff in connection with the hospital, and a new home is being built for its accommodation. This will complete the hospital extension. The wards are a delight to enter; the arrangement of side wings broadening out the top of each ward give a delightful sense of light, air, and space. The nurses' quarters are excellent. Each nurse has a room to herself, heated by a radiator. The sisters' and the nurses' sitting-room each have a grand piano, and there is a library of books supplied by a legacy. The reputation of the University School is evinced by the fact that the sisters are invariably snapped up at the end of their engagements to fill superior posts. Most of the nurses at this hospital are gentlewomen.

Charing Cross was amongst the first hospitals to start reforms in its nursing system. Moved by the good example of its near neigbhour in the Strand, King's College Hospital, it placed its nursing under the control of St. John's House in 1866, and vigorous measures were taken to enforce order and discipline in the wards, and to improve the standard of nursing. This arrangement continued until 1883. Subsequently the hospital got in its own nursing staff and trained probationers on the three years' system.

Changes in the direction of efficiency have taken place under the matronship of Miss Heather-Bigg, who in 1903 introduced a new system. After a personal interview and three months' trial, candidates are received for four years' training. The first year they attend lectures by the home sister on elementary anatomy and physiology, and demonstrations on practical nursing. They are examined by the matron or one of her friends. A probationer who does not pass this preliminary examination is required to terminate her engagement, but, at the discretion of the matron, she may present herself again for examination at the end of six months. During the second and third years, probationers who have passed the first examination receive regular teaching from members of the medical staff—second year, anatomy and physiology; third year, surgical and medical diseases. At the end of the third year they are required to pass a second examination, prior to receiving a certificate of efficiency. If they fail to pass this second examination, they are not allowed to come up for a fourth year of service, unless the matron considers them so far eligible as to permit them to come up again for examination at the end of six months. For the first and second years the pupils are called staff probationers, third year staff nurses, and the fourth year are eligible for sisters' posts. Promotion to posts in the hospital are gained by merit. There is no salary the first year. Afterwards, salaries rise from fifteen pounds to forty-five pounds annually. Special probationers are received for one year's training at a fee of fifty-two guineas.

Miss Heather-Bigg comes of a talented family well represented in the medical world. She was trained at University College Hospital, and has great ideals for her profession. Most of her nurses are drawn from the professional classes, and she seeks to inspire them with the desire for efficiency united to practical usefulness. While looking to State registration as the solution of the difficulties and unsatisfactoriness of nursing in many particulars, Miss Heather-Bigg relies greatly on the tone of the surroundings amidst which a nurse is trained as a factor in producing a class of women who will be real servants of the State, and welcome in the homes of the people.

A well-arranged Nurse's Home in Agar Street has been built in connection with the hospital. When King's College Hospital has removed from the vicinity of the Strand, Charing Cross will have extra demands laid upon it. The way in which it can rise to meet an emergency was exemplified at the disaster at Charing Cross Railway Station in December, 1905, when the matron made such prompt provision for the reception of the sufferers, and the nursing staff rendered invaluable service at the scene of the disaster.

The claims of that admirable institution, the hospital for sick children, Great Ormond Street, Bloomsbury, as a pioneer in nursing reform are apt, in the present day, to be overlooked. Not only was it the first hospital in the United Kingdom devoted to the reception of sick children, but at a time when nearly all the great general hospitals were still in the slough and mire of a disreputable class of nursing, Ormond Street was started on good lines. It was founded by that large-hearted philanthropist, Dr. Charles West, and one of his chief objects was the training of nurses. The hospital was opened in 1852 with twenty beds. The first superintendents were Miss Willey and Mrs. Rice successively, and under them special attention was given to securing respectable young women and training them for work in the hospital. Also ladies, who so desired, could send their nursery-maids to receive a course of instruction in the application of simple remedies, and in the handling and general management of sick children. As years went by, and the standard of nursing rose after the Crimean period, it was found impracticable to continue the training of hospital nurses and of nursemaids in one establishment, and the latter was abandoned.

The development of the nursing at Great Ormond Street proceeded on modern lines, and Dr. Howship Dickinson thus describes its condition in 1862, when he joined the hospital, "the nursing was conducted much as at present, and was excellent. The head of the nursing was an unpaid lady superintendent, Miss Budd, while there was a lady nurse at the head of the girls' ward and the boys' ward respectively. There were ordinary paid nurses under these ladies, but they were of a superior class to what is often met with, and altogether the nursing was such as could not be improved upon."

The excellence of the system was chiefly due to Dr. Charles West, and he found in Miss Budd, the third lady superintendent, an admirable coadjutor. Such training as was given at this period was necessarily informal and purely practical, but educated women were being drawn to the work, and the Ormond Street Hospital was conducted on lines which would attract them. Among the names connected with it none is more honoured than that of Miss Catherine Wood, who there began her nursing career in 1863 as sister of the girls' ward. She was connected with the hospital for twenty-five years, being superintendent from 1878–88. The system of admitting lady pupils was introduced by her successor, Miss Phillippa Hicks, 1888–90. Among other reforms introduced at Ormond Street, was the visiting by sisters of the out-patients in their own homes, before the advent of the district nurse. A mortuary chapel was also provided, and formed a marked contrast to the dirty squalid cellars which were thought good enough for the dead of hospitals in the past. When a little sufferer died at Ormond Street, the nurse or sister of the ward went with the body to see that it was decently and reverently laid out, and subsequently handed it over to the undertakers.

There are now two hundred beds in the hospital, which contains six large wards of over twenty beds each, in addition to smaller separate wards, and an isolated building for diphtheria and for fever cases arising in the hospital, and a ward with sixteen beds has been opened for whooping-cough. The number of in-patients treated during last year was 2537. There is an extensive out-patients' department where two thousand patients are treated weekly. The convalescent home at Highgate receives patients from the hospital for a period of three weeks. Last year two hundred and sixty-eight children enjoyed this privilege. The hospital is under the patronage of the King and Queen. The Duke of Fife is president, and with the Princess Royal takes a deep personal interest in the little sufferers. Mr. Stewart Johnson is secretary, and Miss G. Payne, matron.

The course for nurses at Great Ormond Street now extends over three years. Probationers, who must not be less than twenty-one years of age, pay a premium, although some vacancies are reserved for probationers without payment. Lectures are given by the medical staff, and instruction in practical nursing, cookery, and massage by the matron, home sister, and ward sisters. Certificates are granted upon the satisfactory completion of the three years' engagement and passing examination. The nursing of sick children peculiarly appeals to most women, and the popularity of this branch of the profession is attested by the fact that the applications at Great Ormond Street number three thousand yearly.

In 1881 a private nursing staff was started in connection with the hospital, and the nurses are available for adult as well as for children's cases. Nurses from this pioneer hospital are scattered all over the world, and have been sent into the families of most of the crowned heads of Europe.

The Middlesex Hospital laid the foundation of its nursing school as early as 1867, and the scheme originated with Major Ross, the chairman of the weekly board. The hospital is an old institution, having been founded in 1745, when it began its career in Windmill Street, Tottenham Court Road, where two houses, rented at thirty pounds a year, for the reception of sick and lame patients were opened as "The Middlesex Infirmary." In 1747 one-third of the beds were devoted to lying-in married women, and a rule was enacted that no "woman-midwife be permitted to act as midwife to this hospital." This did not look very promising for the training of women nurses. Evidently sex bias ran high in those early days at the Middlesex; but the authorities could not get away from the long association of a feminine term with this branch of work, and we find in 1763, Dr. Thomas Cooper set down as "physician man-midwife" to the hospital.

Meantime the institution had removed to new

premises erected 1755-57, under the auspices of the Earl of Northumberland, on its present site, Mortimer Street, W., then known as Marylebone Fields, a salubrious district on the outskirts of London. A survival of the rustic period of the Middlesex is the old garden which still remains a grateful retreat for nurses and patients alike, though now surrounded by buildings which mark the various stages of the hospital's extension. In days gone by the garden was devoted to the cultivation of vegetables, and later was converted into a "medicine garden"; then it fell into frivolous uses, was the scene of local flower-shows, and has been used on occasions for evening *fêtes*. One wonders if it ever entered into the imagination of those who tilled the soil of the old garden in its vegetable period (1769) that a century later nurses in dainty uniforms would be studying the latest surgical treatment under its trees.

Some recognition of the claims of the nursing staff was made in 1848, when the extensions and improvements to the hospital included "new rooms for the superior nurses." It was not, however, until 1867 that the nursing department was reorganized by the weekly board under the chairmanship of Major Ross, with the co-operation of the honorary medical and surgical staff. In May of that year, Miss Catherine Martyr, who had trained for the post at University College, was appointed the first Lady Superintendent of Nursing under the new *régime*, and in 1869 a comfortably equipped Nurses' Home was opened by Princess Mary of Cambridge. Miss Martyr was not strong, and during periods of enforced rest her work as superintendent was undertaken by Miss Thorold—a name destined to become a tradition at the Middlesex. She had been a fellow-probationer with Miss Martyr at University College, and was devoting herself to nursing in her father's parish of Umberleigh, North Devon. In 1870, Miss Martyr being no longer able to continue her duties, Miss Thorold was invited by the chairman of the weekly board to fill the vacant post of lady superintendent, and to carry on the work of reform in the nursing department, which had been so ably initiated. She remained at her post for thirty-five years, and before her retirement in 1905 had long been the doyen amongst hospital superintendents and matrons.

During Miss Thorold's long term of office many new schemes and reforms took place in the nursing department of the Middlesex. In 1870 lady probationers were added to the nursing staff, who, on payment of a guinea a week, were employed in the service of the hospital for a given time of not less than six months' training, to fit them for work, philanthropic or otherwise, which they desired to take up. Two years later, with a view to improve the position of the nurses on the hospital staff, and to induce them to remain in the service of the institution, the fees paid by the lady probationers were devoted to the formation of a Nurses' Pension and Gratuity Fund. In 1878 a new Nurses' Home was built, and the day-room tastefully furnished by Miss Cavendish Bentinck. Lectures to the nurses by members of the medical staff were provided for out of the Lady Probationer Fee Fund, and still continue with signal success, certificates being granted to such nurses as have attended the course. In 1886 an institution for private nurses was started, and a building erected contiguous to the Nurses' Home. After five years', or in some cases three years' training in the hospital, nurses may join the Private Nurses' Institute, and obtain a comfortable home, remunerative occupation, and a pension for old age. In 1892, at Miss Thorold's suggestion, lady probationers of promise were, at the completion of their term of training, enabled to enter the service of the hospital as staff nurses. The following year the nurse's dietary was rearranged and improved. In 1904 the Nursing Home was extended by a new building adjoining the institute. The three years' course of training was introduced by Miss Thorold.

In the hospital she saw changes also. The outpatients' department was reconstructed; a children's ward opened; a cancer wing added; new operating-theatres built; electric light installed; a modern laundry established at Hendon; and a convalescent home erected at Clacton. In spite of this extension of work and interests, Miss Thorold's energies never flagged. To the last she adhered to her old custom of visiting the wards twice daily, and making herself acquainted with the needs of each patient. She was the ever accessible friend of nurses and patients alike, and her example inspired an *esprit de corps* throughout the hospital. The place which she occupied in the esteem of all connected with that institution was admirably expressed by the editor of the *Middlesex Hospital Journal*, who thus comments upon Miss Thorold's retirement: "We have lost a good example of how to serve the hospital. Miss Thorold's retirement is still so recent that to many of us the place seems strange without her. That is a testimonial worth having—to be missed when one goes. She loved the hospital, and for five-and-thirty years gave herself to its service. Infinite kindness she had for every one of its patients: it is an impenetrable wonder how she never failed of a smile or a pleasant word, every day, year in, year out, for each of the bedridden folk whom she saw on her rounds through the wards. She must have walked many thousands of miles of wards, always gentle, always kind. Very few men could have done that. To all of us she showed true good-will, and meant it. No protestations, no affectations—just quiet, simple, incessant courtesy and loyal friendship. In her judgment the feminine spirit was not an accident of nursing, but nursing was an accident of the feminine spirit: and seeing to what high excellence, under her just and peaceful reign our sisters and nurses have attained, it is probable that she was right. She has the affection of a host of friends inside and outside the hospital, and the happy certainty that her work was good."

Miss Thorold was one of the earliest supporters of the Royal British Nurses' Association, and one of its vice-chairmen. She was not, however, able to sympathize with its advocacy of the State Registration of Nurses, and in consequence retired from an active participation in its affairs, though feeling great sympathy with its philanthropic aims. The work accomplished by Miss Thorold at the Middlesex forms a remarkable record in the nursing world.

Her successor, Miss Vernet, formerly matron at the National Hospital for the Paralyzed and Epileptic at Queen's Square, Bloomsbury, and a sister at the Middlesex, is a true disciple of Miss Thorold, and under her able management the hospital will maintain its reputation as a training-school.

The largest and most important training-school in Scotland is attached to the Royal Infirmary, Edinburgh, and was founded in 1872. Edinburgh is a city of professors and students, and its atmosphere of learning imparts distinction and gives tone to its great nursing school. Young Scottish women come to Edinburgh to train for nursing with almost the same serious purpose and enthusiasm as their brothers come up for divinity, law, and medicine, and seem to possess the same tenacity and grit and the ability to achieve advancement in their profession. The number of "headships" held by Edinburgh nurses is as proverbial as the political posts held by Scotchmen.

The Royal Infirmary has nearly one thousand beds, and a staff, including five assistant-superintendents, of two hundred and forty nurses. It is situated high up beyond the old town, and when founded in 1728 was beyond the smoke area of Auld Reekie. The Edinburgh Infirmary seems to have been well in advance of the times in its early nursing rules. The head of the nursing and domestic department was, according to quaint Scottish usage, termed "the mistress," and her powers were comprehensive. "She shall have the charge of all the plenishing and furniture in the hospital," runs a rule of 1728, "the trust of buying all provisions, overseeing the patients and servants, ordering their diet, administrating the medicines ordered by the physicians, the trust of buying all house necessaries, the care of keeping the chambers, beds, cloaths, linnens, and all other things within the hospital neat and clean, and to her all the servants and patients within the hospital are to be submissive and obedient." The mistress's "accounts" were to be revised every week by the physician and surgeon attending, " whereby they may judge of the diet provided by her to the patients."

The staff under the "mistress" consisted first of "ordinary nurses," who did the usual ward work, gave the patients their medicine as ordered and their "diet when brought from the kitchen." The rules "enjoin" her on matters of cleanliness and sanitation according to the ideas of that day. After dinner each day she made a round of the ward with a "basket," and collected the "boxes, pots, glasses, etc., belonging to each patient into the box of her basket, where the name of such patient is affixed, and to carry them all to the apothecary, from whom she is to receive back what boxes, pots, etc., should have remained in her ward, which she is to put again into the closet of each patient, and is then immediately to bring back her basket to the apothecary, who shall appoint the time for her returning to receive it with the new medicines."

The second order were "supernumerary nurses," who were called to attend certain patients at night as the doctors judged necessary. Night nursing was then only deemed needful for special cases. The female relations of the patients were often admitted as supernumerary nurses.

The precautions in case of contagious diseases are thus complacently set forth in 1778. "The nurses are to give due attention to the bedding of the patient, especially when they labour under contagious diseases. In such

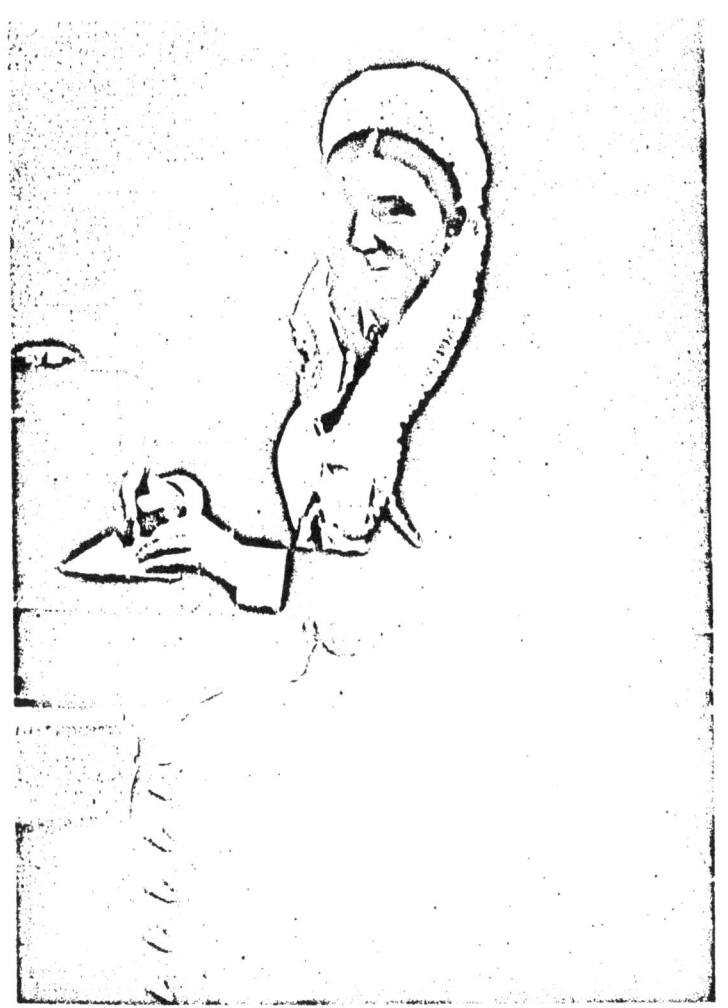

MISS G. M. THOROLD.

Matron, Middlesex Hospital, 1870-1905; Founder and Superintendent of the Nurse Training School.

[*To face p.* 128.

cases the mattresses ought to be exposed to the open air in the wooden frame erected for that purpose, and the blankets and bed-linen washed before they be put to use for other patients." In such manner were things managed in the "good old times," before people's minds were disturbed by a knowledge of germs and microbes and antiseptic treatment !

The modern system of trained nursing was introduced into the Edinburgh Infirmary in 1872 by Miss Pringle, of St. Thomas's Hospital, who, aided by sisters from that institution, reorganized the nursing department on the Nightingale plan. Miss Nightingale followed the work with keen interest, and has always felt a special bond of association with the Edinburgh School. The sisters wear the Nightingale cap of spotted net. Miss Pringle, after her arduous and successful labours at Edinburgh, returned to St. Thomas's Hospital as matron, and was succeeded at Edinburgh by Miss Spencer, the present superintendent (1906), who also was a Nightingale probationer at St. Thomas's, and has ably carried on the system introduced by Miss Pringle. She has a valuable chief-assistant matron in Miss Walker, who trained at the infirmary, and has passed all her professional life within its walls. The average number of probationers at Edinburgh is eighty-six. After a month's trial, applicants are received for a course of three years' training on passing a preliminary examination. Lectures are given by the medical and surgical staff upon medical, surgical, and gynæcological nursing, and examinations held at the end of each course. The first year is devoted to the daily work of a probationer in the wards, then six months' night duty and six months' day duty alternately until the end of the three years' term, when a certificate is granted to those who have satisfactorily completed their engagement. The salaries are—first year, eight pounds; second year, twelve pounds; third year, twenty pounds; head nurses, thirty to forty pounds per annum. There is a pension fund for the sisters, to which the managers of the infirmary pay three-fourths, and the sisters one-fourth of the premium. Each nurse must join when she becomes a sister, and on compulsory retirement at the age of fifty-five, she receives twenty-five pounds a year. Should she leave the service of the infirmary before that time, she receives back the money which she has invested, and also a proportion of that contributed by the managers, according to her length of service.

The quarters provided for the nurses at Edinburgh Infirmary are excellent, and comprise spacious dining and recreation rooms, and an exceptionally good library and reading-room supplied with medical works, current literature, as well as lighter reading, and an abundant supply of periodicals. Each probationer and nurse has a separate bedroom. Cosy sitting-rooms are provided for the sisters close to their wards, where they take meals, with the exception of dinner. There are thirty-three of these rooms, which are a unique feature of the Edinburgh School. Another arrangement peculiar to this institution are the tea-lockers arranged down one wall of the dining-room. There is one for each nurse, furnished with a tea-pot, sugar-basin, milk-jug, cup and saucer and plate, together with a week's supply of tea and sugar. By this arrangement each nurse makes her own tea for breakfast, and in the afternoon at the time most convenient for her "duty"; and the plan is extremely popular.

The nursing accommodation was further extended by the opening in 1892 of the New Nurses' Home, originated by the late Charles Hamilton Fasson, deputy surgeon-general, to whose memory a tablet has been erected in the vestibule. The new Home is built round four sides of an open court, which forms a pleasant outdoor lounge, and is approached by a long corridor converted into a delightful conservatory by one of the sisters skilled in horticulture. As they pass to and from the wards the nurses inhale fragrant perfume, and are refreshed by the sight of beautiful flowers. The recreation and music-room in the new wing is luxurious and palatial. To complete the generous and thoughtful provision made for its nurses by the Edinburgh Infirmary is the Holiday Home at Colinton, three miles from the city.

To the efforts of Lady Augusta Stanley is due the excellent Training-School and Nurses' Home connected with the Westminster Hospital, which was established in 1874. The hospital was founded in 1719, and removed to its present position in the Broad Sanctuary facing the venerable Abbey in 1734. Like other old London hospitals, its nursing system had grown up when Sairey Gamps and Betsey Prigs were the tolerated types of hospital nurses, and though from time to time superior nurses such as those trained by St. John's House were introduced into the hospital, the system remained unsatisfactory. In 1872, Lady Augusta Stanley, who as a visitor took great interest in the poor sick people in the hospital, made an experiment in reform by bringing at her own expense some trained nurses from the Royal Infirmary, Liverpool, to work in the Westminster Hospital.

The experiment was so successful that two years later (1874), Lady Augusta founded the Westminster Training-School and Home for Nurses, at Queen Anne's Gate near to the hospital. Associated with her in this work were Sir Rutherford Alcock, the late chairman of the board, Canon Troutbeck the late treasurer, Lady Lothian, and other friends of the hospital. When the Home was opened it was regarded as one of the most beautifully equipped institutions of the kind in the country, and still compares favourably with more modern ones. In the entrance hall is a bust of Lady Augusta presented by L. M. Rate, Esq., and on the first staircase is a large stained glass window having portraits of Lady Augusta and Dean Stanley. The object of the institution was to train probationers for the service of the Westminster

Hospital, provide them with a home during the period of training, and also to provide a home for the private nurses working under the hospital.

Miss Merryweather, of the Royal Infirmary, Liverpool, was the first matron of the new *régime*, and for six years laboured to realize the high ideal set by Lady Augusta that the nurses and probationers should not only be well trained, but surrounded by Christian influences.

An important era opened when, in 1880, Miss Pyne became matron of the hospital, and Miss Kirwan matron of the home. For eighteen years they worked at organizing and developing the school on modern lines, until 1898, when they resigned together, having accomplished a most important piece of nursing reform. Miss Pyne is still a name to conjure with amongst old "graduates" of Westminster. In those days the senior physician and the matron held their classes at the Home. Now the probationers attend classes and lectures at the hospital, with the exception of the weekly cookery class, which is still held at the Home. In 1873, when Lady Augusta was starting her new scheme, there were only twenty-five nurses at the Westminster and no probationers, now (1906) there is a nursing staff of eighty, including thirty probationers. Candidates are received for four years' training. There is no salary during the first year. The second year it is £20; third year £22, and the fourth year £24.

Miss Cave, the lady superintendent, was trained at the London Hospital. A special feature at the Westminster is the ward for incurables, where one sees poor women with twisted and distorted hands and helpless paralytics doing beautiful needlework. From a nursing point of view such patients are less interesting then acute cases, but Miss Cave devotes herself very specially to brightening the lives of these unfortunate people. She also takes a deep interest in the philanthropic agencies connected with the hospital, and acted for a time as honorary secretary of the Ladies' Association for looking after the welfare of the poor patients and providing the necessitous with garments. Miss Cave was one of the two matrons of civil hospitals appointed on the council of Queen Alexandra's Imperial Army Nursing Service.

Miss Crawford, the matron of the Nurses' Home, is an old Westminster probationer trained under Miss Kirwan, and was invited to take the post in 1905. Miss Crawford spent her early life in America, and was for five years matron of the hospital in Bermuda.

The Training School and Home are managed by the Nursing Board, of which Sir J. Wolfe Barry, K.C.B., is chairman. Amongst members of the board, the names of the Honourable Maud Stanley and Miss Edith Troutbeck recall early promoters of the Westminster Training School.

CHAPTER X

HOSPITAL TRAINING-SCHOOLS (*continued*)

St. Bartholomew's Hospital—Guy's Hospital—Royal Infirmary, Glasgow—Sir Patrick Dun's, Dublin—Steeven's Hospital—St. George's Hospital—St. Mary's Paddington—The Royal Free Hospital—Summary of Hospital training to-day.

ST. BARTHOLOMEW'S, London's most ancient hospital, the early history of which has been sketched in the opening chapter, began the reorganization of its nursing in 1868, but did not adopt the modern system of training until 1877.

Between those periods there was a gradual process at work in eliminating the unsatisfactory material and substituting a better class of nurses. The movement was originated and organized by the lay authorities. Mr. Cross, whose name has become a tradition at "Bart's," had recently been appointed "clerk"—a term surviving from olden times—and he was active in promoting reforms in connection with the nursing staff. Mr. Cross remained at his post until 1904, a period of thirty-eight years. Although appreciating the advance made in the substitution of the trained for the untrained nurse, Mr. Cross bears testimony to the good qualities of the old-fashioned nurse as he found her at St. Bartholomew's in 1866. She was for the most part clean, honest, and kind and diligent in her attendance on the sick, and did rough work and laboured long hours with heroic fortitude. Of course there were occasional moral lapses, which the authorities promptly punished. Not at that period, at any rate, was "Betsey Prig" a fair type of a St. Bartholomew's nurse, whatever she might have been in Dickens' day.

The first step in reform was in 1868, when the nurses were relieved of scrubbing the floors of the wards, and regular scrubbers appointed. Next the mealing was arranged. Under the old system the nurses cooked their own food, and had their rations served out to them daily—one pound of bread, three-quarters of a pound of potatoes, half a pound of meat, and ale. The on and off duty time was systematized. The nurses then did day and night work, every third night a nurse being on night duty. Every third period she was on duty for twenty hours. The following memoranda made by Mr. Cross of the nurses' hours in 1869 will be read with interest:—

In the course of every three days (*i.e.* seventy-two hours) a nurse had twenty-four hours' rest, as follows: She rises at six o'clock (say on Monday morning), goes to bed at five p.m., rises at ten p.m., sits up all night, and goes to bed as soon as she likes after tea is finished on Tuesday evening (this may certainly be by seven o'clock); she rises at six o'clock on Wednesday morning, goes to bed at ten in the evening, and rises at six on Thursday morning. The above course is then repeated.

The seventy-two hours will have been spent as follows:—

Up	In Bed
11 hours	5 hours
21 ,,	11 ,,
16 ,,	8 ,,
48 ,,	24 ,,

During the time that a nurse is up she can be said to be "on duty" only in the sense in which a domestic servant is "on duty," from the time of her rising in the morning to that of her going to bed at night. She has time for taking her meals, and has leisure for reading, needlework, etc. And during the *daytime*, after she has been sitting up at night, she has the opportunity (of which nurses frequently avail themselves) of an hour or two's (or more) sleep while sitting in the ward.

"Every nurse is allowed the following leave from the hospital :—

"Every third Sunday—say from ten o'clock in the morning till nine at night ; one week-day in the course of every three weeks for the same time ; and one hour on two days in every week ; thus in the course of every three weeks a nurse may have twenty-eight hours' leave.

"In addition to the above, every nurse who has been in the service a year has one week's holiday, and those who have been in the service four years have a fortnight's holiday in the year ; in all cases wages being paid during holiday time."

The systematic training of nurses and the reception of probationers at St. Batholomew's began, as we have stated, in 1877. The matron at that time was Mrs. Drake, who, though not herself a trained nurse, sympathized with the new movement and helped it by all means in her power. She resigned two years later, and was succeeded by Miss Machin, who had been trained at St. Thomas's, and brought with her to St. Bartholomew's the traditions of the Nightingale School. The next matron was Miss Manson, who subsequently became the wife of Dr. Bedford Fenwick, and is known as the eloquent advocate of the Registration movement amongst nurses. She was trained at Nottingham, and had been a sister at the London Hospital. During her matronship at St. Bartholomew's Mrs. Bedford Fenwick was energetic in promoting reform. Miss Isla Stewart, the present matron, came to the post in 1891. She was trained at St. Thomas's under Mrs. Wardroper, and believes in the strict discipline which she enjoyed (?) when a probationer.

It is difficult to say to which of the foregoing matrons most credit is due in developing the trained system at St. Barthlolomew's. All performed their duty zealously and successfully. Miss Stewart is a woman of great experience and capability, who has introduced new methods, and is an admirable lecturer. She is a strenuous advocate for the state registration of nurses, and a leader in the movement. Miss Stewart has recently initiated a post-graduate course of lectures for nurses.

St. Bartholomew's has long had a first-rate reputation as a training-school, and the number of important posts held by its graduates is remarkable. Its probationers enter into a four years' agreement, three of which are spent in training. There is no preliminary school, but probationers are required to pass an examination in elementary anatomy, physiology, and hygiene, before being accepted as probationers. At the end of the first year's training the probationers are examined in such matters as they have had an opportunity of becoming acquainted with since entering the hospital. Those who pass satisfactorily are employed as staff probationers for the next two years, and receive instruction in medical and surgical nursing from members of the hospital staff. At the end of the third year a second examination takes place, and a certificate is granted to those who pass and who have given satisfaction in ward work. A gold medal, given by the Clothworkers' Company, is presented to the probationer who passes first in the final examinations. Special probationers are received for not less than three months at a premium of thirteen guineas a quarter. There is a private nursing institution connected with the hospital. Though so well to the front in its training, St. Bartholomew's is behind the times in nursing accommodation. A hospital of such eminence and historic traditions should have a Nurses' Home on a par with those of other institutions. Possibly a modern Rahere may arise to supply this deficiency. Considerable building alterations are now taking place at the hospital.

"Bart's" has a noble record of great surgeons and physicians who have ministered within its walls. The name of Abernethy at once suggests itself, but, to come to modern times, that of Sir James Paget recalls many memories. Writing in 1885, Sir James thus refers to wards for a two months' preliminary trial, and if satisfactory, are received for a course of three years' training in medical and surgical nursing. The fee for the preliminary course, including six weeks' board and residence, is six guineas, payable in advance. A pupil's day is arranged as follows: breakfast 7.30 a.m., after which tidy own room and do some general housework in the home; 10.30 to 11.30 a.m., attend theory class by one of the sister-instructresses; 11.30 to 12 a.m., practise the making of dressings, padding of splints, etc.; 12.15 p.m., dinner; 1 to 2 p.m., study for lectures; 2 to 5 p.m., cookery classes, stock work—being the making of dressings, splint pads, etc.—and on two afternoons a bandaging class, when the pupils practise on each other, a method preferred to the use of dummies; 5 p.m., tea; 5.30 p.m., attend lectures by one or other of the sister-instructresses on anatomy, hygiene, or physiology: 7 to 9 p.m., study for lectures; 9 p.m., supper; 9.30 p.m., prayers in chapel; 10 p.m., go to rooms; 10.45 p.m., lights out.

Should the probationer fail in her examination at the end of her six weeks' preliminary course she leaves, but if successful enters upon the second stage of preliminary training as a ward probationer. If at the end of two months in the wards she does badly in practical work, she has to give up; but if satisfactorily, she attends the various lecture courses, and continues her training in the wards. The curriculum is thus arranged: nursing and practical instruction in the wards by the sisters; lectures on elementary anatomy and the nursing of surgical cases by Mr. R. P. Rowlands, April, May, and June; lectures on nursing by the sisters, July, August, and September; lectures on elementary physiology and the nursing of medical cases by Dr. Bryant, October, November, December; lectures on the elements of pharmacy and dispensing by the pharmacist of the hospital, January, February, and March. After each course the probationer must present herself for examination, and it is compulsory that she pass each examination, or otherwise she ceases to be a probationer. This course of study occupies her first year, after which she continues to work in the wards for two years. A probationer can, if she wishes, take a special course in midwifery—at the lying-in charity of the hospital—or massage. A certificate is granted at the end of the three years' engagement. There are various prizes to stimulate proficiency. Proud is the probationer who carries off the Cazenove gold medal with the immortal Guy in flowing wig on the face. Next in honour comes the silver gilt medal, and the silver medal of similar design. These are awarded to probationers who obtain the highest average marks at the examinations during the year. The Keogh prize (nursing instruments) is awarded to the probationer who obtains the highest marks in the surgical examination; the hospital prize (books) to the probationers who obtain the highest marks in the medical and nursing examinations respectively; and the Raphael gold medal for massage. The Butterworth silver medal, instituted by Joshua Butterworth, a governor of the hospital in 1889, is given to every nurse on the completion of five years' service.

Some thirty lady pupils are received for a twelve months' course of training, and are required to attend the lectures given to the ordinary probationer, and present themselves for examination. Certificates are granted for one year's training. The premium for paying probationers is thirteen guineas each quarter, payable in advance. They are lodged in the matron's house.

The hospital has an institution for trained private nurses at 14, St. Thomas's Street, a short distance away. The nurses, after obtaining their three years' certificate, are eligible to join the institution, and are required to bind themselves for one and a half years. In addition to their salaries, which rise from £8, as first-year probationers, to £40, the nurses receive 10s. 6d. per week when engaged in nursing mental or maternity cases. Each year a certain proportion of the profits arising from fees is set apart as a bonus fund, from which nurses, in their fifth year of service receive benefit. All nurses, whether on the private or hospital staff, are expected to take out a policy of not less than £7 10s. per annum, the hospital taking out a similar po   on their behalf of £11 5s. per annum, payable at fifty years of age.

It is by no means all work and no play at Guy's. Off duty is arranged on a liberal scale. Probationers have one and three hours on alternate days, two half-days and one whole day in four weeks; Sunday, two and a half hours every week, and an additional three hours every other week. Head nurses have, in addition to the above, one Sunday to precede or follow the whole day. Annual holidays are from two weeks at the end of the first year to a month at the end of the third and subsequent years.

A very pleasing feature of this hospital is the Nurses' League, which all probationers are required to join at a small yearly subscription. The president is Mrs. H. Cosmo Bonsor, and among the many patrons and patronesses one may mention the never-failing interest shown in its work by the Countess of Bective. The objects of the league are to promote social and professional intercourse amongst past and present nurses, provide for present nurses increased facilities for mental and physical recreation, and to keep a register of nurses who have been trained at Guy's Hospital. Whatever a nurse's talents or hobbies may be, the league provides her with an outlet in its various sections, which embrace the musical society, the cycling club, the debating society, the photographic society, the tennis and croquet club, the library, and the swimming bath. The musically gifted nurses form a choir in the beautiful old chapel, and entertain at various social gatherings. Christmas is a great season at Guy's, when excellent entertainments are arranged for the patients, and doctors and nurses give generously of their time and talent.

The hospital, in spite of continual extension, still retains the beautiful old garden with the immemorial trees, a pleasant breathing-space for nurses and patients, and a most convenient place for summer *fêtes*. It is one of the few gardens left in the heart of London, and affords a cheerful prospect from the hospital windows. If the worthy founder were to come forth from his tomb in the chapel crypt, he would speedily be in need of an ambulance, such would be his amazement at the great organization for the relief of the suffering poor which has sprung from the seeds he planted nearly two centuries ago.

The Royal Infirmary, Glasgow, has a particularly well-organized school of nursing, which dates from 1879, and has developed under the management of Mrs. Strong, who has held the post of matron for a period of twenty-seven years. Mrs. Strong entered St. Thomas's Hospital as a probationer in 1867, and received her training under Mrs. Wardroper. She remained connected with St. Thomas's until 1873, when she was appointed matron of Dundee Royal Infirmary. In 1879 she came to Glasgow, and from that date a three years' residence for nurses was made compulsory, and classes were introduced. It was found, however, that this seriously interfered with the discipline of the house and the working of the wards, probationers having to be taken away at irregular hours to attend the lectures. Neither was it found practicable to provide them with time for study, and consequently the majority derived little real benefit from the lectures, only a few being able to stand the double strain. This led to the adoption of a long-projected scheme for a preliminary course, which came into operation in January, 1893. Mrs. Strong received the cordial support and co-operation of the medical staff and the managers of the infirmary in effecting the change. The scheme for the preliminary course was worked out by Sir William Macewen of Glasgow University, who was the first to suggest to Mrs. Strong the system of preliminary classes for nurses before they entered upon practical work in the hospital. The Glasgow Royal Infirmary is the pioneer of the system of preliminary training.

Candidates are received of from twenty to thirty years of age, and height not less than five feet three inches. The latter restriction does not support the fact that short women often make admirable nurses, as instanced by more than one distinguished matron of the present day. The preliminary education consists of twelve lectures and demonstrations each on elementary anatomy, physiology, and hygiene. Only the candidates who pass the examination in those subjects are eligible for further instruction. The second course consists of twenty lectures and demonstrations each on surgical cases and medical cases, and twenty practical lectures by the matron and housekeeper on ward work and cookery. The fee for the first course is two guineas, and for the second course three guineas. The classes occupy three months, during which time the pupil provides board and lodging at her own expense. Having successfully passed the preliminary examinations, she becomes a hospital probationer, and continues her training and residence for three years, receiving a rising salary from £12 to £22, with board, lodging, and laundry. At the end of that period, after passing a final and practical examination, she receives a certificate.

The Glasgow Royal Infirmary School is arranged in such a manner that it can at any time adapt itself to legislative demands without interfering with its ordinary routine. Mrs. Strong has for many years looked forward to the establishment of a central examining body for nurses, with a curriculum fixed by the state as the goal to be attained.

In Ireland the first general hospital to start the training of nurses under a trained lady superintendent, was Sir Patrick Dun's Hospital, Dublin. The first probationers were received about 1879. This hospital has a very interesting history. Patrick Dun was body surgeon to William III., and dressed a wound in the shoulder which that monarch received on June 30, 1690, the eve of the battle of the Boyne. It is said that afterwards William knighted the clever surgeon.

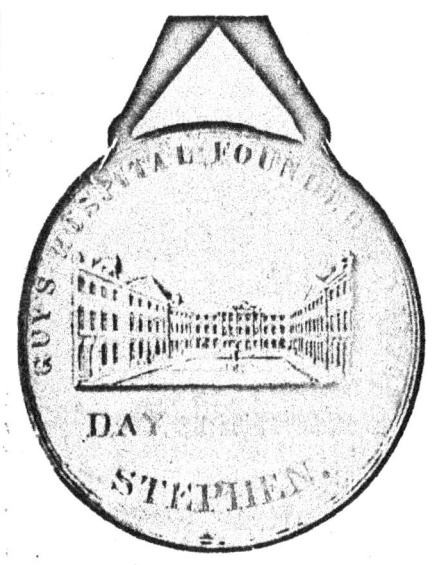

MEDAL WORN BY THE HEAD NURSES AT GUY'S HOSPITAL UNDER THE OLD RÉGIME.

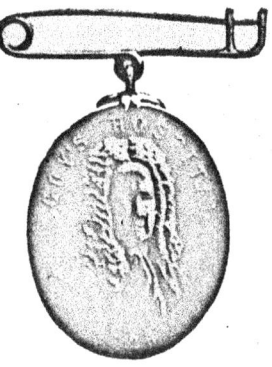

RAPHAEL GOLD MEDAL FOR MASSAGE, GUY'S HOSPITAL.

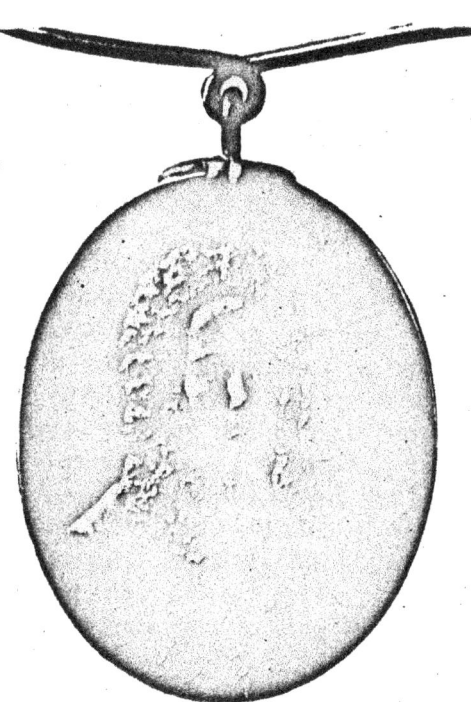

CAZENOVE GOLD MEDAL, GUY'S HOSPITAL.

Sir Patrick Dun settled as a physician in Dublin, and took an active part in procuring the second Charter of the King's and Queen's College of Physicians, and was appointed the first president of that renewed body in 1690. He died childless in 1714, and after the death of Lady Dun disputes arose regarding the disposition of his property, which terminated in a portion of the profits of his estate in Co. Waterford being applied to the maintenance of an hospital in Dublin, to be called Sir Patrick Dun's Hospital. Until 1866 it was devoted to the reception of medical cases and medical students only. The cholera epidemic of that year showed the defects of the hospital in regard to its nursing arrangements, and a reconstitution was effected. In 1867 surgery and midwifery were placed in the work of the hospital, on the same footing as medicine, and arrangements also made for improving the skill and training of nurses in the hospital, for which the governors owe special gratitude to the Countess of Meath and the Hon. Mrs. Chenevix Trench. The system of modern training for probationers was not, however, adopted until 1879.

The school has now attained a high state of efficiency, and has an average of twenty-seven probationers in training. The hospital is small, having only one hundred and four beds, including a separate wing with twenty beds for infectious diseases. Candidates must be between the ages of twenty-one and thirty, and after a personal interview and three months' trial, are received for four and a half years' training and service. They pay an entrance fee of twenty-five pounds in quarterly instalments. The first three years are spent in the hospital, and the last year and a half either in the hospital or acting as a district or private nurse, as the lady superintendent may direct. The probationers attend the lectures of the Dublin Metropolitan Technical School for Nurses, on anatomy and surgical nursing, physiology and medical nursing, hygiene and invalid cookery, in which they have to pass examinations. During the third year their

L

practical knowledge of nursing is tested by examination. The certificate is not granted until the nurse has satisfactorily completed her four and a half years' engagement. Paying probationers are received for not less than three months, but receive no certificate for less than three years' continuous training. The Nurses' Home is in Lower Mount Street, and has been recently enlarged for the accommodation of the private nurses when off duty.

The name of Miss Margaret Huxley is much honoured at Sir Patrick Dun's, for the long years of service in which she laboured as lady superintendent to bring the nursing school up to modern requirements. She is recognized as the pioneer of trained nursing in Ireland. Miss Huxley has been succeeded by Miss L. V. Haughton, who is efficiently carrying on the work through a difficult period of straitened finance. The old hospital, which has done such magnificent work in the past—during the famine years of 1826-28 and 1846-48, no less than 10,132 cases of fever were treated in the wards of the hospital—is feeling the strain of greatly reduced income, owing to the depreciation of the rents from the Patrick Dun's estate, and has now to rely chiefly on the gifts of the charitable. Its private nurses are much sought after, and nursing fees are an increasing and important item in the income of the hospital.

The Steeven's Hospital, Dublin, started its training school in 1880, under the able management of Mrs. Louisa M. Franks, who had been a sister at St. Thomas's Hospital, and introduced the Nightingale system into Ireland. Mrs. Franks trained a large number of nurses during the time that she was matron at Steeven's Hospital. It is of interest to note that she had charge of the bodies of Lord Frederick Cavendish and Mr. Burke after their terrible murder in the Phœnix Park.

The largest training-school in Ireland is attached to the Mater Misericordiæ Hospital, Dublin, managed by Sisters of Mercy. The staff of nurses numbers one hundred and ten, including forty-five probationers. It has a private staff of thirty nurses. Candidates are received for four years' training and service. Premium, twenty pounds. Applications average five hundred. This hospital was founded in 1861, and the Training Institution for Nurses opened in 1891. The Superioress is Sister M. B. Barry.

St. George's Hospital, originally founded in 1719 in the locality of the city known as Petty France, was established on its present site opposite Hyde Park Corner in 1733. Then the old turnpike gate was standing, and there were few houses between it and the village of Brompton. It is difficult to realize that the hospital which now looks on the whirl of West End traffic originally stood in a lonely road frequented by footpads.

The first mention in the hospital records of the admission of a nurse, is dated November 30, 1733, when one Elizabeth Graves was engaged by the weekly board at six pounds a year, with a gratuity at Christmas. As the matron only had ten pounds a year wages, Nurse Elizabeth Graves no doubt thought herself well off. In those days the apothecary was the important functionary of the hospital, and was largely concerned with the nursing department. At the outset, when the hospital contained only thirty beds, there were ten nurses, a proportion of one to three as now.

The potmen used to go the rounds through the wards touting for orders from the head nurses, who selected their favourite tap. In 1782 this was forbidden, and the nurses received their beer in the hall. Rules were also made against provisions and strong drink being brought to the patients, and it was found necessary to fasten down the window-sashes of the ground floor to prevent victuals and drink being handed through the windows to the patients.

When the hospital was rebuilt in 1828-30, the era of trained nursing had not dawned. The first probationer for training came to St. George's in 1844, from Mrs.

Fry's Institution of Nursing Sisters. In 1849 another probationer was received. At this period the nurses were under no particular authority save that of the head nurse of the ward in which they worked. They dressed as they pleased, wore no uniform, and took their meals promiscuously.

Mr. Todd, who has been secretary to the hospital since 1861, has witnessed many changes. When he first came there was the usual untrained matron at the head of the female staff, who managed the housekeeping and visited the wards. There was a head nurse to each ward, and one or two nurses under her. The nurses scrubbed and cleaned the wards and cooked the patients' meals. The assistant nurses had board wages, and provided their own rations and drink, the latter an important item in the *menu!* In those days the convalescents helped to nurse the patients.

In 1869 came a great change. The first trained superintendent of nurses was appointed. She was Miss Veitch, a St. John's House sister, who had trained at King's College Hospital. She made short work of the old staff, dismissing the incompetent, and superannuating the old. The nurses now were required to wear a uniform, and were provided with a dining-room. Although the nursing was reorganized up to a certain extent, and practical teaching given, no course of theoretical instruction was begun until 1884, when Mr. Clinton Dent, F.R.C.S., now senior surgeon, volunteered to give a course of lectures, which he continued in subsequent years. In 1889 two physicians started courses of medical lectures. The first examination for probationers was held in 1894.

Nothing, however, which could be dignified by the name of a "school" existed at St. George's until the present efficient system of training was organized by Miss Smedley, who has filled the post of matron since 1895. Miss Smedley was trained at St. Bartholomew's, and introduced at St. George's a similar curriculum to that of her *alma mater*, and has laboured most assiduously at her task, supported by Mr. Clinton Dent, Mr. Todd, and the members of the nursing board. Probationers enter for four years' service, three of which are passed in training. Certificates are granted after the final examination, and classified under "qualifying," "with credit," and "with honour." St. George's gives a pension to nurses on the permanent staff for faithful service. The Nurses' Home is in Montpelier Street, at some little distance from the hospital, but the first-year probationers live in the hospital. Apart from the good reputation which St. George's is acquiring for its training, the delightful situation, overlooking Hyde Park, makes it attractive alike to patients and nurses. A private nursing institute has recently been started.

St. Mary's, Paddington, has been developing its nursing school since reforms were first instituted by Miss Williams, who was matron until 1883. Miss Medill, who succeeded her, carried on the development on extended lines. Miss Medill had been a sister at St. Bartholomew's. She recently resigned her position at St. Mary's. During the thirteen years that she was matron, the hospital was greatly enlarged, and the staff of nurses almost doubled. In 1902 she made some alteration in the system, and instituted a *viva voce* and a written examination at the end of the first and of the third year of training. The engagement of probationers is for four years, and the certificate is not granted until the end of the fourth year. A new Nurses' Home is shortly to be opened at St. Mary's, and has long been needed. The hospital has fifty-six ordinary and nine paying probationers in training. Miss M. E. Davies has succeeded Miss Medill as matron: Miss Davies was trained at King's College Hospital under Miss Monk, was ward sister and assistant-matron at University College, and matron of Queen Charlotte's Lying-in-Hospital, 1904–6.

The Royal Free Hospital, Gray's Inn Road, started

its training-school in 1888, and has modified the regulations from time to time. Probationers are admitted for training between the age of twenty-three and thirty-five, on three months' trial. At the end of that period, if the probationer is considered suitable, she signs an agreement to serve the hospital for four years, viz. for three years as probationer, and for the fourth year on such duty as may be prescribed by the matron. Probationers are provided with board, lodging, washing, and uniform. No salary is given for the first year, £15 for the second year, £20 for the third, and £25 for the fourth year.

Princess Christian is president of the hospital, and Her Royal Highness's daughter, Princess Louise Augusta of Schleswig-Holstein, is president of the ladies' association. The Earl of Sandwich is chairman of the committee, and Charles Burt, Esq., treasurer. Princess Christian inaugurated in 1905 new additions to the hospital, which include further accommodation for the nursing staff. The nurses' new sitting-room has access to a promenade roof, which affords a pleasant outlet.

Miss Wedgewood, under whose superintendence the training-school was developed, resigned her post as matron in 1905, having held it for thirteen years. She has been succeeded by Miss Cox Davies, formerly matron of the new hospital for women. The total number of the nursing staff, including probationers, is fifty-six. The medical staff have recommended a further addition, and the whole subject of the nursing of the hospital is at present under consideration by a special sub-committee of the weekly board.

Nursing at the Royal Free derives a special interest from the fact that the wards are "walked" by women students. The London School of Medicine for Women, inaugurated in 1877, is associated with the hospital, which forms the training-ground for its graduates. The increasing demand for the services of duly qualified medical women is testified by the fact that they have obtained forty-three resident appointments during the past year, several of these being posts in hospitals and infirmaries not previously held by women. Six medical women, former students of the school, have been appointed by the London County Council as assistant medical officers, and two by the Central Midwives' Board as examiners in midwifery.

It is impossible to follow further the spread of training-schools for nurses in London. Practically every hospital now trains probationers, but special prestige naturally attaches to the old London hospitals which have the advantage of being associated with famous medical schools. Such centres command lectures by the first physicians and surgeons of the day, and have the most up-to-date appliances.

In the provinces training-schools are connected with all the chief hospitals. The Royal Infirmary, Liverpool, as we have seen, was the pioneer. Its progressive neighbour, Manchester, has followed suit, and schools maintaining a high standard of nursing are to be found in the leading cities and towns of the kingdom. The reform in the nursing in provincial hospitals was not rapid, and the first trained matrons appointed to the smaller institutions had a difficult task to perform. An old Nightingale probationer, when she first went as sister to a Midland hospital, was asked to "walk out" by one of the porters, and invited to meet him, in an evening, at the "Royal Arms"—a select public-house. He was much surprised at the manner in which the "new nurse" met his proposal. In the same hospital the porters had been in the habit of coming into the wards at all hours. So recently as 1890, in a small hospital where untrained women had been employed, the new matron found that the nurses were in the habit of inviting the young men patients, who had been discharged from the hospital, to little select beer parties in the back garden.

To summarize modern training, each hospital remains at present a law unto itself. There is no uniformity of education, no general test or examination of fitness and competence. Nursing certificates are granted, but each certificate stands on its own merit. There is much rivalry between the various schools, "healthy rivalry," say some, while more strenuous reformers look to the time when a State diploma shall fix the standard of minimum efficiency. Three years have been almost universally adopted as the standard length of training. Education consists of practical work in the wards under the head nurses or sisters, lectures and demonstrations on practical nursing by the matron and home sister, and sick-room cookery by sisters or special teachers. The medical staff give lectures on elementary anatomy, physiology, and hygiene, and on the theory of nursing, an examination following each course. In an increasing number of hospitals a preliminary course is arranged for probationer candidates, and the London and Guy's have special preliminary schools. The latest advance in education is a movement in favour of a post-graduate course to keep trained nurses in touch with the latest methods. A nurse's education, in these days of new discoveries and new appliances, is never finished; while there is division of opinion as to details and methods of education, there is happily none regarding the need of practical and skilled training for nurses. What had been a trade, and a bad trade, has become a skilled profession. So far, at least, has opinion advanced in fifty years.

The London Hospital, which has developed its great school on lines peculiarly its own, is dealt with in a separate chapter.

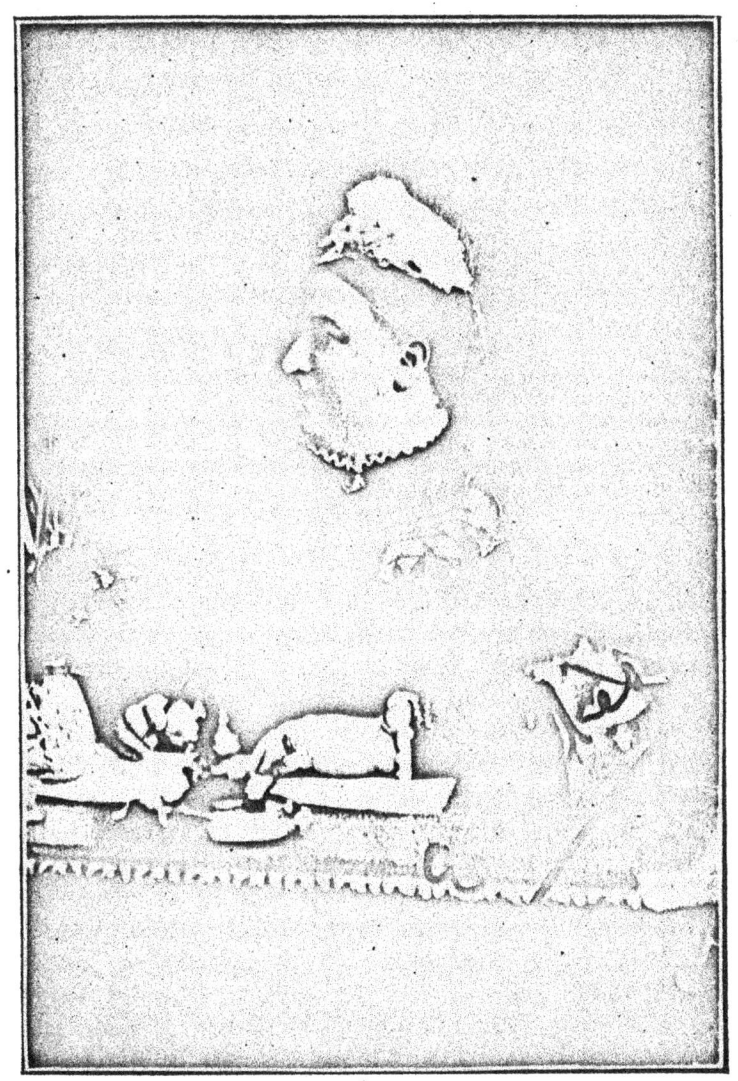

MISS EVA LÜCKES.

Matron of the London Hospital since 1880; Founder and Superintendent of the Nurse Training School.

(*Photograph by C. Vandyk, London, S.W.*)

[*To face p.* 152.

CHAPTER XI

THE LARGEST TRAINING-SCHOOL

The London Hospital—Miss Eva Lückes appointed matron—Her splendid work—Gradual reforms—Founds the London training-school—Preliminary training at Tredegar House—A probationers' day—Ward probationers' examinations—Two years' certificate—Maternity wing—Scale of payment—The nurses' quarters—The Lückes Home—The Honourable Sydney Holland—His work for the hospital and nurses—Work of the London Hospital—Tragedy and humour—Queen Alexandra as president—The King honours his nurse.

THE London Hospital, which to-day has the largest training-school in the kingdom, and is remarkable for its splendid system and organization, was rather backward in setting its house in order. The St. Thomas's School had been in existence twenty years, and other hospitals had followed suit in the adoption of a system of trained nursing before the "London" awoke to its needs and necessities. Established in 1740, this great general hospital, situated in Whitechapel, in the midst of the teeming population of the East End, presented an anxious problem to the reformer, and the gigantic task delayed solution. Like many another big undertaking, it waited the coming of the competent person. The psychical moment arrived in 1880, when Miss Eva Lückes became matron of the London, and was the first trained head to preside over that vast institution for suffering humanity.

In 1905 Miss Lückes celebrated, amidst universal felicitations from the governing body and past and present nurses of the hospital, what might be termed her "silver nursing wedding." Those twenty-five years of persevering work, during which the nursing department has been changed and reorganized until the topmost cobweb of inefficiency has been swept away, constitute one of those records of personal achievement which are the glory of a noble profession. To-day Miss Lückes rules a staff, counting all grades, of five hundred and sixty-six nurses, a little army requiring no small amount of skill in generalship. She is voted " a matron of matrons," ever kind and thoughtful, untiring in dealing with detail, a master of organization, an inspiring teacher, and preserving to those countless visitors and candidates, who yearly pass through her office, an even front of smiling good temper. It is a happy coincidence that the year which has seen the completion of the reorganization and rebuilding of the London Hospital should find Miss Lückes in her old place, capable and vigorous as ever. Little could she have imagined twenty-five years ago that such advances would have been made as those effected by the new improvements. The most important of these are the new out-patients' department to accommodate fifteen hundred people ; the elaborately fitted X-ray and light department; the new blocks for infectious diseases ; the thirteen new operating theatres, where forty anæsthetized operations take place daily ; the Hebrew wards and special kitchen ; the beautifully arranged maternity wards, with baby's cosy cot slung at the foot of mother's bed ; new classrooms for the nurses ; the training-home of Tredegar House for probationers ; and the new and luxuriously fitted Nurses' Home, appropriately named the " Eva Lückes."

When Miss Lückes was appointed to her important post in 1880, she was only twenty-six years of age and the youngest matron in London. The old-fashioned notion had prevailed that a matron, like a bishop, should be a person ripe in years and experience. The more seasoned indeed the better. · That idea is dying down in ecclesiastical circles, and hospital authorities have also come to see that the vigour and freshness of comparative youth are valuable assets in the holder of an arduous post. The appointment of so young a woman to be matron of a great institution was a new departure in the history of nursing.

It is pleasanter to rejoice in the present than moan over the past, and Miss Lückes would doubtless fain forget the "London" as she knew it, but from the historical standpoint the steps of progress are the points of interest. Her first care on being appointed matron was the reorganization of the "mealing," no separate arrangement then existing for the food of patients and nurses. Indescribable confusion, too, reigned in the wards, where an army of "scrubbers" came every Saturday to clean floors and turn out the patients' lockers. Nurses who could afford it would pay the "scrubbers" to do some of their ward work for them. Miss Lückes did away with the "scrubbers," and introduced wardmaids, to whom was committed the cleaning of the floors and some of the more menial work which had hitherto devolved on the nurses, thus setting them free for increased attention to the patients.

The off-duty time was a matter which early engaged the new matron's attention. At that time a nurse was only allowed one hour twice, and two hours once a week, and no off days at all. Frequently, too, if there was no one forthcoming to relieve the nurse, she lost even the small off-duty time. The committee furthered Miss Lückes' efforts by increasing the nursing-staff of the hospital, in order that the off-duty might be reorganized on a more liberal scale. The extra time given was made compulsory in the interest of the nurses' health. No sister might stop off-duty time, and no nurse elect to give any part of it up. There was, at first, difficulty between patients and nurses over this matter; a good-natured nurse sometimes being unwilling to leave a patient who wanted her services.

The development of good nursing-quarters early

occupied Miss Lückes' attention, and in 1886 the first nurses' home was opened, with comfortable accommodation for one hundred and two nurses. The private nursing staff was next started. It had occurred to Miss Lückes that the people whose generosity supported the hospital were often worse off in time of illness than the poor in the wards, and the system of trained nurses for private families was started with great and increasing success, only nurses up to the hospital standard being sent out.

In the year of her appointment, 1880, Miss Lückes founded the London training-school, and started the modern system, with the help of sisters from other schools, until she could train her own. The nurses had been largely drawn from the domestic class, and the new matron made a point of obtaining others of superior education. It is noteworthy that she started a two years' training system from the first, at a time when the general standard at hospitals was only one year. The first certificate was granted for the two years' course in November, 1882. The first lectures given to the probationers were by Mr., now Sir Frederick, Treves, and by Mr. Sandson. These gentlemen are gratefully remembered by all old "Londoners." For many years Sir Frederick never missed giving his appointed lecture, and no nurse would be likely to miss, if she could help it, the opportunity of listening to the lucid and captivating instruction of this eminent surgeon.

Matrons' lectures on practical nursing, which are now a feature of every hospital training-school, were originated by Miss Lückes at the "London." In volume form, the lectures given by her at various periods have helped many not within the fold of her staff. She further instituted the matron's Tuesday evening "At Homes," which remain such pleasant and helpful occasions for social intercourse between the head and her sisters and nurses, and old "Londoners" also.

Tutorial classes by the home sister were early adopted

as part of the "London" curriculum, and resulted in a marked improvement in the work of the probationers. In 1893 an important step was taken by the house committee, on the suggestion of Miss Lückes, when an outside examiner was appointed, it being felt that it was fairer to the nurses that they should be examined by one who had not been brought into contact with them in hospital work.

The next important scheme initiated by Miss Lückes, and sanctioned by the committee, was the establishment of a preliminary training-school for probationers, where they should receive six weeks' training in theoretical and practical work before passing into the wards of the hospital to begin their regular two years' course. It was a unique departure in the history of London nursing, and has so far only been followed by Guy's Hospital, although other hospitals have plans under consideration.

Tredegar House, the "London" preliminary training-school, was opened June, 1895. It is situated in Bow Road, within easy walking distance of the hospital, and is a prettily furnished and most comfortably arranged Home with a pleasant garden. The classroom is detached from the house, and has a range of windows looking on to the garden, where lawn and trees supply refreshing green as a relief to eyes intent on white bandages and dressings. It is superintended by Miss Hosking, assisted by Miss Hunt, and is under the control of the matron of the hospital. The following rules and a description of an ordinary day's work will convey some idea of the routine observed.

Candidates for pupil-probationers are eligible between the ages of twenty-three and thirty-three years. After having been supplied with a set of the rules, the candidate is seen by the matron, and by one of the physicians, Dr. Francis Warner, who respectively report on her personal fitness and health. If the report is satisfactory, she comes into residence at Tredegar House on a Saturday evening as one of a company of twenty-eight pupils, who all begin work together. The first evening, as they sit round the supper-table, comradeship begins and friendships are formed. It is the aim of the superintendent to make the probationers feel that they are a family party. Talk on a variety of subjects is stimulated, and "shop" is strictly taboo at meals. Nevertheless, strict order and discipline reign at Tredegar House, and the raw nursing recruit is taught obedience, order, and punctuality.

After breakfast at 7 a.m., and prayers, the work of the day begins by each probationer doing an allotted portion of housework—sweeping, dusting, washing-up, etc.—to fit her for such tasks as will fall to her lot in the wards. Next the pupils walk or ride to the hospital and attend lectures on anatomy, physiology, or hygiene in the special lecture-room provided for their use. At 11 a.m., after a light lunch, they return to Tredegar House, and receive instruction in practical nursing from the superintendent. A demonstration is given in the changing of sheets for helpless patients, the preparation of a taking-in bed for a surgical case with the aid of a dummy, whose agonized countenance must be an excellent preparation for encountering the faces of real sufferers. At other times the application of dressings and poultices, placing of water-beds, the taking of temperatures, reading measure-glasses, and the names of surgical instruments are taught.

The lesson over, the probationers troop off in a merry company to the garden classroom, where a demonstration is given in the bandaging of dummy arms, legs, shoulders, and heads. The pupils practise the skilful methods first demonstrated by Miss Hosking, and are strictly timed in their operations, and marks given accordingly. Five minutes are allowed for the bandaging of head, leg, or arm, three minutes for the knee, four for the ankle, and five to seven for the shoulder. The tendency of the pupil is to take too long in her anxiety to neatly adjust the folds of the bandage, but the superintendent's reminder, "How would a suffering patient feel under your leisurely movements?" hastens operations. On some mornings an ambulance class is held, and first aid to the wounded is taught on the much-suffering dummy, whose fractured limbs are put into splints improvised by pieces of wood, walking-sticks, umbrellas, and any odd thing which would be to hand in a street accident. The classroom contains a skeleton in a cupboard, who lends his bones for the study of anatomy. Mothers are sometimes anxious about the propriety of the skeleton. One lady taking a preliminary view of the classroom, thus resigned herself to the inevitable—

"As my daughter will have to see the skeleton, I had better do so first."

At 1.30 p.m. dinner is served in the pleasant dining-room, and the pupils answer the roll-call as they enter. Talk and merriment help digestion; an agreeable contrast to the merciless decorum of the early nursing-institutions, when probationers were forbidden to talk at meals.

Next bonnets and cloaks are donned, and the pupils set off again for their special classrooms at the hospital, and in the model kitchen attend a cookery demonstration by Miss Apperley. In the spacious dressing-room connected with the classrooms, each probationer has a locker for her walking-out things, and her own key and number. Cooking has been taught at the "London" since 1897, but the model kitchen is of recent date. Its rows of sinks, cooking-stoves, and utensils are a marvel of neatness and order, while the white-tiled walls give it a delightfully clean, fresh look. Over the cooking-stoves is a glass roof and arrangement by which smell and fumes are carried off, and the heat goes out at the window of the roof. The dressers have ventilated cupboards.

There are two demonstrations and two practice classes a week, which the probationers attend in relays. Each pupil has a cookery-book in which she makes notes and neatly transcribes the recipes under the headings, "ingredients," "food value," "method." The pupils are taught to cook both at a kitchen-range and at a gas-stove. At the long tables in the centre of the kitchen they manipulate dishes under strict time allowance, and the results when cooked are critically inspected by the teacher. At the end of the class the pupils clean and polish the sinks, scrub down their own part of the table, and do everything required to leave kitchen and utensils in perfect order, except cleaning the floor and the stoves. Each probationer, on completing her six weeks' course, goes through examination. She has learned all the recipes on the school list, and draws lots for which she is to make from the dishes selected by the examiner. She receives a copy of "Cookery for Invalids and Convalescents," by C. Herman Senn, on passing the examination. After the pupil probationers have passed to the hospital, they may come back to refresh their memory at the cooking-classes, a useful advantage for those intending to take up private or district nursing.

The cooking-class over, the probationers return to Tredegar House for tea. In the evening they attend a two hours' class on elementary hygiene, anatomy, or physiology, also given by Miss Apperley. They take notes, which are carefully corrected and given back to them, to ensure that the lectures have been individually understood. There is a quiet hour for study until supper at 8.30 p.m. At 9 p.m. prayers, and at 10 p.m. the probationer retires to her room, and lights are out by 10.30 p.m.

Each pupil probationer has two hours per day off duty, when she may go out or receive her friends. She has four hours off duty on Saturdays and Sundays, and is at liberty to attend any religious service she likes, and her hours for study are arranged so as not to encroach on off-duty time.

On the completion of the six weeks' preliminary course, which is given together with board and laundry free of expense, the pupils are examined by Dr. Hadley in

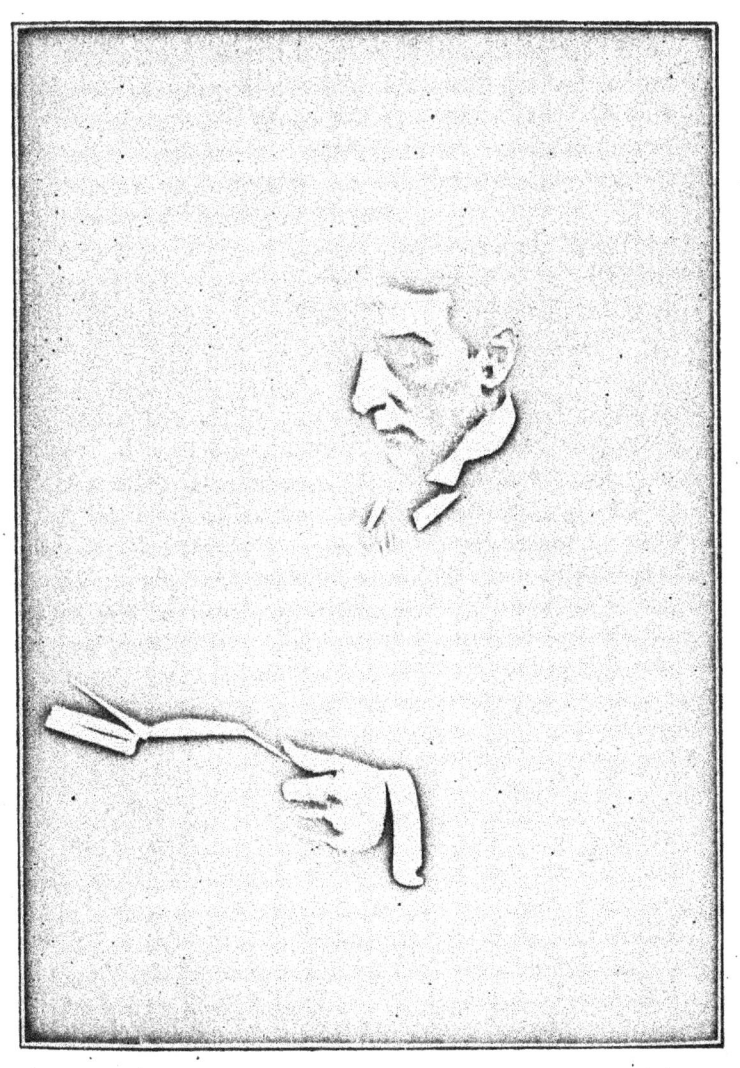

THE HON. SYDNEY HOLLAND.
Chairman of the London Hospital.
(*Photo: Enid Wigram*)

[*To face p.* 160.

hygiene, Dr. Dawson in physiology, the senior assistant-matron in practical nursing, and by an examiner from the National Training School of Cookery in sick-room cookery. Those who appear suitable personally, as well as being successful in the examinations, are transferred to the hospital, and a new set of twenty-eight pupils take their place at Tredegar House.

We will follow the progress of the pupils who, the preliminary course over, enter the hospital and have their first experience of ward work. No more dummies to bandage and dress, but living patients to deal with now. The work, however, is not so strange as if the probationer had come straight from the parental fireside to the wards. Those six weeks at Tredegar House have taught her what to expect, and she enters upon the duties of ward-probationer with a corresponding degree of confidence and facility. The theoretical training now begins afresh, and she attends one lecture a week until she has passed her final examination. In addition to the lecture, she attends one instruction-class and two study-classes a week, in order to help her to assimilate and to test the knowledge imparted by the various lectures. These classes are a part of her working-hours. There are three courses of lectures in the year, one by the matron, one by a member of the surgical staff, and another by a member of the medical staff. Instruction is continued in ambulance work, and every nurse at the "London" becomes proficient in dealing with accidents and emergencies, the probationer also receives instruction in practical work from the sisters and staff nurses under whom she works in the wards.

At the end of each course of lectures there is an examination by an outside examiner. Dr. Hayward, of Haydock, St. Helens, Lancashire, has for many years been examiner. He sets the questions after each course of lectures, and the papers are sent to him. At the end of the third course Dr. Hayward comes to London, and in addition to the written examination, holds a *viva voce* examination with each probationer for a quarter of an hour, and subsequently takes sets of four of these probationers together for twenty minutes for a practical examination in the wards. This completes the first year of training.

The second year is spent in work in the wards, consolidating and putting into practice the knowledge acquired in the lectures and classes, and in continuing the training in practical work under the sisters and staff nurses. Special care is taken that each probationer has experience in men's, women's, and children's wards, and that she gains a thorough knowledge of medical and surgical nursing. She has also invaluable experience in the receiving-room, out-patient, and special departments. During their two years' training, probationers take night duty for periods of three months.

At the end of the first year a probationer's certificate is filled up in accordance with the result of the examinations, but the full London hospital certificate is not given until the end of the two years' training, when further entries are made with regard to the conduct and practical work, which may be different to the standard of the examination. It is a feature of the London certificate that it takes character much into consideration as well as theoretical efficiency. The certificate is signed by the chairman and matron of the hospital, by the surgeon and physician who have given the lectures, and by the examiner. There can be little doubt about the thorough training given under the "London" system, and though the period is only for two as against the now almost universal term of three years, the authorities claim that the variety of cases in their great hospital, and the carefully arranged experience for each nurse, make the two years' training adequate.

The new maternity department, started at the "London" in 1905, affords its nurses training in midwifery, and the pupils also train in the district. Dr. Lewers and Dr. Russell Andrews supervise this department, and give the necessary lectures. Miss Sleight is in charge of the maternity wards, and two sisters acting as district midwives accompany every pupil to her outside cases. The greater part of the money for the erection of this new wing came in response to fifty thousand personal letters sent out to the women of England. Five out of every hundred responded, and the result was a total of fourteen thousand pounds. Mr. James Hora gave ten thousand pounds in memory of his wife "Mary Celeste," after whom the wards are named. They were opened on the twenty-fifth anniversary of the day that Miss Lückes became matron of the "London."

The engagement of a nurse to the hospital is for four years. On the joyful day that she obtains her training certificate, she takes a month's holiday, and returns for her final two years, either on the hospital or the private nursing staff. Frequently these last two years are divided between the hospital and the private staff. Not until her four years are completed is her certificate fully filled up. She can then continue in the service of the hospital or seek another engagement.

The scale of payment at the London Hospital is as follows—Probationers receive £12 the first year, and £20 the second. If they become staff-nurses, £24 the third year, and £25 the fourth. If they become holiday sisters, £30 the third year, and £35 the fourth, rising to £40 the next year if they remain in the service of the hospital. If a newly certificated nurse is placed on the private staff, she receives £30 for the third year, £35 for the fourth, £40 for the fifth year, and £45 for the sixth year, with laundry and everything found, including about £4 for uniform.

After six years from the date of entering the London Hospital as a probationer, every member of the nursing staff receives an additional £5 per annum, which brings a private nurse's salary up to £50 per annum. After twelve years in the service of the hospital, a second addition of £5 a year is given, so that a private nurse, by the time she has reached, say, thirty-seven years of age, receives £55 per annum.

After being eighteen years a member of the London Hospital nursing staff, she may, if she is disposed, retire at the minimum age of forty-five, receiving a pension of £55 per annum, without having had to set aside any of her salary in order to secure this.

Paying probationers are received at the London Hospital between the ages of twenty-two and forty, and are admitted for periods of three months on payment in advance of thirteen guineas. They may renew their engagement indefinitely upon the same terms; and by special arrangement a paying probationer, who is within the limit age of twenty-two to twenty-three years, may, after a period of training, be transferred to the list of regular probationers. Paying probationers attend all lectures, and may present themselves for examination, but they do not receive the hospital certificate unless they have gone through the regular two years' course, including night duty.

It is a rule of the London Hospital that its nurses shall have proper time allotted for everything, study included, and there is no wasting of the strength and working power of the staff by rushing and driving. The off-duty time is on a liberal scale. We have already given the "time" for pupil probationers, and after they pass to the hospital they get three hours off duty each day, and a whole day once a fortnight, a week's holiday at the end of each period of six months, and a full month on completion of the two years' training.

The nurses' quarters form a succession of three homes connected by bridges—the "Old," the "New," and the "Lückes." The last, opened in 1905, is a model of comfort, refinement, and artistic arrangement. It accommodates two hundred and fifty nurses with separate rooms, and twenty-six sisters with bed sitting-rooms. The nurses' sitting-room is a luxurious apartment decorated in a tasteful scheme of oak, red, and green. Opening out of it is a smaller room said to be sacred to snoozing. It is divided from the principal room by

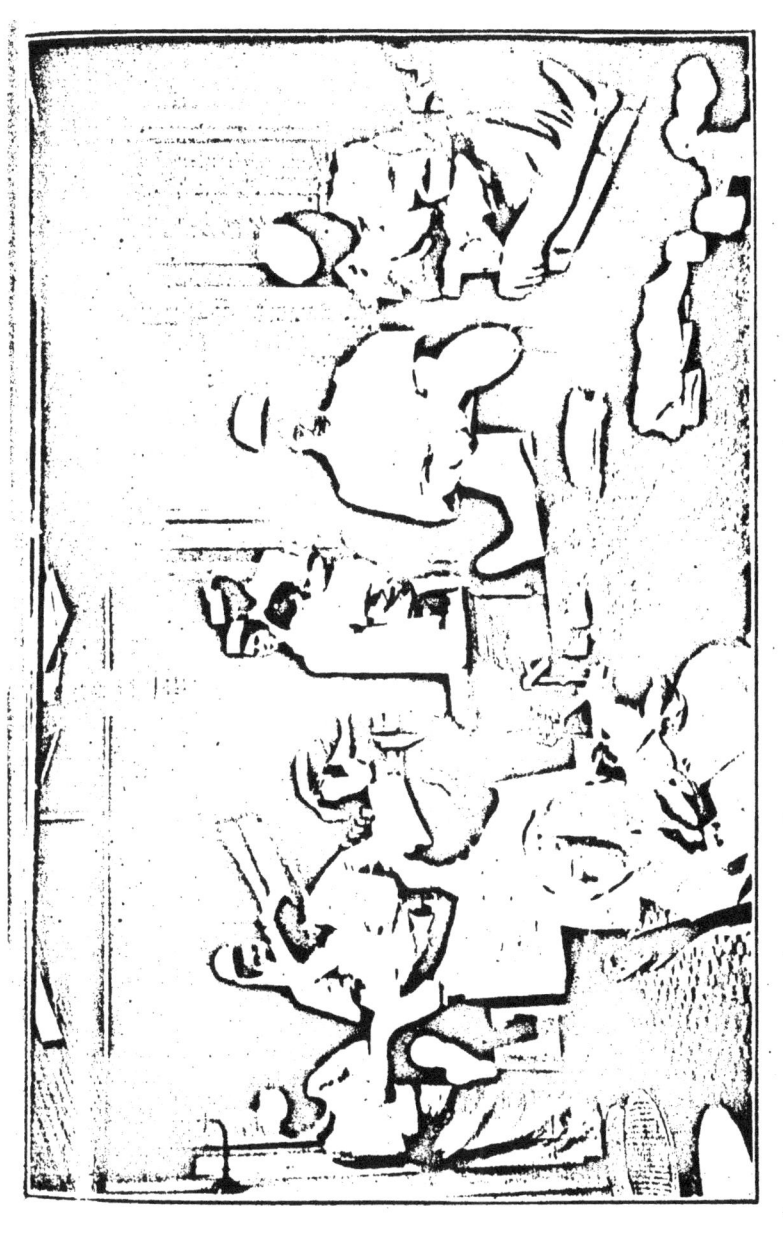

A BANDAGING CLASS AT TREDEGAR HOUSE.
The Preliminary Nurse-Training School of the London Hospital.

pillars made out of the oak taken from the old chapel. There is also a visitors' room, where nurses receive their friends. A tablet in the sitting-room records the fact that the Home is named the "Lückes," as a tribute of respect to Miss Eva Lückes, who at the time of its erection had been matron of the London Hospital for twenty-five years.

. Close to the nurses' quarters is a private recreation ground, tastefully laid out with trees and grass and flowers, and provided with abundance of seats. It is called the "Garden of Eden," but the planting of apple trees has, I believe, been carefully avoided. Sick nurses have the advantage of the "Herman de Stern" Convalescent Home at Felixstowe, under the kind care of Miss Wamsley.

The religious refreshment of the nurses is not forgotten at the "London," and beautiful services are arranged for the staff by Mr. Vatcher at St. Philip's Church. Special preachers, including the Archbishop of Canterbury, officiate at these services.

If the "London" nursing staff has been fortunate in its matron, it has also been exceptionally privileged in having a chairman like the Hon. Sydney Holland. Ever since he entered upon that position in 1897, the conditions for the nurses have been rapidly improving, and the whole hospital, structurally or otherwise, has been altered for the better with great discernment and wonderful rapidity. "I am proud, nurses," said Mr. Holland, in one of his delightful "talks" at the end of his first year of chairmanship, "of being at the head of what I believe to be one of the best nursed hospitals in England, and it is an added joy to me to be associated in the work with a woman whose life's work it has been to perfect hospital nursing, and whose single aim and ambition in life has been to see round her happy workers doing good work. It will be a great pleasure to me if, by my work, I can help our matron to see her aim and ambition fulfilled." In the years which have elapsed since he uttered those sentiments, Mr. Sydney Holland has more than redeemed his promises. "We are very proud," wrote Miss Lückes, recently, "to have Mr. Sydney Holland's name associated with our work, and during my long years of hospital experience, I have never met with any one who so fully shares my ideals of what trained nurses and nursing should be, and who has laboured so unselfishly and indefatigably to give them practical shape." Prominent amongst Mr. Holland's labours has been his generous efforts on behalf of the Nurses' Pension Fund.

The amount of work accomplished by the London Hospital is enormous. An average of eight hundred people are daily nursed within its walls, and a large number are daily seen in the out-patients' department. Last year 1750 private cases were also nursed, and, what is more wonderful still, only twelve complaints were made to the hospital. The "London" nurses have certainly been drilled in the art of making their services agreeable as well as skilled. The hospital does its work without State aid or rate aid, but in Mr. Sydney Holland it possesses a chairman who has a genius for rousing the sympathy of the charitable public.

Tragedy and humour are pathetically mingled in the experience of the medical and nursing staff of this great hospital for the suffering poor of the East End. Sir Frederick Treves relates a touching story of the gratitude of a Norwegian sailor, who had come under his care in the hospital. An operation had restored the man to health and working power, and some time after being discharged from the hospital he sought the great surgeon's house. He looked ill and poor, and Sir Frederick supposed he had come to ask for help. But no, he produced a gold coin, a twenty-kroner piece, and thus related its history: "Before I sailed from home, my wife sewed this coin into my belt, and made me promise not to part with it unless I was starving. For three years it has stood between me and hunger. Since I left the hospital I have been in great want, but I have managed to keep the coin, and now that I have found a ship I want you to accept it." Sir Frederick took the gift in the spirit in which it was offered, and counts it amongst his most treasured possessions. It speaks of rare and simple gratitude.

The out-patients' department affords many pathetic incidents, of which the following may serve as an example. One evening a little girl, thin and poorly clad, came asking to have a tooth drawn. After the operation was over, the nurse in attendance, touched by the little one's half-famished look, gave her a cup of tea and some bread and butter. Next evening the child presented herself again, and, being asked what was the matter, eagerly replied, "Please can I have another tooth drawn?" The operation from which most children shrink with fright was this poor mite's remote chance of getting something given her to eat.

Queen Alexandra, as president of the London hospital, takes a great interest in its work. Nurses selected from the hospital private staff by Sir Frederick Treves nursed the King through his memorable illness. At the "London," the Queen first installed the light treatment for lupus, discovered by the late Dr. Finsen of Copenhagen, who sacrificed his life in the cause of medical science. In appreciation of the Queen's unfailing interest in the cause of human suffering, a statue of Her Majesty is to be placed within the hospital. The King recently conferred a unique honour on the nurse who had attended him since his last illness. One day, when she was binding his ankle, he said, as she knelt before him, "Nurse, I have a present for you," and gave her the M.V.O.—an honour never before conferred upon a woman.

CHAPTER XII

NURSING IN MILITARY HOSPITALS

Florence Nightingale and the Crimean War—The old army nurses unsatisfactory—Evidence of the Duke of Newcastle—Mr. Russell of the *Times* makes an appeal—Florence Nightingale responds—Letter from Mr. Sidney Herbert—Nursing at Scutari—Value of Miss Nightingale's work—Reorganization of military hospitals after the Crimean War—Nursing sisters first employed at Chatham—Death of Lord Herbert of Lea—Royal Victoria Hospital, Netley—Increase of sisters in military hospitals—System extended to India in 1888—Military hospitals lacked nursing organization—Superfluity of nurses—Story of soldier in South African hospital—Soudan and Egyptian campaigns—Queen Victoria institutes the Royal Red Cross—Nursing in the South African campaign—Sir Frederick Treves' testimony—Tommy's appreciation of the sisters—Queen Alexandra's Imperial Military Nursing Service—Miss Monk's work in organization—Rules of the service—Nurses' Home, Millbank—Miss Sidney Brown, R.R.C.; Miss C. H. Keer, R.R.C.; Miss Annie B. Smith, R.R.C.—The Army Nursing Service Reserve—The British Red Cross Council.

THE history of modern military nursing dates from October, 1854, when, in the midst of the throes of the Crimean campaign, the War Office issued a proclamation to the effect that "Miss Nightingale, a lady with greater practical experience of hospital administration and treatment than any other lady in this country, had undertaken the arduous work of organizing and taking out a band of nurses to the succour of the wounded soldiery." The *Times* also notified the fact that "Miss Nightingale had been appointed by Government to the office of superintendent of nurses at Scutari," the great barrack hospital on the Bosphorus placed at the disposal of the British commander by the Turkish authorities.

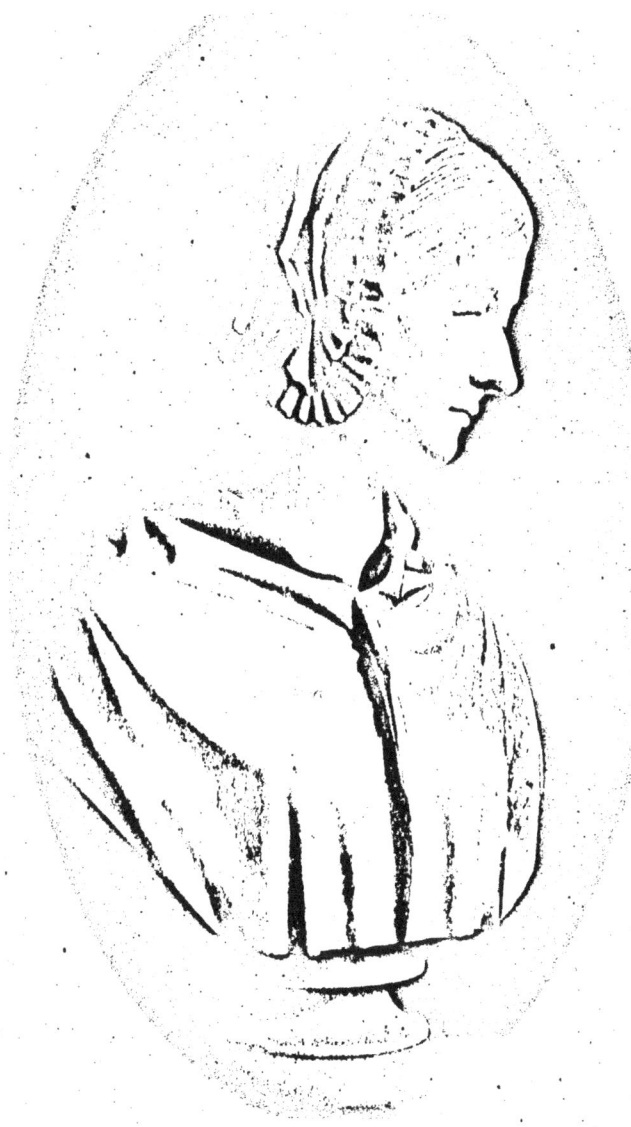

Miss Florence Nightingale.
(From the bust at Claydon.)

This bust was presented to Miss Nightingale by the soldiers after the Crimean War, and was executed by the late Sir John Steele.

The harrowing events which led up to the first official recognition of women as army nurses is a thrice-told tale. When the army was despatched to the Crimea in the spring of 1854, no provision worthy of the name was made for tending the sick and wounded. Beyond the small body of women in training at St. John's House and the Institution of Nursing Sisters in Devonshire Square, there were no trained nurses in the country, and the authorities would hardly have ventured to suggest that the highly respectable members of those institutions should go and nurse in a military hospital. Hitherto the women employed in time of war were the limited number of married women allowed to accompany their husbands' regiments and the unfortunate class known as camp-followers. In times of stress and emergency, the ministrations of these two classes had been utilized for the sick in the same way that their services were requisitioned for cooking, washing, and other domestic labour.

The conditions under which married women lived in camp were revolting to a woman of any sense of propriety. Married couples would be allotted a corner in a barrack-room, where a number of single men slept. A woman of the highest respectability who accompanied her husband to the Crimea, has related to the present writer that she and her husband occupied a tent in which nine soldiers were quartered. When ill with fever in the trenches before Sebastopol, she was nursed by men. On one occasion, when it seemed probable that they would be separated, the husband prepared to shoot her sooner than leave her to the fate which the withdrawal of his protection would involve. Finally, this woman was sent home on a troopship, where, thanks to Florence Nightingale, some nurses were on board.

In such ill odour was life in camp or military hospital held, that the idea of sending respectable women as nurses was out of the question, and the available class were so undesirable that the authorities decided to dispense with female nurses altogether. The situation was thus explained by the Duke of Newcastle, secretary of state for war, when, in 1855, he gave evidence before the War Commission. Asked "When did you first determine on sending nurses to Scutari?" the Duke replied, "The employment of nurses in the hospital at Scutari was mooted in this country at an early stage, before the army left this country, but it was not liked by the military authorities. It had been tried on former occasions. The class of women employed as nurses had been very much addicted to drinking, and were found even more callous to the sufferings of soldiers in hospitals than men would have been. Subsequently, in consequence of letters in the public press, and of recommendations made by gentlemen who had returned to this country from Scutari, we began to consider the subject of employing nurses. The difficulty was to get a lady to take in hand the charge of superintending and directing a body of nurses. After having seen one or two, I almost despaired of the practicability of the matter until Mr. Sidney Herbert suggested Miss Nightingale, with whom he had been previously acquainted, for the work, and that lady eventually undertook it."

It was the popular outcry raised after the battle of the Alma at the privations and neglect to which the wounded soldiers were subjected, which brought matters to a crisis. The wounded lay uncared for on the battle-field, the dying unconsoled, and those who, after the prolonged agony of a voyage with wounds undressed, at length reached the hospital at Scutari, found themselves in a hotbed of pestilence, without the necessaries or the decencies of life. The medical staff were insufficient to cope with the endless procession of wounded and suffering men who were disembarked at Scutari, and there were no nurses except untrained orderlies and patients who were a little less ill than their fellows.

Then came the stirring appeal of Mr. (now Sir) William Howard Russell, the war correspondent of the *Times:* "Are there no devoted women amongst us able and willing to go forth to minister to the sick and suffering soldiers of the East in the hospitals at Scutari? Are none of the daughters of England, at this extreme hour of need, ready for such a work of mercy? . . . France has sent forth her sisters of mercy unsparingly, and they are even now by the bedsides of the wounded and the dying, giving what woman's hand alone can give of comfort and relief. . . . Must we fall so far below the French in self-sacrifice and devotedness, in a work which Christ so signally blesses as done unto Himself? 'I was sick, and ye visited me.'"

That call was heard and responded to by Florence Nightingale. The letter in which she offered her services, by a curious coincidence, crossed that of Mr. Sydney Herbert (afterwards Lord Herbert of Lea) the War minister, who, authorized by Government, invited Miss Nightingale to organize and take out a band of nurses to Scutari, believing that she was the one woman in all England who had the training and ability to grapple with the task.

In less than a week Miss Nightingale had mobilized her force of thirty-eight nurses drawn from St. John's House, the Institution of Nursing Sisters, Devonshire Square, and from Roman Catholic sisterhoods, and on the evening of October 21, 1854, left London *en route* for the East. The company arrived at Scutari, November 4, and took up their quarters in one of the towers of the great Barrack Hospital. Next day, before lint and bandages were unpacked, the lady-in-chief and her staff were called upon to cope with the most gigantic nursing problem ever faced. The wounded poured in from Inkerman, until every inch of the space in the huge building was crowded with sufferers. For twenty-four hours they continued to arrive in appalling numbers, and for many there was no resting-place but on the muddy ground outside. Several days had elapsed since the men had left the battlefield. The majority had wounds undressed and limbs unset. The hospital was devoid of the " needful " in almost every particular, and the insanitary conditions were beyond description. The labour of the next few months, which reduced this scene of misery and disorder into a comparatively well-ordered military hospital, is known wherever the English language is spoken. The pen of Kinglake has paid no unstinted tribute to the lady-in-chief and her " Angel Band ; " the Crimean veterans wax eloquent to-day at mention of their name, and not a soldier went out from that Barrack Hospital who did not raise his hand in parting salute to the nurses' tower. The fitness of women to minister to the sick and dying soldier was settled for all time by that object lesson at Scutari.

Before the long-delayed Peace came, Miss Nightingale had organized the nursing of the General as well as the Barrack Hospital at Scutari, and, proceeding to the seat of war, inspected the camp hospitals before Sebastopol, and carried her nurses even to the heights of Balaclava. Miss Stanley, the sister of the late Dean, had also, in the early part of the war, brought out a party of nurses, and did some useful work at the little hospital at Kullali, but shortly returned home.

The great value of Miss Nightingale's work as affecting the position of women as army nurses was, that she held a direct mandate from the War Office, and conducted her organization of the nursing service, not as an irresponsible philanthropist, but as a Government servant. The heroine of the Crimea was something more than an efficient nurse or the " soldier's friend ; " she possessed that commanding genius which enabled her to govern, control, initiate, and organize, and one such woman, whose personality arrests attention and defies patting on the back, is of more value to a movement than hundreds of nonentities, useful as their work may be.

The immediate outcome of the Crimean War was the reorganization of the military hospitals' nursing system at the instance of Lord Herbert of Lea, who was the mainspring of the royal commission to inquire into

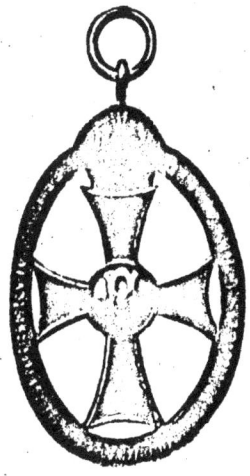

BADGE OF
QUEEN ALEXANDRA'S
IMPERIAL MILITARY
NURSING SERVICE.

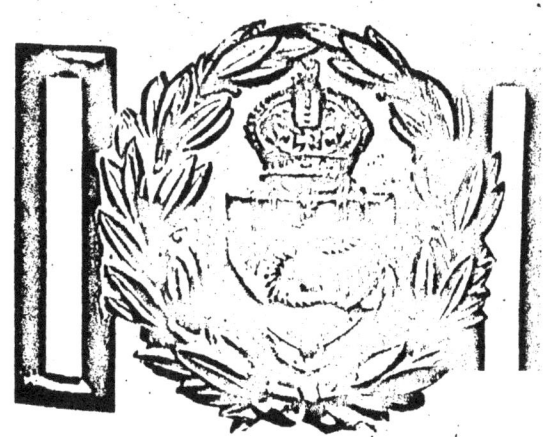

BELT CLASP OF QUEEN ALEXANDRA'S IMPERIAL
NAVAL NURSING SERVICE.

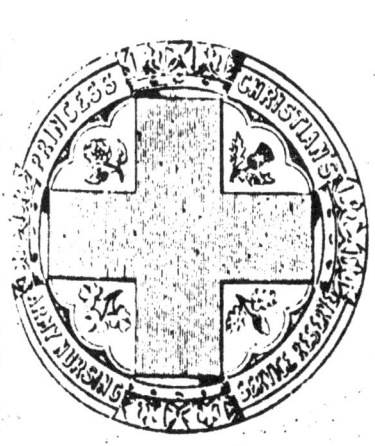

BADGE OF THE ARMY NURSING
SERVICE RESERVE.

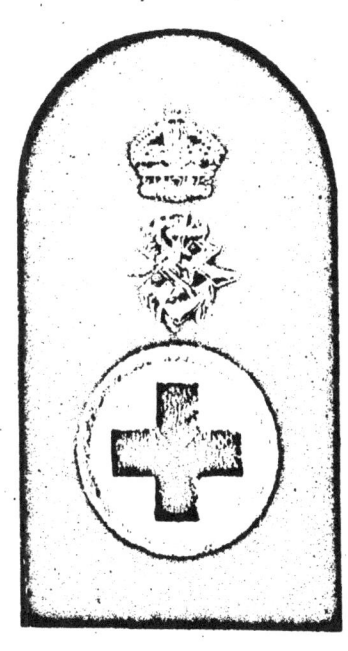

BADGE OF QUEEN ALEXANDRA'S IMPERIAL
NAVAL NURSING SERVICE.

[To face p. 172.

matters, and eventually took office as Secretary for War. Until his death in 1861, this brilliant statesman and great philanthropist found a valuable helper in Miss Nightingale. He took counsel with her continually in matters relating to the army medical department. Reforms were instituted at the military hospital at Chatham, and there nursing sisters were first employed. They were also introduced into the new hospital at Woolwich, which Lord Herbert of Lea had planned as a model military hospital, and which was ultimately transformed into the present large building now known as the Royal Herbert Hospital. It was by a sad coincidence opened August 2, 1861, the day on which Lord Herbert died.

Queen Victoria had taken a deep interest in the army nursing reforms, and when the Royal Victoria Hospital at Netley, erected under her auspices and those of the Prince Consort, was opened, provision was made for a staff of nurses under Lady Jane Shaw Stewart, the matron or lady superintendent. She was succeeded in 1869 by Mrs. Deeble, R.R.C., who for a period of twenty years was lady superintendent at Netley, and saw great developments in the nursing system. Mrs. Deeble was succeeded by Miss H. C. Norman, R.R.C., who had charge at Netley for thirteen years, and did most arduous work during the South African War when the great hospital was filled to overflowing with the sick and wounded from that terrible campaign.

Although as early as 1866 the War Office made provision for the appointment of nursing sisters to any military general hospital, for a long time only a few were employed at Chatham, Netley, and Woolwich. Then in 1882 a staff of nursing sisters was appointed to the Guards' hospital in London, and subsequently to the hospitals in Egypt and Aldershot. In 1884 it was decided to appoint a nursing staff of ladies to every military hospital of one hundred beds and over, such as Gosport, Portsmouth, Devonport, Dover, Shorncliffe, Canterbury, Dublin, Curragh, Gibraltar, and Malta, and from that time forward there was an increase in the number of hospitals having nursing sisters. In 1888 the system was extended to the Indian army, and has been worked with great efficiency.

Nursing in military hospitals lacked, however, the organization which had grown up in civil hospitals. The number of sisters was small, and the orderlies were untrained and subject to be drafted into the wards from doing outside work in the barracks. Many of the orderlies, like the old untrained nurse of the civil hospitals, had learned much by experience. They were kind and sympathetic to their sick comrades, and it would not have been easy to persuade an orderly who had had fever himself, that he was not qualified to nurse a comrade similarly afflicted. In time of peace military nurses were somewhat at a discount. One has heard of a hospital where there were fourteen nurses to three patients. Those unfortunate three must have been almost in as perplexing a condition as the soldier in a base hospital during the early stages of the Boer War, when ladies volunteered in overwhelming numbers to tend the sick soldiers.

"What can I do for you, my poor man?" said a lady visitor; "shall I wash your face?"

"Thank you kindly, ma'am," replied embarrassed Tommy; "but I have already promised fourteen ladies that they shall wash my face"!

In the Soudan and the Egyptian campaigns, the army sisters rendered good service, and several received the Royal Red Cross from a grateful Sovereign. Queen Victoria instituted that Order in 1883, and proud is the sister to-day who is entitled to R.R.C. after her name. The Royal Red Cross is the blue riband of the nursing world. The decoration was designed as a reward for women who had shown zeal and devotion in providing for and nursing sick and wounded sailors, soldiers, and others with the army in the field, on board ship, or in hospitals. The list was headed by Queen Victoria, the

Princess of Wales, and other royal ladies. Lady Wantage received the honour for her efforts on behalf of Red Cross work.

In the year of its institution the Red Cross was bestowed on twenty-nine nurses, headed by the name of Florence Nightingale. On the occasion of her Diamond Jubilee (1897), Queen Victoria bestowed the Red Cross on nine Crimean "veterans"—Sister Mary Aloysius, Sister Mary Stanislaus Jones, Sister Mary Anastasia Kelly, Sister Mary de Chantal Huddon, Sister Mary Elizabeth Joseph, Mrs. Hely, Miss Sarah Anne Terrot, Miss Susan Cator, and Miss Emma Halford. After the South African War, the roll of the Red Cross reached a total of two hundred and eleven, and was represented by nurses who had done special service in the Crimean, Egyptian, Transvaal, Soudan, and South African campaigns, and in minor wars. The roll included a few ladies not in the nursing profession, who had aided in organizing work on behalf of the soldiers.

The South African campaign, 1899-1901, saw the service of women utilized for military nursing on a widely extended plan. One saw contingent after contingent depart for South Africa during that thrilling time, and the sister's cloak with the magic red cross stirred the heart of the people more even than the khaki-clad soldiers. On hospital ship and hospital train, the sisters plied their gentle ministrations. They formed part of the staff of every field hospital, and bore their share of privation out on the open veldt under blinding dust or scorching sun, jolting in ox-waggons for weary hours, through country where no water was, snatching fitful slumber on the bare floor of a looted house, or cheerfully giving up their sleeping hours to minister to the suffering heroes, who poured into the field hospitals in a continuous stream of ambulances and stretchers after Colenso, Spion Kop, or Maggersfontein, with heroic courage.

Military and medical officers alike have borne testimony to the work done by women during the South

African War. There were, of course, critics and scoffers who singled out frivolous exceptions in the hospitals at the base, and made them a type of army nurses, but against such criticism we would set the testimony of that great surgeon who valued their services so highly. Of the nurses on the staff of his Field Hospital, who shared the privations at Chieveley, Sir Frederick Treves wrote, in "The Tale of a Field Hospital"—

"These ill-housed women" [the sisters had no choice between a night in the open, or in a bare railway waiting-room used as a stable by the Boers], "as a matter of fact, were hard at work all Friday, all Saturday, and all Saturday night. They seemed oblivious to fatigue, to hunger, or to any need for sleep. Considering that the heat was intense, that the thirst which attended it was distressing and incessant, that water was scarce, and that the work in hand was heavy and trying, it was wonderful that they came out of it all so little the worse in the end.

"Their ministrations to the wounded were invaluable and beyond all praise. They did a service during those distressful days which none but nurses could have rendered, and they set to all at Chieveley an example of unselfishness, self-sacrifice, and indefatigable devotion to duty. They brought to many of the wounded and the dying that comfort which men are little able to evolve, or are uncouth in bestowing, and which belongs especially to the tender, undefined, and undefinable ministrations of women."

When trained women nurses were first employed in military hospitals, many people were quite sure that the soldiers would rather not have them. Tommy has settled that question for himself. The men who wept like children at Scutari, because the nurses made them feel so "homelike," was eloquent tribute enough. True, when the soldier is convalescent, he is quite satisfied with, and often prefers being tended by, an orderly; but "when pain and anguish wring the brow," the suffering man leans on a woman's sympathy, her voice soothes, her

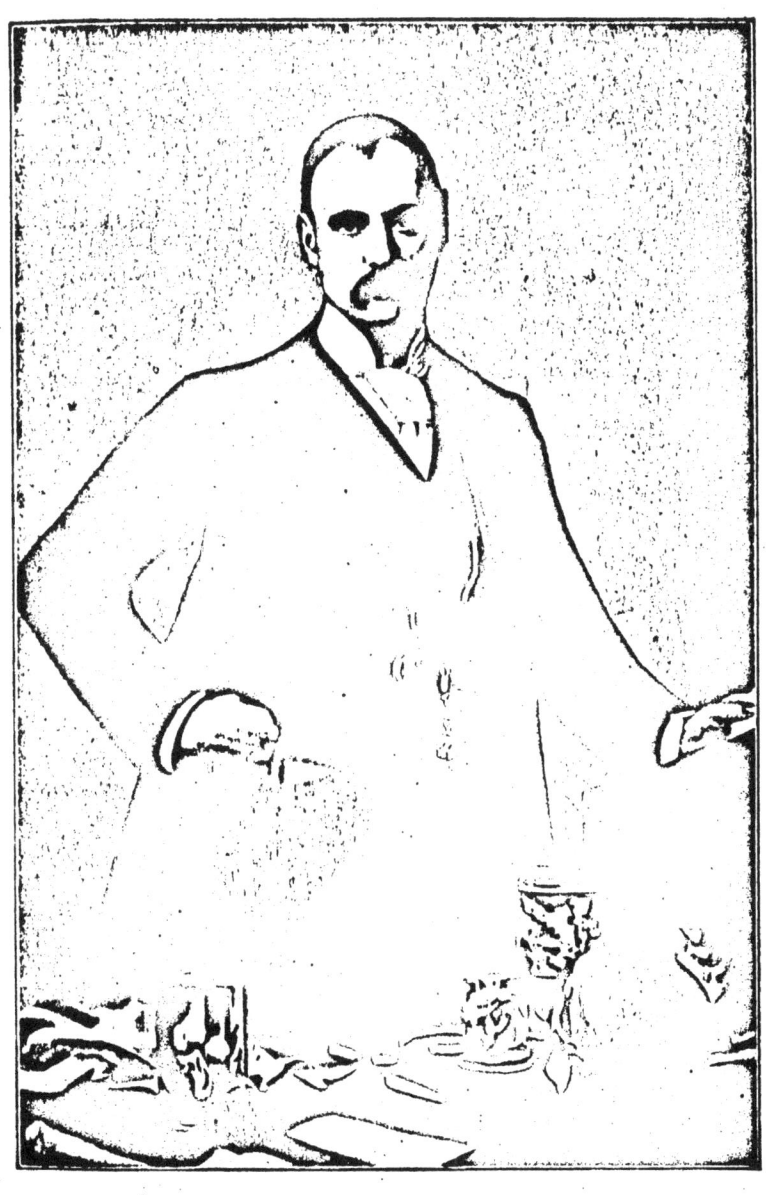

SIR FREDERICK TREVES.

hand calms and comforts. "Sister, won't you dress me?"
is the frequent request of the soldier who has struggled
back to life, a shattered wreck after fever or dysentery.
And when the shadows deepen, and the hour of passing
approaches, it is to the sister that Tommy confides his
farewells to mother, sister, or sweetheart. He dies in
happy confidence that the cherished belt worked by
loving hands, or the trinket he has worn next his heart, in
the heat of battle, will be reverently buried with him.
He does not mind breaking down, because the woman at
his bedside weeps too.

The British soldier, so brave and fearless in battle, is
full of sentiment. Beneath his rough exterior there is a
fine chivalry towards good women, and the big burly
fellow who is unruly in the hands of his mates, will be
docile to the nurse who tends him. He places her little
lower than the angels, and is often amusingly considerate
of her feelings. A dying soldier in a field hospital in
South Africa was dictating a letter to his mother. He
shyly intimated that he would like to include a message
for "his girl." "What shall I say to her?" asked the
sister. Poor Tommy searched his vocabulary for a
correct sentiment, one which in his chivalrous judgment
would not shock the sensibilities of a lady. "Will you,"
said he, "please say I send my kind regards." One feels
sure the sister substituted "love," and perhaps "kisses"
too!

Sir Frederick Treves relates that, when going through
the wards of the hospital at Pietermaritzburg, he noticed
a paralyzed man treasuring under his pillow an extremely
dirty handkerchief. The great surgeon suggested that
he should ask for a clean one. But the man replied,
"I am not going to give this one up; I am afraid of
losing it. The sister who looked after me at Chieveley
gave it to me, and here is her name in the corner."

"Pretty sentiment, but not of much practical use in
sick-nursing," may be the hasty cynicism of some critics,
but the sentiment points to the influence wielded by a nurse

over her patient. To quote Sir Frederick again, there was the case of Kelly, the Irish soldier who had had his arm smashed on Spion Kop, and passed two nights on that hill of carnage, keeping himself alive until succour came by crawling from one dead comrade to another to get the water left in their bottles. When he at length reached the hospital, it was necessary to amputate the whole upper limb, including the shoulder-blade and collar-bone. It is small wonder that after his fearful experiences he was difficult to manage. However, he grew to have a great veneration for the sister who looked after him, and in her hands became docile as a lamb.

There is hardly a nurse who has tended the wounded in war time, who could not give touching instances of Tommy's docility and gratitude. No further evidence is in these days needed to prove a woman's fitness for military nursing. The dying Marmion on Flodden Field was cheered by the draught of water ministered by gentle hands, and Scott's immortal lines beginning, "O Woman! in our hours of ease" has become a soldier's psalm of thanksgiving for the institution of army sisters.

During the progress of the Boer war, Queen Victoria and her advisers recognized that the Army Nursing Service needed reorganization. The revered Queen, who took such a deep personal interest in the welfare of her soldiers, did not live to see the reforms accomplished. After the conclusion of the war, the King gave his sanction to a scheme for the inauguration of a new military service in the special Army Order of March 29, 1902, from which the subjoined is an extract :—

"EDWARD, R.I.

"Whereas we deem it expedient to further provide for the nursing services of our army, Our will and pleasure is that an Imperial Military Nursing Service, to be designated the Queen Alexandra's Imperial Military Nursing Service, and comprising our Army Nursing Service, shall be established."

NURSING IN MILITARY HOSPITALS

Queen Alexandra's Imperial Military Nursing Service was established to extend the scope of the duties of the woman nurse in the hospitals of the Royal Army Medical Corps. Although the male nurse is of paramount importance in time of war, it had become apparent to military authorities, based on the experience of the valuable aid of women in the South African campaign, that a more extended organization of nursing by trained women in the army was desirable to elevate the general standard of nursing, both in time of peace and war. It is managed by a Nursing Board, of which the Queen is president. The vice-president is Countess Roberts, C.I., R.R.C., who devotes much time to the work; the chairman is the Director-General of the Army Medical Service. Members of the Advisory Board are Sir Frederick Treves, Bart., and the Deputy Director-General; the first matron-in-chief, Miss Sydney Browne, R.R.C., Queen Alexandra's Imperial Nursing Service; two matrons of civil hospitals —Miss Monk, of King's College, and Miss Cave, of Westminster Hospital; and two members nominated by Her Majesty—Viscountess Downe and Hon. Sydney Holland. The secretary is Lieut.-Colonel Skinner.

Miss Monk rendered valuable assistance in organizing the service, her skill in such work having been demonstrated by the manner in which she reorganized the nursing at King's College Hospital. To the great regret of the Queen and the Nursing Board, Miss Monk was compelled, through ill health, to resign her position early in 1906. Miss Isla Stewart, matron of St. Bartholomew's Hospital, was appointed a member of the Board on the retirement of Miss Monk.

The headquarters of Q.A.I.M.N.S. are at the War Office, 68, Victoria Street. There are three grades in the service—matrons, sisters, and staff nurses. At the head is the matron-in-chief. There is a principal matron for South Africa. A lady, on appointment, is usually graded as staff nurse. A candidate must be between the ages of twenty-five and thirty-five years, and possess a certificate of not less than three years' training and service in medical and surgical nursing in a civil hospital recognized by the Advisory Board. She must be of British parentage or a naturalized British subject. If accepted for service, a staff nurse is appointed provisionally for a period of six months. A special report furnished by the matron of the hospital is laid before the Nursing Board, and on this provisional report the final acceptance depends. The pay of a staff nurse is £40 a year, rising by annual increments of £2 10s. to £45; of a sister £50 a year, rising by annual increments of £5 to £65; of a matron £75 a year, rising by annual increments of £10 to £150 a year. A principal matron receives on appointment £175, and the pay rises by annual increments of £10 to £205. The matron-in-chief's pay is £300 a year, rising by annual increments of £10 to £350. All grades receive in addition certain allowances; charge pay is granted to a matron or sister in charge of a hospital containing more than one hundred beds. All members of the nursing service are entitled to a pension on attaining the age of fifty. The uniform is grey faced with scarlet. The Queen's Badge is always worn by members when in uniform. It is on a cross pattee (as borne in the Royal Arms of Denmark) surmounted by an Imperial Crown, the letter A within a circle, and surrounded by an oval band bearing the inscription, "Queen Alexandra's Imperial Military Nursing Service," and the motto "Sub cruce candida."

Queen Alexandra's nurses are employed in all military hospitals, at home and abroad, of one hundred beds and upwards. Service abroad is limited in duration to from three to five years, according to climate, and is taken in rotation in the several grades of matrons, sisters, and staff nurses. The foreign stations in which military nurses work are Egypt, Gibraltar, Malta, South Africa, Canada, Bermuda, Ceylon, Hong Kong, and Singapore.

The members of the nursing staff of a military hospital live together in quarters provided by the State.

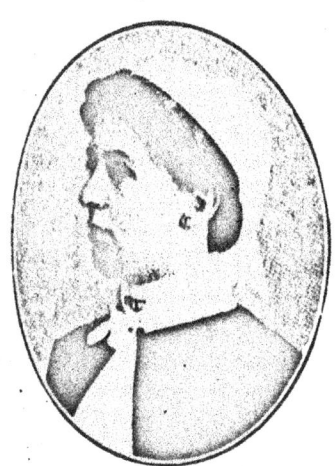

Miss Chadwick, R.R.C.
Matron, the Curragh, Ireland.

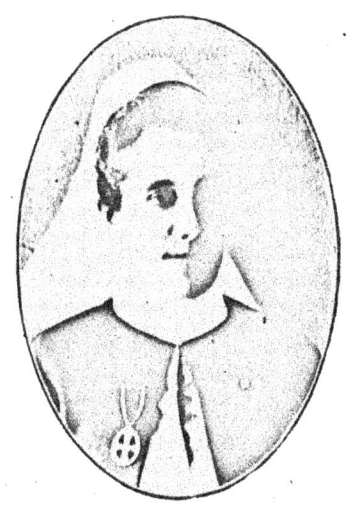

Miss Addams-Williams, R.R.C.
Principal Matron, South Africa.
(*Photo: Elliott & Fry.*)

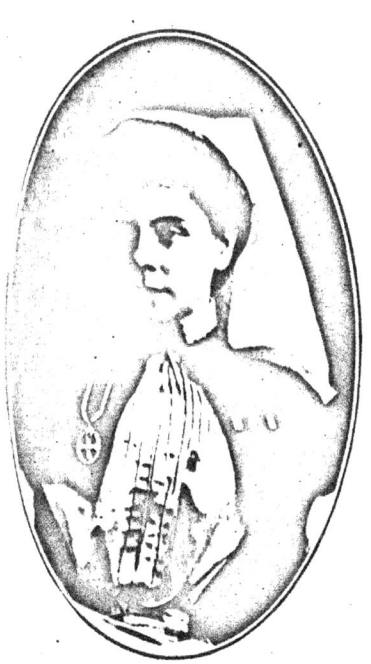

Miss Annie B. Smith, R.R.C.
Matron of the Royal Victoria Hospital, Netley.

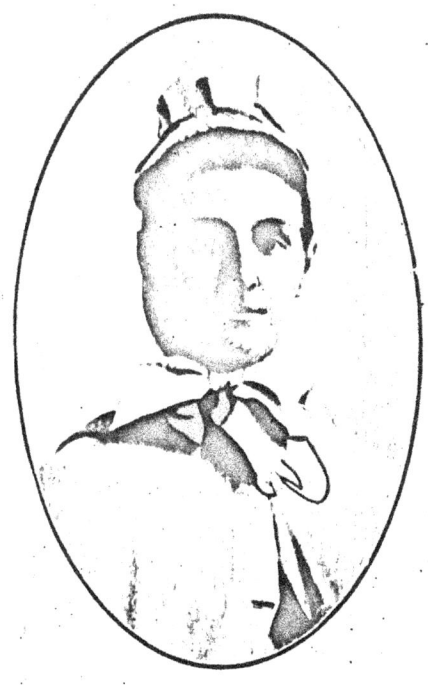

Miss Garrock, R.R.C.
Matron of the Royal Herbert Hospital, Woolwich.

There is an allowance for board, and the arrangements of the mess are undertaken by the head of the nursing staff, and not, as in civil hospitals, as part of the hospital administration.

An important change in the status of the army nurse is shown by the duties which she performs under the new organization. In addition to the charge of wards by day and by night, under conditions similar to those of civil hospitals, matrons and sisters give lectures and practical demonstrations to those men of the Royal Army Medical Corps who are selected for training in nursing. The day of the untrained orderly will soon happily be passed. The training of the orderlies is now conducted by the sisters on a similar plan to that of probationers in civil hospitals, with a three years' course of study and examination. The part played by the army sister to-day is one of enlarged usefulness and responsibility, and the key-note of the service is efficiency. The abolition of the ward-master from military hospitals, and the placing of the orderlies under the tuition of the sister, have occasioned a little friction in some quarters, but this is dying down.

In February, 1906, a new order was issued by the War Office to the effect that "Sisters of Queen Alexandra's Imperial Military Nursing Service will not be promoted to the rank of matron until they have passed an examination." To enable sisters to qualify for the necessary certificate of administrative capacity, sisters of four years' service and over in that rank may at their own request undergo a two months' course of special instruction in matron's duties.

A central military Nurses' Home in London is in course of erection (1906), in connection with the hospital at Millbank, of which Miss Beatrice Jones is matron, and from it nurses will be sent as required to smaller military hospitals and institutions of under one hundred beds.

The progress in army nursing which has followed the reorganization may be judged from the fact that when the Boer war broke out in 1899, there were only eighty-seven sisters from military hospitals available for duty; now there are close upon four hundred.

Miss Sidney Browne, R.R.C., who was appointed matron-in-chief of the new service, filled the office with marked ability and distinction for four years until her compulsory retirement in accordance with the age regulations in April, 1906. To her is due the credit for the smooth manner in which recent changes have been effected. Miss Browne is a picked woman in her profession, and it is interesting to note that she bears for a first name that of Sidney, like Lord Herbert of Lea, who sent Miss Nightingale to the Crimea, and the Hon. Sydney Holland, who, as chairman of the London Hospital, has devoted so much time to the question of nursing.

Miss Browne was drawn to enter the profession through attending a course of lectures on nursing by Miss Florence Lees (Mrs. Dacre Craven). As was usual in those days, her friends tried to dissuade her from undertaking the work. However, she felt it to be her vocation, and, in 1879, entered the Guest Hospital, Dudley, and later went to the West Bromwich Hospital. In 1882 she became a staff nurse at St. Bartholomew's Hospital, an institution with which she is proud to have been associated. A year later she came to the Royal Military Hospital, Netley, and worked henceforth in the service of which she was destined to become matron-in-chief,

Miss Browne has served in Egypt, the Soudan, Malta, and South Africa, and her decorations include the Egyptian medal and clasp, the Khedive's Star, the South African medals, the Coronation Medal, and the Royal Red Cross. During the Boer war she rendered invaluable service in the superintendence of hospitals, and while in camp at Pretoria received the cablegram offering her the chief post in Q.A.I.M.N.S. She returned home to pursue with tact, vigour, and a cheery optimism, all her own, the arduous work of that office.

During the fruitful years that she held the post of matron-in-chief Miss Browne had the satisfaction of seeing army nursing placed upon a level which it had never before approached. Miss Browne is a member of the Nursing Board, and of the Advisory Board at the War Office. The Queen received Miss Browne in private audience before her retirement to specially thank her for the work which she had accomplished, and the R.A.M.C. staff at the War Office entertained her to a farewell dinner. The War Office is said to be the grave of great reputations, but Miss Sidney Browne, the first matron-in-chief, has cheated Fate by retiring with a greatly enhanced reputation.

Miss C. H. Keer, R.R.C., who succeeded Miss Browne as matron-in-chief, was, like her predecessor, called from Pretoria to the highest post in the service. Miss Keer was principal matron of Q.A.I.M.N.S. in South Africa. She has had a varied life and career. Born in India, the daughter of an English officer, educated in England, she went to Boston City Hospital for training in her profession. Returning to England, she entered the Army Nursing Service in 1887, and the following year was ordered to Egypt, where she remained until 1894. Subsequently she was stationed at Dover, and was ordered to South Africa at the beginning of the war, 1899. At the conclusion of the war she returned home, and was stationed at Colchester. In June, 1903, she was appointed principal matron in South Africa. Miss Keer has arduous work before her, for much yet remains to be done in consolidating the Army Nursing Service on its new basis, but her past record gives hostage for her future success.

Miss F. E. Addams-Williams, R.R.C., formerly matron at Netley, where she did valuable work in reorganizing the nursing of that great hospital after the institution of Queen Alexandra's Service, has succeeded Miss Keer as principal matron in South Africa. Miss Addams-Williams was trained at the Royal Infirmary, Edinburgh, and became a sister in the Army Nursing Service in 1890. She has been superintendent of the military hospital, Canterbury, and of the Connaught Hospital, Aldershot.

Miss Annie B. Smith, R.R.C., who has been appointed to Netley, was trained at St. Bartholomew's Hospital, and held there the posts of theatre sister, night sister, and ward sister. In 1899 she joined the Army Nursing Reserve, and served in South Africa until 1902, when she returned to St. Bartholomew's, and remained until, in 1903, she was appointed matron in Q.A.I.M.N.S., and was stationed in Dublin until appointed to Netley in March, 1906.

The Army Nursing Service Reserve

It had long been felt by far-seeing people that the nursing, like the fighting army, should have its reservists, ready for mobilization when war broke out. Sir John Furley had always been an advocate for being ready for the outbreak of war. Mrs. Bedford Fenwick was also an early advocate for the formation of a nursing reserve, and Surgeon-General Evatt, late A.M.S. to the *British Medical Journal*, proposed in 1885 the formation of a corps of reserve nurses.

In 1886 Her Royal Highness Princess Christian founded the Army Nursing Service Reserve. Candidates were received under the following regulations. They must be between the ages of twenty-five and thirty-five, have a certificate of three years' training in a general civil hospital, and in addition must produce testimonials of efficiency in medical and surgical nursing from registered practitioners under whom they had worked. Candidates were also required to produce guarantees that their social position, character, and education were such as to fit them to enter a service of ladies, and they were required to sign a declaration of willingness to accept service in a military hospital if called on to do so in time of war. The badge chosen by Princess Christian for her nurses was in the form of a silver brooch,

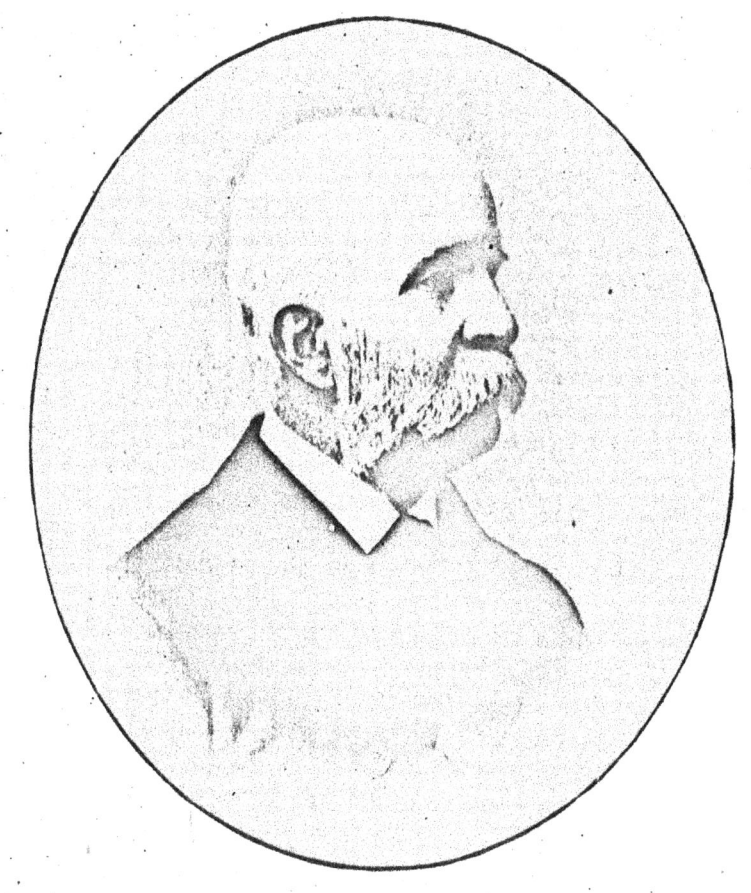

SIR JOHN FURLEY.

ornamented with a Geneva cross, with a crown at the end of each arm of the cross, and between the arms representations of the rose, shamrock, and thistle. The badge bore the inscription, "Princess Christian's Army Nursing Reserve."

When, in 1899, war broke out in South Africa, Princess Christian had the satisfaction of being able at once to call up a reserve of one hundred trained women to take the place in the military hospitals of the army sisters going to the front. During the winter of 1899–1900, some eight hundred more nurses were enrolled in the reserve and were drafted for duty at the home hospitals, and those at the seat of war as required. The machinery for providing these supplementary nurses was, thanks to commendable foresight, in working order. Day after day, during the stress of that terrible time, Princess Christian worked indefatigably as president of the committee, and herself inspected the testimonials of applicants.

During the height of the nursing-fever which seized women at that period, much discretionary power was needed to repel the unfit. The self-made testimonials laid before the committee were often amusing. One lady naïvely wrote inquiring when the *untrained* nurses were going to be sent to the front, as she was ready to join them!

After the close of the Boer war, some alterations took place in the Army Nursing Reserve, by which it was brought into closer touch with the War Office and the permanent service. In time of peace it works under a specially constituted committee, of which Princess Christian is president. Candidates are admitted according to the regulations formerly laid down. Some new rules have been issued with the aim of more closely assimilating the regulations of the permanent and reserve services. Members of the reserve, when not doing military duty, are not bound by any rules as regards dress or uniform, but are expected to wear the badge of the Army Nursing Service Reserve on the right breast. When members are doing military duty, they are supplied with a regulation uniform, similar to that worn by Queen Alexandra's Imperial Military Nursing Service, with the exception that the cape is of grey material, with a border of scarlet cloth two and a quarter inches wide, and that the badge of the reserve is worn instead of that of Queen Alexandra. Reserve nurses, when called up for service, are graded as matrons, sisters, and staff nurses, and receive the same rates of pay as the members of the permanent service.

The pay is now the same for the reserve as for the permanent service, which ends a grievance much felt since Queen Alexandra's Imperial Military Nursing Service was established. The headquarters of the Army Reserve are at the War Office, Army Medical Department, 68, Victoria Street. In time of war the members of the service who are called up for duty are under the command of the Army Council, and are amenable to the ordinary regulations of Queen Alexandra's Imperial Military Nursing Service. There are now six hundred and twelve nurses in the reserve. Mr. Haldane, Secretary of State for War, has expressed himself regarding the desirability of mobilizing the reserve, and plans may at any time be brought under consideration.

The British Red Cross Council

An important movement in relation to military nursing was the institution of Red Cross Societies, which, by affording protection to those engaged in succouring the wounded in time of war, enabled the military authorities of all countries to employ women nurses without the fear of exposing them to the fire of the enemy or to molestation.

That beneficent movement began in gallant little Switzerland, in the year 1863, when some benevolent men, moved by the appalling revelations of the scenes of human anguish on the battlefield of Solferino, made by M. Dunant in his pamphlet "Un Souvenir de Solferino," met in the city of Geneva to consider whether anything could be done to mitigate the horrors of war. The following year an international conference was held, and the treaty known as "The Geneva Convention," was drawn up on August 22, 1864, by the representatives of sixteen governments. Within four months it was signed by eight European powers. Others speedily followed. The British Government attached its signature February, 1865. To quote Sir John Furley, "The treaty was designed to remove soldiers when sick or wounded from the category of combatants, and to afford them relief and protection without regard to nationality. This protection is also extended to all persons officially attached to hospitals or ambulances, and to all houses, so long as they contain invalid soldiers. Inhabitants of a country occupied by a belligerent army, and who may be engaged in the care of the sick and wounded, enjoy the same privilege. Provision is also made for the return of invalid soldiers to their respective homes. The distinctive mark of hospitals and ambulances is a white flag with a red cross upon it—the colours of Geneva reversed—and individuals wear a white armlet with a red cross. Every red cross flag must be accompanied in time of war by the national flag of those using it.

At first the societies were called National Aid Societies, but by degrees became known by their emblem, the red cross. Holland was the first to adopt the name. They spread round the civilized world, and came into action as war demanded. The red cross on ambulance waggon and tent, on the arm of surgeon and nurse, or hoisted above sufferers on the battlefield, became a recognized sign of neutrality amongst combatants.

> "Wheresoever lay the wounded,
> Hospital, or church, or shed,
> Waved therefrom the glorious symbol—
> Waved the white flag crossed with red."

Although Great Britain was one of the early signatories to the Treaty of Geneva, six years elapsed before it started a national society, and its formation was largely due to Sir John Furley, who has devoted the greater part of his life to Red Cross work.

Sir John, then Mr. Furley, attended the conference of Red Cross societies at Berlin in 1869, and when it was pointed out that England had not started a society, he rose and gave his undertaking that if a great war broke out in Europe it should be found that England was not behind other countries in this particular. Little did he anticipate that his promise would be put so quickly to the test. Scarcely a year had elapsed before the Franco-German war broke out. Sir John now rallied his friends. A meeting was held at Willis's Rooms, and in the month of July, 1870, the "British National Society for Aid to the Sick and Wounded in War" was formed. The scheme was substantially aided by that distinguished soldier, the late Lord Wantage, who headed the subscription list with a thousand pounds. Soon, three hundred thousand pounds was subscribed, and the women of the country, from Queen Victoria to the humblest of her subjects, laboured to supply lint, bandages, and comforts for transmission to the seat of war. Sir John Furley acted as commissioner abroad, and his adventures during the siege of Paris and on the battlefields of that sanguinary campaign are graphically and modestly described in his entertaining book of recollections, "In Peace and War." Sir John effected an entrance into Paris during the siege by dressing in the livery and passing for the coachman of a distinguished official. He was thus able to bring relief to the starving people.

The British Society, having sprung into being under private enterprise, was not organized by military authority, as were those of France and Germany, and afforded little outlet for the employment of women nurses. There were a few brilliant examples, notably Miss Florence Lees (now Mrs. Dacre Craven), who had been a probationer at St. Thomas's. She volunteered for service, and with the benediction of Miss Nightingale upon her set out for the seat of war. Subsequently Miss Lees made an adventurous journey across the lines, and at special request took charge of the Crown Princess's lazarette before Metz.

The war of 1870 brought military nursing much to the front. The Red Cross work in Germany was splendidly organized under the late Empress Augusta, and her daughter-in-law, the Crown Princess (the late Empress Frederick), and her daughter, the Grand Duchess of Baden, aided in the work. Under the protection of the Red Cross women nurses were employed more freely in the vicinity of battlefields than they had ever been before. Branch societies were started throughout the German States, each working independently in time of peace, but all owing obedience to the central committee in Berlin in time of war. In 1883 the German societies were in a position to place at the service of the central committee six hundred female and one hundred and twenty male nurses, besides a large number of trained hospital attendants. France, too, which was the first state to sign the Convention of Geneva, developed a good system of Red Cross work, which materially aided the country in its reverses. After 1870 the French society did not relax its efforts. It paid great attention to the improvement of ambulance material, and established schools in Paris and other towns for the instruction of *brancardiers* and nurses. The Russian society was also active in pioneer work, and during the wars in the Balkan provinces, 1876-78, its *personnel* included five hundred sisters of mercy and five hundred male nurses.

An important outcome of the British National Aid or Red Cross Society was the utilization of the income arising from the large balance left in its exchequer after the Franco-German war, in the training of "female nurses" at the Royal Victoria Hospital, Netley.

It was not until the outbreak of the South African war that the British Red Cross Society was called upon to extensively deal with work on behalf of our own soldiers. In January, 1899, a new body, the Central British Red Cross Council, was, with the approval of the War Office, appointed to deal with Red Cross work throughout the empire, and was composed of representatives of the original National Aid Society to the Sick and Wounded in War, of the St. John Ambulance Association, the St. Andrew Ambulance Association, the headquarters for the work in Scotland, the Army Nursing Reserve, and of the Admiralty and War Office. Queen Alexandra, then Princess of Wales, was president of the Council; Lord Knutsford, chairman; Sir John Furley, hon. treasurer; and Major T. McCullock, hon. secretary. The rapid enrolling of nurses by the Reserve, the vast shipments of "comforts" for the wounded, and the general enthusiasm of all classes in furthering Red Cross work, are well remembered.

The *Princess of Wales* hospital ship was the first which had ever sailed under the magic symbol. I see it in memory as it lay at anchor in Tilbury docks flying the Red Cross flag beside the Union Jack, and the cross on its white sides gleaming through the murky atmosphere of the Thames. Queen Alexandra had just concluded her visit of inspection, and had left evidences of her special thought for the ship's nurses as well as for the prospective patients. There were piles of soft red cushions carried on board, and the Queen (then Princess of Wales) said to superintendent-nurse Chadwick, "We made these at home (Sandringham). I thought they might be useful." Voyage after voyage was the ship destined to make, bringing home to Netley, Woolwich, Portsmouth, and Chatham the wounded and suffering soldiers from the battlefields of South Africa.

The Princess Christian hospital train, planned by Sir John Furley, was another novel Red Cross equipment which did admirable service at the seat of war. Sir John, who had gone to the Cape in charge of the train, was, on his arrival, called upon by the War Office to act as general superintendent of Red Cross work in South Africa. Lady Furley remained at the Cape during her husband's absence in the Transvaal, superintending the forwarding of supplies for the sick and wounded at the front. In recognition of her unselfish and arduous service, Lady Furley received the Royal Red Cross.

After the war there was a reconstruction of the Red Cross Council. It, like the Nursing Reserve, works independently under its own committee in time of peace. The Queen is president of the Council, and presides over the meetings of the committee. Her Majesty is anxious that the Red Cross movement should be more widely taken up by the women of the country, and that local branches under their own committees should be established throughout the kingdom. In the event of war, local societies would pass under the control of the central board, and be worked under War Office regulations. The training of military nurses is a special object of the Council.

CHAPTER XIII

THE NURSING IN NAVAL AND SEAMEN'S HOSPITALS

Jack as a patient—The handy man—Story of Admiral Sir Harry Keppel—In the old days—Admiral Sir Edward Parry's appeal—Naval sisters appointed, 1884-85—"Queen Alexandra's Royal Naval Nursing Service," 1902—Its rules and regulations—Training of male attendants—Duties of the sisters—The Seamen's Hospital, Greenwich—Nursing on the *Dreadnought*—Training-school at Greenwich—Branch hospital at the Royal Albert Docks—The tropical school—Oriental patients—Amusing story—"The Hobson Jobson"—Characteristics of seamen—A hot and a cold pipe—A land and a sea age—Popularity of naval nursing.

THE early history of nursing in the navy lacks the element of romantic interest which the Crimean episodes have woven around nursing in the army. The introduction of sisters into naval hospitals is, too, of considerably more recent date. Jack is a most popular patient, and reciprocates the privilege of nursing by the gentler sex to the full. " Why can't we have the ladies to look after us when we're in sick berth ?" exclaimed a jolly old tar, when sisters were first introduced into military hospitals. "Think as how we don't know what's manners before a lady ?" continued he, as he folded his tatooed arms with complacent dignity. Jack had no occasion for apprehension on that score. Some of the most distinguished pioneer nurses would have deemed it a privilege to be a sister at Haslar, or Plymouth, had circumstances permitted.

The sailor, after rough life on board amongst his mates, is specially sensitive to feminine influence, a fact which Miss Agnes Weston has proved in her Sailors'

Rests, where a kind word and a smile from a good woman is the best deterrent from evil Jack knows. People who have studied his temperament as thoroughly as Miss Weston know what they are about when they hang pictures of pretty modest girls about lounges and reading rooms for sailors. If the presence of refined women improved the tone of military hospitals, of equal benefit was their presence likely to be in naval institutions.

The "handy man" waited long for his privilege because he was so handy. There was little he could not do for a sick mate on board ship, and experience thus gained made him a useful and intelligent nurse, when drafted into the wards of a hospital. A sailor, too, is so much accustomed to the exercise of skill and ingenuity at sea, that it serves him well on land. The sarcasm cast at a clumsy man who blunders at things, "You have never been to sea!" elucidates the point. Jack is impatient, too, of doctoring, and accustomed to take his own case in hand. The popular Admiral, Sir Harry Keppel, was a notable example in an officer. In his old age he was tormented with an aching tooth, and went to a dentist to have the offending molar extracted. The dentist declined to operate, thinking it unnecessary, as the tooth was in good condition. Sir Harry, in high wrath, trudged back up the numberless steps to his London chambers, and sitting in front of his mirror, summarily extracted the tooth, sailor fashion. When he appeared smiling at the dinner-table, his daughter supposed that the visit to the dentist had brought relief, but the "Little Admiral" undeceived her with language strong and to the point.

Nelson, dying in the cockpit of the *Victory*, had tender and devoted nurses in his brave comrades, who knew how to minister to his needs in the last hour as they had rallied to his call for England's sake and duty when the guns boomed and bullets flew. The sailor, though disliking to be fidgeted about minor ailments, often shows sublime courage in facing the operation table. "What makes you sailor men so brave to face pain?" asked a nurse of a patient, whose heroism during an operation had astonished her. "Sister," said the suffering man, simply, "there is no back door to a ship!"

In the olden days a few women of the lowest type were employed to nurse in naval hospitals, and were assisted by some of the convalescents, and a few old sailors on regular duty. Admiral Sir Edward Parry, who had been favourably impressed by the work of the sisters in the naval hospitals of France, made an effort to improve the nursing at our Royal Naval Hospital, Haslar. In June, 1847, he drew up an appeal to the Christian public, pointing out the impossibility of obtaining any but the lowest type of women to attend the sick sailors. He begged "all good Christians" to try and induce three or four respectable women to volunteer their services, and to undergo a special training such as Kaiserswerth provided. The appeal was signed by five medical officers. It did not, however, elicit a single volunteer, in such low estimation was nursing in a naval hospital regarded by women.

Respectable nurses not being procurable, the old staff of women were gradually eliminated from the hospitals, and the nursing passed almost entirely into the hands of elderly men, naval or marine pensioners, some of whom, after a little training in the methods of modern nursing, were fairly satisfactory. They were under the supervision of the medical and hospital authorities.

A new departure was made in 1884-85, when the Admiralty appointed sisters to take charge of the nursing in the chief naval hospitals. Each head sister had a staff of sisters under her. Only eighteen in all were appointed and were thus distributed:—

Royal Naval Hospital, Haslar, head sister and 10 sisters.
„ „ Plymouth, „ „ 6 „
„ „ Chatham, „ „ 3 „

The experiment proved successful and the number of sisters was gradually increased in each hospital, and the system extended to other naval hospitals at home and abroad. In 1905–06, the appointments stand thus :—

Haslar, head sister and 14 sisters.
Plymouth, ,, ,, 10 ,,
Chatham, ,, ,, 8 ,,
Malta, acting head sister and 5 ,,
Hong-Kong, ,, ,, ,, 2 ,,
Deal, 2 sisters.
Queensferry, ,,
Shotley, ,,
Bermuda, ,, for six months only.
Osborne Cadets, sick quarters, 3 sisters.

The three head sisters have equal rank. Miss Florence Cadenhead came to Haslar in September, 1902, having been two years previously made head sister at Chatham. She is the junior of the three head sisters, though her hospital is accorded first-rank importance. Haslar, built in 1745, is the oldest and largest of the naval hospitals, and is to the navy what Netley is to the army. It has nine hundred and fifty beds, and in an emergency, two thousand can be arranged. Next in order comes Plymouth, of which Miss A. French is head sister. She began as head sister at Chatham in 1893. Plymouth is also a most interesting old hospital. It was built in 1760–62, and was then considered a marvel of architecture, having been one of the first built in the block system. Miss French became acquainted with it in January, 1885, three months after the arrival of the first sisters. There was then accommodation for between six and seven hundred patients. When the process of reconstruction which Plymouth is at present undergoing is completed, it will bring up the total to one thousand beds. Miss Grace Mackay has been head sister at Chatham since 1892, and had previously worked as such at Plymouth and Haslar.

In 1902, the naval like the military nursing service

was reorganized, and has since been designated Queen Alexandra's Royal Naval Nursing Service. The headquarters are the medical department of the navy, 18, Victoria Street, under control of the director-general. The Queen is president of the naval as of the military service, and takes a deep interest in all connected with it.

The service consists as formerly of two grades, head sisters and nursing sisters, the head sisters being, as a rule, appointed by selection from the list of nursing sisters. Candidates must produce certificates of training for at least three years, at a large civil hospital in the United Kingdom, in which adult male patients are received for medical and surgical treatment, such hospital being also provided with a matron and staff of nursing sisters. Candidates must be of British parentage or naturalized British subjects. The limits of age for appointment is from twenty-five to thirty. All nursing sisters will be required to undergo twelve months' probation before they are confirmed in their appointment. Should they then be reported upon as fit in every respect for H.M. Service, they will receive an appointment signed by Queen Alexandra, and their seniority will count from date of entry. Foreign service is obligatory.

The salaries and allowances are as follows—

HEAD SISTERS.

At Haslar, Plymouth, and Chatham: £125 to £160 by annual increments of £5.

At Malta and Hong Kong: None borne, but an allowance of £10 a year will be made to the sister acting as head sister for the time being.

At Gibraltar, Deal, Dartmouth, Osborne, Queensferry, and Shotley: None borne.

NURSING SISTERS.

£37 10s. to £50, by annual increments of £2 10s. Each head sister and nursing sister at home is allowed in

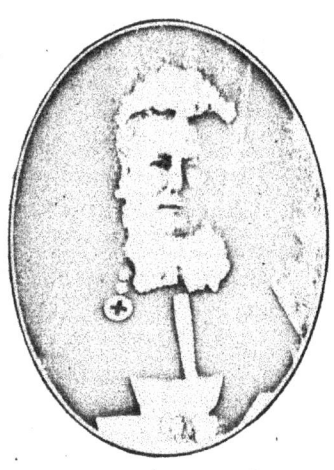

MISS CADENHEAD.
Head Sister, Royal Naval Hospital, Haslar.

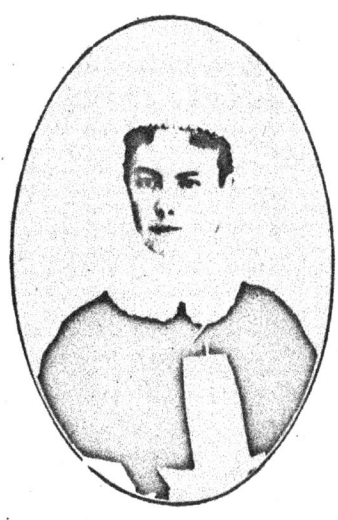

MISS FRENCH.
Head Sister, Royal Naval Hospital, Plymouth.

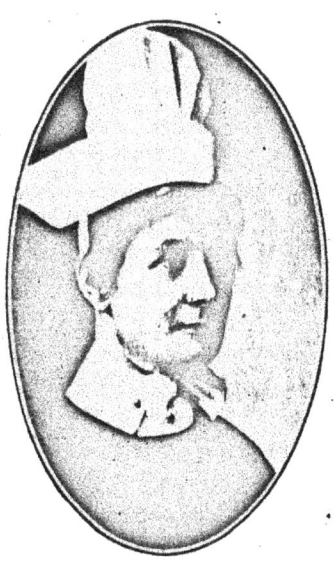

MISS ALICE MARY HALL.
Lady Superintendent, Seamen's Hospital, Greenwich.

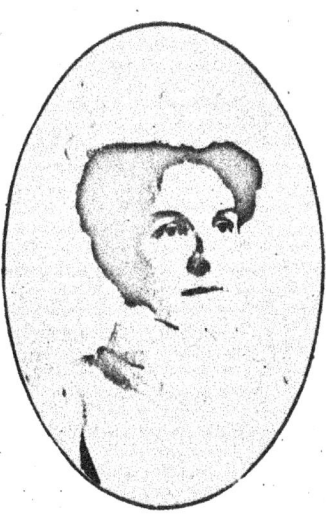

MISS GRAHAM KNIGHT.
Lady Superintendent, Seamen's Hospital, Albert Docks.

[*To face p.* 196.

addition 15s. a week in lieu of board, and for her personal laundry, except at Deal, Dartmouth, Osborne, Queensferry, and Shotley, where an allowance of 19s. a week is made. At Malta and Gibraltar, each sister is allowed £1 1s. a week in lieu of board and washing, and at Hong Kong the temporary allowance is £1 15s. a week to each sister for this purpose. The charge pay to senior sister in charge of a hospital ship is 1s. 6d. per day.

The quarters provided for the nursing staff of each hospital, include a mess-room, reading-room, kitchen, and offices; a sitting-room and bedroom for the head sister, a joint sitting-room for the sisters, and a separate bedroom for each nursing sister. Fuel and lights are provided. The head sister is president of the mess, and is responsible for the maintenance of order and regularity. It is obligatory on all members of the staff to join the mess. Maid-servants are appointed for attendance on the staff at each hospital.

The head sisters and nursing sisters are regarded as officers of the hospital and take rank after the surgeons. Their uniform consists of navy blue serge dresses with scarlet cuffs, and a cape to correspond. White muslin caps, collars, cuffs, and aprons are worn. The out-door uniform is a navy blue straw bonnet, trimmed with navy blue ribbons, and a navy blue tweed cloak with sleeves. A variation in the uniform is made for sisters serving in hot climates. The badge of the naval service is a red Geneva cross on a white ground in a gold border, and above Queen Alexandra's monogram, two A's in red, interlacing an anchor and cable, the whole surmounted by the Imperial crown. The badge is worn on the right breast. Belts are not compulsory, and if worn are of white Petersham, provided by the sisters themselves. The white metal clasp is designed with an anchor surrounded by leaves, and surmounted by the Imperial crown.

The sisters of the naval service are entitled to a pension which is calculated solely upon salary. After ten years' service, the rate is thirty per cent. of the salary for the preceding year, and rises two per cent. for each additional year's service, to a maximum of seventy per cent. of salary for the year preceding the grant of the pension. A head sister compulsorily retires on her pension at the age of fifty-five, and a nursing sister after fifty. Both grades may be called upon at any time to retire on the pension or gratuity, earned by their service, should the Admiralty so determine, and they are eligible to retire on pension after ten years' service, if rendered unfit for hospital duty, through injury or disease. A sister pensioned for disability is liable to be recalled to the service, should such disability cease. The regulations as to pension and retirement apply only to nursing sisters who have entered the service since February, 1901. Those who entered previously may continue until the age of sixty, and their rate of pension is calculated on the scale allowed by the regulations under which they entered the service.

The nursing in a naval hospital is still largely done by male attendants (sick-berth staff), who receive their instruction from the sisters, after the manner of probationers in a civil hospital, being taught practical duties—handling of patients, applying dressings, administering medicines, diets, and "extras," and sick-room cookery. This has become an important part of the sister's duty under the reorganized service. No longer are old pensioners, who have picked up a little nursing knowledge, deemed fit attendants on the sick. The male staff must be trained nurses. They join as probationer attendants, and rise to be second and first class sick-birth stewards respectively, and then ward masters, and serve in the hospitals, and on board the ships. The head wardmaster is a warrant officer, who is in charge of the rest, and details them their duty under the principal medical officer. There are a varying number of sectional wardmasters, who have charge of stores, and are responsible for the cleanliness of the wards, and for the discipline of the men—attendants and patients alike.

The number of male attendants in a naval hospital varies according to the requirements of the ships, to which they are often despatched at short notice, but a usual average is one steward or attendant to five patients, irrespective of the probationers under instruction, who though they assist in the wards have numerous classes to attend, given by the surgeon in charge of them, the dispenser, cookery instructress, and by the sisters and stewards who teach practical nursing.

A naval hospital is in charge of a senior medical officer, styled the "Inspector-General," whose time is chiefly taken up with administrative work, while the treating of the patients is performed by the medical staff, each principal medical officer having charge of a section, assisted by the more recently qualified young surgeons. The head sister exercises general control and supervision over the nursing sisters, visiting the wards where they are employed at any time she may think proper. She allots specific duties to the nursing sisters, and sees that they carry out the orders and instructions of the medical officers, and arranges the detail of night duties, for the sisters and sick-berth staff under instruction.

A nursing sister supervises a larger number of wards than she would be called upon to do in a civil hospital, because, in the first place, while there are a fair proportion of cases who are really ill, a considerable number suffer from trivial ailments, which simply render them unfit for duty, and in the second place she is, strictly speaking, only responsible for the nursing, and not for the charge of linen, crockery, or for the cleanliness of the wards, and this to some extent minimizes her duties. However, although a sister is not vested with authority in regard to the keeping of the wards, she can make her influence felt, and by taking a helpful interest assist in maintaining nice order.

A day sister takes charge of from four to six wards of fourteen beds each, and is assisted by a steward (corresponding to a staff nurse in a civil hospital) and attendant in each watch ward, as well as "specials" for critical cases, and one, either steward or attendant, in each convalescent ward. The term "watch" signifies that there is always a man on duty night and day, and these wards are devoted to the more serious cases, while the convalescent wards are only visited after the day steward is off duty.

The night sisters, of whom, to take Plymouth Hospital, where the new scheme has been so ably inaugurated by Sir John Watt Reid, as an example, there are two, each takes charge of half the hospital, one medical, one surgical, and visits the patients, frequently being responsible for medicines, stimulants, feeding, and applications, and personally assists the stewards and attendants as she finds it necessary, especially with the more serious cases. The sisters, of whom in this hospital there are ten, take night duty for a month at a time in rotation. Each sister has a small cabin near her ward for the convenience of her work while on duty. The matrons in the naval service have charge of the laundry, and are not trained nurses, neither have they any connection with the sisters.

But to pass from the Royal Naval Service, a most interesting example of the nursing of sailors by a trained staff of women is afforded at the Seamen's Hospital at Greenwich. It is in this respect a pioneer institution, and the introduction of its nurses preceded the advent of sisters in the Royal Naval hospitals by fourteen years. It has no help from Government, being entirely supported by public subscriptions to the Seamen's Hospital Society, founded for the benefit of sick seamen in 1817–18, when the victories of Nelson were fresh in the public mind. In 1821 the society founded a floating hospital on the Thames on board the *Grampus*, moored off Greenwich, for the exclusive use of sick and diseased seamen. In 1830 the hospital was transferred to more extensive accommodation on the old gunship *Dreadnought*, but that vessel becoming unhealthy another change was made in 1857 to the *Caledonia*, re-christened the *Dreadnought*. In 1870 the patients were moved ashore, and established in the old infirmary of Greenwich Royal Naval Hospital, which received the name of the Dreadnought Hospital for Seamen. To-day the great fireplaces, with the cheerful coal fires, the light over each man's bed, and the general air of comfort and homeliness which pervades the wards, to say nothing of the smiling faces of the trim nursing staff, form a remarkable contrast to the happy-go-lucky style in which Jack was nursed when Trafalgar was fought and won.

When the hospital was afloat, the patients were tended either by those of their own sex or by such women as could be found to face the inconveniences and insanitary conditions of the old *Dreadnought*, and the malaria arising from the Thames mud. After removal ashore a trained matron and staff were introduced, a nursing school gradually established, and to-day, with the exception of two orderlies for work in certain cases, the hospital is nursed entirely by women.

"Do you like the change?" I asked an old seafaring man in one of the wards. He attentively surveyed the tattoed monster on his wrist, and turning his weather-beaten face, with a knowing smile replied, "Give me the ladies." He recalled the old days on the *Dreadnought* ship, when there were no trim figures in blue and red dresses, and snowy caps and aprons flitting from bed to bed, and life in hospital was dull, dreary, and hard. "They called her the *Dreadnought*," continued the old salt, "and I reckon them as manned her dreaded nought when she was in the fightin' line; but when you lay aboard her sick, there was a something to dread. I knew a mate as had his leg took off by candle-light, and lor! the fever and the cholera as raged on that 'ere old ship was a treat!"

The ancient mariner scarcely overstated the case. The wards of the *Dreadnought* had become saturated with septic poison. Ventilation could only be obtained by opening the ports, which, being a little above the beds of the patients, had to be kept shut in foggy and gusty weather. There was a great want of light, especially during the winter months, when surgical operations had frequently to be performed by candle-light. The ship had three wards, containing from sixty to seventy beds each. The nursing was on a par with the sanitary (?) arrangements.

The *Dreadnought* ashore, appropriately situated in Nelson Street, Greenwich, and having pleasant grounds near the river, accommodates about two hundred and twenty-five patients. There are eighty-eight small wards, the majority containing only three beds, situated on both sides of a corridor which runs down the centre on each floor. In these the patients get equable temperature, quietude, and privacy, without loneliness. Sick seamen of *every nation* are received on presenting themselves at the hospital, their sick condition being sufficient to obtain admission. And as sailors are often without homes or friends who can take them in, the hospital allows a patient to remain after convalescence until he has regained his health and strength, and in the interim an opportunity is afforded him of obtaining employment.

The difficulty of women nurses keeping order amongst convalescent as well as sick male patients has been most successfully solved at Greenwich, and also at the branch hospital at the Albert Docks. It is a speaking fact, that one sister and a staff nurse on night duty manage fifty-three patients without any trouble or disagreeable incidents.

The nursing staff at Greenwich consists of a matron and fifty nurses, including the sisters. Miss A. M. Hall was appointed matron in 1894, after holding a similar position at the Albert Docks' Hospital. She keeps everything ship-shape at the *Dreadnought*, and is enthusiastically devoted to seamen. Miss Hall shares Florence Nightingale's belief in the effect of colour on the mind, and in order to please Jack's love of cheerful colours originated the pretty uniforms worn by her nurses. The sisters' dresses are blue, and the nurses' pale red cotton, and combined with white caps (Sister Dora) and aprons, form the national scheme of red, white, and blue.

The hospital trains its own nurses. Probationers are received on a four years' engagement—three years at Greenwich, and one year at a London hospital for women and children, to gain experience not afforded by male patients. Systematic courses of lectures are given during the winter and spring by the medical and surgical staff, and include courses in medicine, surgery, gynæcology, and tropical diseases, unrivalled opportunity for studying the latter being afforded by the number of oriental patients passing through the hospital, while at the Albert Docks' branch is the world-famous school for tropical diseases. Practical nursing lectures are given by the matron. Examinations are held at the end of each course, and certificates are given upon satisfactory completion of the four years' engagement. The school is very popular, applications averaging two hundred, and vacancies eleven yearly. It supplies sisters to other hospitals and to the Indian and Army and Naval Services, and its nurses are specially fitted for colonial and foreign work. The study of foreign languages is specially advised, and many of the sisters are good linguists.

Mr. W. Johnson Smith, F.R.C.S., who was principal medical officer 1882–1905, has taken great interest in the development of the trained nursing. He was assistant surgeon on board the *Dreadnought* in 1869, became surgeon soon after the removal ashore, and in 1882 was appointed principal medical officer. For many years Mr. Johnson Smith was visiting surgeon to the branch hospital in the Albert Docks. He has served the Seaman's Hospital Society for thirty-six years, and his retirement in 1905 caused universal regret.

The branch hospital at the Royal Albert Docks was built in 1890. It was intended to contain twelve beds and a small out-patient department; but it rapidly outgrew the accommodation provided. More beds were added and a new wing subsequently built, which brought the number of beds up to fifty. A new out-patient department and isolation wards were added.

Connected with this hospital is the London School of Tropical Medicine, which attracts students from all parts of the world. It was founded upon the initiative of Mr. Chamberlain in 1898, and carried through with the assistance of the Indian, Colonial, and Foreign Offices. The laboratories and the museum are most interesting to visit. The specimens of organs attacked by curious tropical diseases in the museum recall the story of the matter-of-fact Glasgow waif. · A benevolent gentleman, meeting a destitute lad, inquired if he had no parents.

" I've nae faither, and ma mither's deid," replied the boy.

" But have you no one belonging to you ? " queried the gentleman.

" I hae a brither," said the boy, dubiously.

" A brother ! " persisted the kind man. " Where is he ? "

" In the Glasca University."

" At the Glasgow University ? Then he must be in a position to help you ? "

" He canna," replied the lad, stolidly. " He's corkit in a bottle—he was born wi twa heids ! "

The Tropical School Museum contains many curious things " corkit in bottles," the most arresting to the casual visitor being a foot and part of the leg of a patient from Barbadoes, swollen with that dreadful Eastern disease, *Elephantiasis*, until it more nearly resembles the foot of an elephant than that of a human being.

The Albert Docks' Hospital is nursed entirely by women, under the same regulations as the parent institution at Greenwich. The work is most interesting, by reason of the novel cases, and it is a great education to be in touch with the Tropical School, especially for nurses going to India and the Eastern colonies. Lady doctors for India also come for a special course. The hospital has a very able matron in Miss Graham Knight, appointed in 1898. Miss Knight had formerly been a sister at Greenwich, and was trained at the London Hospital.

Women are supposed to be specially gifted with intuition, and an appreciation of the picturesque, and nursing in the wards of the hospitals for seamen is calculated to call forth these faculties. The beds are filled with patients of every clime and every colour, from the fair Scandinavian to the dusky negro. It is a curious sight to walk through the wards and see Japs and Chinese, alert, black, bead-eyed Arabs, and swarthy Hindoos with their distinctive faces silhouetted against the white pillows, and all having that pathetic far-away look of the sea in their suffering eyes. What tragedies, what romances may lie locked in the breasts of these men! They speak in strange tongues, and show no disposition to confide their domestic affairs to Western ears. These Eastern men are mysterious and reticent. They may be dreaming of a dusky maiden in that far-away land which they call home, or of wife or child; but they make no sign, confide no domestic secrets, or even give information. They smile with gratitude, not untouched by astonishment, on the nurses permitted by Western custom to minister to their needs. I recall the dark brown face of a Punjaubee, framed in long black hair, and with eyes rolling like balls of fire beneath his dusky brows. He looked fierce and distraught, but the sister said he was as gentle as a lamb. In her hands, doubtless; for perhaps the most wonderful sight of all was to see the obedience and discipline maintained amongst this motley gathering of patients from many climes and speaking in curious tongues by a nursing staff of women.

In addition to a knowledge of several Continental languages, a sister at Greenwich or the Albert Docks' Hospital finds it advantageous to acquire Pidgin English, which is the medium of communication in the convalescent wards. One feels, however, that there ought to be a professor of Esperanto at the Tropical School. Occasionally a seaman presents himself for admittance who speaks in an obscure dialect unknown even to an expert like Sir Patrick Manson, M.D., senior physician to the Seamen's Hospital Society. However, a woman's intuition assists the trained eye, and the wants of a patient are quickly understood by the nursing staff.

There is a story which the authorities think must be apocryphal; but in any case it does credit to some wag, and, after all, it may be true! A foreign seaman presented himself at Greenwich, and was promptly taken in as a patient. Not the cleverest linguist in the institution could make out a word of what he said. Of course it was assumed that he was suffering with some ailment, and the doctor who examined him decided that the seat of disease was the lungs. Directions were given accordingly, and the patient was washed, put to bed, poulticed, and treated, he all the time protesting. When a few days later he came into the convalescent ward, he discovered a friend who spoke his dialect. Explanations were made, and it was found that the "patient" considered himself a hale and healthy man, and had merely called at the hospital to inquire for his compatriot. Tableaux of doctors and nurses!

The Chinaman is a patient who requires to be watched for more reasons than one. He usually brings into hospital a costume of many pockets, and departs with them well lined if the nurses are not vigilant. One Chinaman, being sent out of hospital rather earlier than he had expected, left under his mattress knives and forks which he had secreted, preparatory to filling his pockets. Another was found departing with a double set of underwear.

A very exciting event to the patients in the Albert Docks' Hospital is the yearly religious festival which takes place in the spring, and is called the "Hobson Jobson." The convalescent patients join their Eastern compatriots from the crews of the ships in dock, and dressed in picturesque Oriental garments, form a grand procession and go through various national religious observances.

Not only the Oriental, but the prosaic Britisher becomes entertaining when he has braved the billows and stood at the mast, and is usually an interesting patient. He has a smattering of several languages, odds and ends of information about foreign countries and customs, always a yarn to tell, and often a romance of his own equal to anything in fiction. He is a patient full of surprises. The sister may discover that the youth with the horny hands but gentle tongue is a boy of good family, who has run away to sea, and may be instrumental in persuading him to let his people know where he is. Jack is not so much given to fancy work as Tommy, he prefers the elegant tracery of a sea-serpent on his arm to marvels in cross-stitch. He loves games, and music, and flowers, is a great reader, and appreciates a nurse who will enter into the plots of Victor Hugo and the humour of W. W. Jacobs. Pain and exhaustion are forgotten under the influence of "Toilers of the Sea," and digestion aided by laughter over "Many Cargoes." Greenwich has a good library in all languages. Pets are a great diversion in a sailor's hospital, and birds of fine plumage and rare song are often brought by the patients. "A wild man from Borneo" has not yet, I believe, been brought either to Greenwich or the Albert Docks' Hospital! Amongst other qualities which swell the total of Jack's ability for adding to the gaiety of a ward is his delicious lying! Still, he is a kind, simple-hearted fellow who, after roughing it at sea, or in the grimy lodgings of sea-port towns, is keenly appreciative of the home comforts he gets in hospital, and it makes him very amenable. Matrons and sisters agree that he is easier to nurse than a landsman. A visitor going over the seamen's hospitals cannot fail to be struck with the good understanding and spirit of friendliness existing between the patients and the nursing staff.

The sisters are sweetly indulgent to the pipe, and there is a standing rule that unless the doctor forbids, the patients may smoke in the wards at certain hours, and on Christmas Day as soon as they wake. "One would never think of robbing a sailor of his pipe," says the matron, and the men smile content under their red and white quilts. But Jack is frail though *gallant*. Nelson had that convenient blind eye to put to the telescope when it was likely to reveal what he did not want to see, and artful Jack keeps a cold and a hot pipe.

"Smoking out of hours," says the sister, as she enters a ward and scents the tell-tale odour. "Is it you, Daddy?" she asks of an old offender.

"Feel my pipe, sister," says Daddy; and with an air of injured innocence presents a perfectly cold "clay."

Sad to relate, a search will probably reveal a hot pipe concealed beneath the bed-clothes.

It is the custom of sailors also to have a land and a sea age. When signing on for a ship, Jack is often tempted to take off ten years. One man in hospital, when the doctor who was making out his certificate asked his age, replied, "Forty-five." The doctor looked incredulous. "That is his sea age," explained the sister; "sailors take off ten years." The patient, overhearing the remark, bowed with great politeness to the sister and said, "Ladies do that sometimes!"

By common consent Jack is a popular patient, and nursing in the Royal Naval hospitals or in those provided for seamen is a very attractive branch of the profession.

CHAPTER XIV

THE POOR LAW NURSING SERVICE

A social blot—Opinion of Lord Shaftesbury—The old Poor Law—Reaction in 1834—Neglect of the sick—Pauper nurses—Mrs. Jameson's exposures—Dr. Joseph Rogers at the old Strand Union—Story of a nurse—Flagrant abuses—Poor houses abroad—The Irish system good for the times—First attempts at reform in England—Dr. E. Sieveking's proposal—Lord Raynham's motion, 1856—Miss Louisa Twining—Her early efforts—The Workhouse Visiting Society founded—Its work—Mr. Gathorne Hardy's Bill, 1867—Dr. Joseph Rogers at the Strand Union—*Lancet* Commission, 1866—Mr. William Rathbone's work at the Liverpool Infirmary—Miss Agnes Jones starts the training of workhouse nurses—Her death, 1868—The movement quickened in the metropolis—Mr. Ernest Hart publishes an account of investigations—Passing of the Metropolitan Poor Law Bill, 1867—Its provisions—The Highgate Infirmary makes an experiment in trained nursing—The Workhouse Nursing Association founded 1879—Mary Adelaide nurses started 1881—Dr. Joseph Rogers reviews the changes during thirty years—The Departmental Committee of Local Government Board appointed 1892—Miss Catherine Wood—Her investigations—The Meath Workhouse Nursing Association—The Countess of Pembroke's nurses started, 1897—Nursing Orders by Local Government Board, 1896-97—Report of the Departmental Committee, 1902—Royal Commission on Poor Law appointed 1904—Decision of the Workhouse Nursing Association to continue its work, 1906—Training under the Poor Law Nursing Service—Marylebone Infirmary—Kensington Infirmary—Need of trained women inspectors in country workhouses—Further action awaited.

THERE is no greater blot on the social history of the middle of the nineteenth century than the neglect and cruelty to which the unfortunate, but in many cases deserving and respectable, sick and infirm poor were subjected in our workhouses. Speaking on behalf of the blind, the late Lord Shaftesbury said, "Many had nothing to look forward to but the Union workhouse, so God knew that for persons in such a condition, it would be better to sit in the dirtiest corner of the dirtiest cellar than to go there." The shocking neglect of the sick and aged pauper was in some measure an outcome of the rigorous rules enforced as a rebound from the old lax discipline.

The old Poor Law, instituted in the reign of Elizabeth, to deal with the poor and helpless left uncared for after the suppression of the monastic institutions, had developed glaring abuses. The poor-houses, originally established as a refuge for the homeless, houseless, helpless, lame, blind, infirm, and for orphan children, became the chosen home of men and women who objected to work. Many labourers preferred "the house" to the pursuit of agriculture. Sir F. B. Head, writing on "English Charity," in the *Quarterly Review*, thus describes the generous *régime* which prevailed in the early part of last century : "The Kentish pauper has what are called three meat days a week, in many cases four, and, in some, five ; his bread is many degrees better than that given to our soldiers; he has vegetables at discretion ; and, especially in the larger workhouses, it is declared, with great pride, ' that there is no stinting, but that we gives 'em as much victuals as ever they can eat!'" Even the Poplar pauper of the present day might envy his brother of the good old times.

The reaction came in 1834, by the passing of a new Act, which established the Poor Law Board as a central authority, and instituted Boards of Guardians. Under the new *régime*, the treatment of workhouse inmates became suddenly and frightfully harsh, and there was no classification of the deserving and undeserving. To be a pauper was to become a victim of unfeeling, often inhuman, tyranny, and the sick, the infirm, the old and bedridden suffered equally with the able-bodied and vicious, and for them there was no escape.

In those days there were no separate infirmaries for the sick. The metropolitan workhouses were huge caravanserais, where the sick, the insane and epileptic, the blind, aged, infirm, and bedridden, and even those suffering from infectious diseases, together with the vicious and able-bodied, were housed under one roof. People, ill from all manner of diseases, languished in comfortless and insanitary workhouse wards, tended for the most part by old pauper nurses, who vented the spleen caused by their own infirmities and troubles on the helpless people committed to their care. Pauper nurses regarded the work as a penance for being in the House, and nursed with the same turbulent spirit as the inmates who picked oakum. They received no pay beyond a few extras in diet, including beer and sometimes gin, and they used measures to extract something from the patients. A bedridden, helpless old lady, allowed sixpence a week by a friend, paid sixpence a month to the nurse to secure attention, yet when she begged in the night to be turned on her pillows was crossly refused. A poor, decent old woman, sinking into death in a ward with twenty-five inmates, wished to be read to, and pathetically offered a "hap'orth of snuff" to the nurse, or any one who would read to her, but could not get it done. The melancholy dulness of the wards was mingled with license and levity.

In 1854, the inmates under medical treatment in the London workhouses, omitting Marylebone, were fifty thousand. They were tended by only seventy paid nurses, and by five hundred pauper nurses and assistants, one-half of whom were above fifty, one quarter above sixty, many not less than seventy, and some more than eighty years old! In one of the metropolitan workhouses a woman between seventy and eighty was in charge of a ward of imbecile old women and those who had fits.

Mrs. Jameson, who in 1855-56 was inspecting charitable and reformatory institutions at home and abroad, relates, in her "Community of Labour," "Never did I visit any dungeon, any abode of crime or misery, in any country, which left the same crushing sense of sorrow, indignation, and compassion—almost despair—as some of our English workhouses. The inmates of some jails had better treatment." Mrs. Jameson's description of the "nursing staffs" would be laughable were it not so sad. "In a great and well ordered workhouse, under conscientious management," she writes, "I visited sixteen wards; in each ward from fifteen to twenty-five sick, aged, bedridden, or, as in some cases, idle and helpless poor. In each ward all the assistance given and all the supervision were in the hands of one nurse and a helper, both chosen from among the pauper women who were supposed to be the least immoral and drunken. The ages of the nurses might be from sixty-five to eighty, the associates were younger. I recollect seeing in a provincial workhouse a ward in which were ten old women, helpless and bedridden; to nurse them was a decrepit old woman of seventy, lean and withered and feeble, and her assistant was a girl with one eye, and scarcely able to see with the other. In a ward, where I found eight paralyzed old women, the nurses being equally aged, the helper was a girl who had lost the use of one hand. Only the other day I saw a pauper woman in a sick ward who had a wooden leg! I remember no cheerful faces; when the features and deportment were not debased by drunkenness or stupidity, or sullen or bloated or harsh. And these are the sisters of charity to whom our sick poor are confided!"

When Mrs. Jameson asked a workhouse matron to point out her most efficient nurse, she indicated a crabbed, energetic-looking old woman, saying, "She is active and cleanly and to be depended on, so long as we keep her from drink." "All the nurses drink when they go out," continues Mrs. Jameson, "and are put to bed intoxicated in the wards which they are set to rule over." It was obvious that the patients hated the nurses, who would do nothing for them without bribery. Some pauper nurses made five shillings a week by fleecing the poor inmates and their friends of pennies and sixpences. Those who could not pay implored in vain to be turned in their beds.

Even when the matron was a kind and conscientious woman, she could do little more than enforce cleanliness and order. She exercised little moral authority. The old hags, her deputies, did as they liked. The sick wards were the perpetual scene of scolding, squabbling, and swearing. Drunken jeers mingled with the groans of the suffering, and the gasps of the dying were drowned by oaths. The gentler patients who had seen better days fared the worse; the "she-bullies" were alone a match for the pauper nurses.

One hears much of the kindness of the poor to the poor, and doubtless in some of the country Unions the respectable sick and infirm, who had passed their lives in the district, elicited sympathy in their misfortunes from the matron and nurses, but in the workhouses of London and other large towns, neglect, cruelty and harshness prevailed. Lady visitors were not permitted in those days to bring the sunshine of their presence into the dreary workhouse ward, and the average guardian of the fifties would have regarded the Brabazon employment scheme as a menace to the nation.

The Poor Law rules were administered in the harshest manner. A respectable old woman driven to end her days in the House often found consolation in bringing a few trifles from her wrecked home to speak to her of better days. The rules, however, forbade paupers to bring in crockery. An old woman of eighty, ignorant of this, arrived at the House with a china tea-pot, which had been her pride, since she received it on her wedding-day. One knows in what a kind way the modern trained nurse would have viewed Granny's treasure, and how sweetly she would have enlarged on its artistic beauty, and if it had to be taken away would have arranged the matter, without distressing the poor old soul. Not so the old-time workhouse nurse, who in this particular case, took the tea-pot from the trembling, withered hands and dashed it to pieces before the heart-broken woman's eyes.

The sick and infirm had no relief from heartless tyranny. The permanent officials of the old Poor Law Board appear to have been careless and indifferent, and often culpably negligent. The guardians, with some exceptions, were ranged against the pauper, whether he were well or sick. The medical officer was under their heel, and there was no independent medical inspection. The workhouse masters and matrons were sometimes no doubt well-disposed if ignorant people, but oftener they were tyrants. The matron visited the wards once a day, in some workhouses only once a week, and for the rest of the time the patients were left at the mercy of the nurses. Occasionally the guardians made tours of inspection, but if an inmate ventured to complain, retribution was swift. A matron of a London workhouse refused for two years to speak to a bedridden old woman because she had complained to a guardian.

The pauper nurses themselves were as much to be pitied as blamed. They were set to do work for which they were totally incapacitated by age, infirmity, or ignorance. They slept and lived in the wards, whether the patients were men or women, and could scarcely be said to be off duty during the twenty-four hours. After hobbling about the ward all day, it is small wonder that exhausted nature or stimulants made these women cruelly indifferent to the patients at night. The cries of the distressed and the entreaties of the dying often went unheeded.

They were nurses, too, in a system which did not provide even homely medical comforts and remedies for the sick. Dr. Joseph Rogers, who made such a splendid fight for the sick poor when medical officer at the old Strand Union in Cleveden Street, and later, at the Westminster Infirmary, relates that, finding he had many consumptive and bronchitic patients, he asked the guardians to supply linseed that the patients might have linseed tea. The idea was scouted by the nurse in the female ward. One Charlotte Massingham, who had been in supreme authority for many years, was usually muddled, and, after the manner of her kind, treated the medical officer with supreme indifference and undisguised contempt. Imbued with the prevailing notions, she regarded a doctor who insisted on paupers "having their physic regular" and being supplied with things necessary to their sick condition as a mild lunatic. When Dr. Rogers informed Charlotte that the guardians had consented to meet his request for linseed tea, she received the amazing intelligence by taking a flying leap into the air, and coming down slapping both sides with her arms, exclaimed, "My God! linseed tea in a workhouse!"

The administration, not the Poor Law, was chiefly to blame for the abuses. According to the rules, paid nurses might be engaged for the sick, but Bumbledom, anxious to line its own pockets and flaunt zeal for economy before the eyes of the ratepayers, relegated the care of the sick to unpaid pauper women and begrudged even mustard poultices and linseed tea. When paid nurses were employed no inducement was offered in wages, food, or treatment to secure respectable women. They were the dregs of womanhood, who having gone the round of the hospitals, undertook workhouse nursing as a last resort. Low, vicious, and repulsive in appearance, they strutted about the wards in dirty finery to show that *they* were not paupers. The sick poor were, indeed, between the devil and the deep sea as regards the pauper and the paid nurses.

Another flagrant abuse of the sick arose out of the custom of the medical officers being required by the board to provide drugs and medicines out of their salaries, which were often very inadequate. The result was that unprincipled officers saved their pockets by dispensing coloured water in lieu of medicine.

While such was the state of things in England, other countries had long had humane, well-managed institutions for the old infirm poor. For more than a century Holland had had an admirable system of poor houses, which favourably attracted the attention of Howard, the philanthropist. In Paris, that gigantic establishment the *Salpetrière de la Vieillesse* was giving asylum to some five thousand aged, infirm, or insane poor, who were tended by *surveillantes*, women specially trained for the work. Paris provided no workhouses for the idle and ablebodied, but the *Hospices* for *des incurables Hommes* and *des incurables Femmes*, containing respectively five hundred and eight hundred inmates, provided for the care of incurable sick people. The nursing was in the hands of the *Sœurs de St. Vincent de Paule*, gentle, trained, dignified women, who presented a remarkable contrast to the pauper nurses in our workhouses. The *Bureaux de Bienfaisance* provided out-door relief for the poor of Paris and was managed entirely by women. In Germany the Kaiserswerth deaconesses were employed in the care of the sick poor.

At this period Ireland had a better system of Poor Law medical relief than England or Scotland. It was administered by the Poor Law Commissioners under the Irish Medical Charities Acts, instituted after the great potato famine and the epidemic of fever which followed. Dr. Joseph Rogers was agreeably surprised by the excellence of the Irish system when, in 1868, he went to study it on the spot. A few years later, he again visited Ireland, and, referring to the North and South Dublin Workhouses with their four thousand inmates, writes, "There is a large staff of visiting physicians and surgeons besides resident medical officers. It is one of the finest hospitals in Dublin, and the arrangements for the efficient treatment of the sick poor were in the highest degree creditable to the Irish Poor Law, now the Local Government Board."

In England the first attempts to rouse the public conscience with regard to the condition of workhouse inmates began about 1847, when the publication of "The Diary of a Workhouse Chaplain" arrested the attention of philanthropic people. Previously, in the last years of her

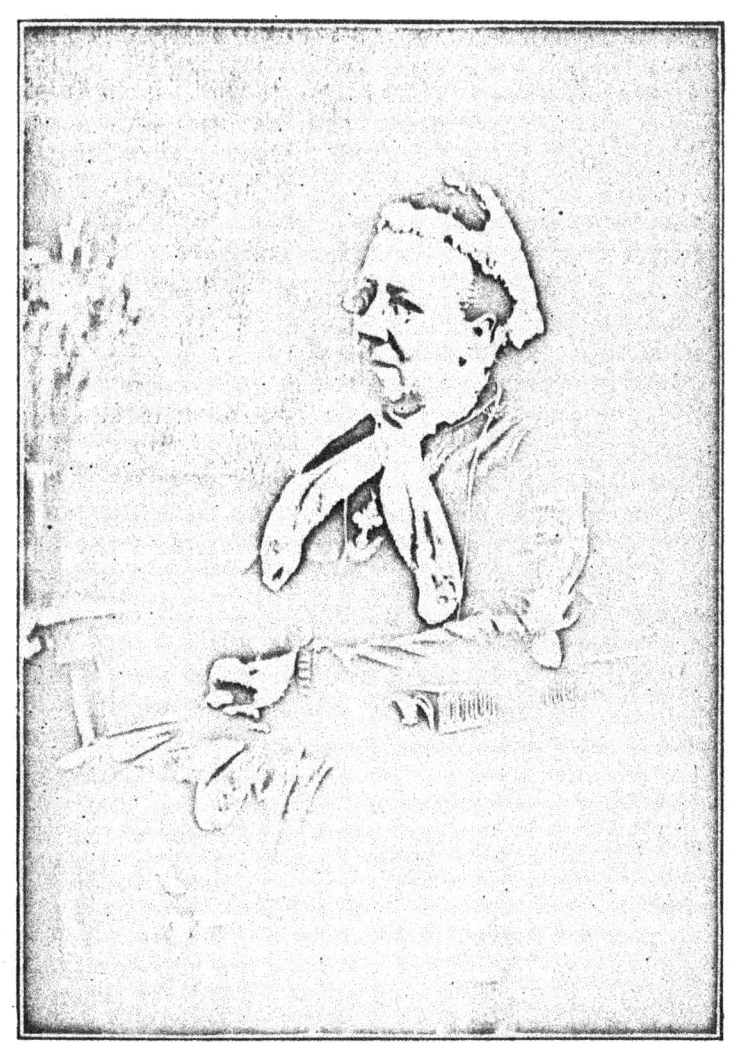

Miss Louisa Twining,
Pioneer of Workhouse Nursing Reform.
(*Photo: Elliott & Fry.*)

life, Elizabeth Fry constantly urged her friends to pray for the amelioration of the workhouse system. In 1850 came a pamphlet by a lady, entitled "A Plan for rendering the Union Poor-houses National Houses of Mercy." In 1853-54, Miss Louisa Twining began her vigorous campaign, of which more later; and about the same period Frederick Denison Maurice, Canon Kingsley, Dr. Sieveking, and Dr. Johnson, of King's College Hospital, Rev. J. Ll. Davies, Rev. J. S. Brewer, and other public men were giving "Lectures to Ladies," with a view to enlisting the co-operation of women in social reforms. In 1855 the Epidemiological Society brought forward the matter of nursing, and Dr. E. Sieveking and several other eminent physicians suggested that the able-bodied women in workhouses should be trained in the infirmary and sent out as nurses. In 1858 the Poor Law Board sanctioned the plan, and instructed the guardians to carry it out. The plan was scarcely likely to have succeeded, considering the low character of the women, and it is fortunate that it was never carried out. Still, it is interesting as showing official acknowledgment of the need for trained nurses.

In June, 1856, Lord Raynham brought a motion in Parliament on workhouse mismanagement. In the following year Mrs. W. Sheppard drew melancholy pictures of the condition of the sick, aged, and infirm in "Experiences of a Workhouse Visitor," which quickly ran through four editions, and was followed by her "Sunshine in the Workhouse;" while Mrs. Jameson's vigorous and illuminating work, "The Community of Labour," kept the subject alive. The public feeling roused at this period on behalf of the sick soldiers during the Crimean War reacted on civilian institutions, and the question of nursing reforms came rapidly to the front. But while considerable effort was being put forth to train nurses for hospital and private work, the same enthusiasm was not shown with regard to workhouse nursing. Bumbledom was a deep-rooted abuse. Canon Kingsley hit the mark when he said that the great need was to have guardians who were gentlemen, and, he might have added, to have women guardians also.

From amongst the group of pioneer workers in the reform of workhouse nursing the name of Miss Louisa Twining stands prominently forward. She has continuously laboured in the cause for more than half a century, and now (1906), at eighty-six years of age, keenly follows the course of events, and never fails to remind the President of the Local Government Board of the yet outstanding abuses in the Poor Law nursing service. Miss Twining served for some years as guardian of the poor at Kensington Workhouse and also at the Tunbridge Wells Union. In 1861 Miss Twining urged upon the Parliamentary Committee the need of women guardians, and had the satisfaction of seeing the first elected in 1875 to the Kensington Workhouse, where she was herself later to do such admirable work. Miss Twining was president of the Society for Promoting the Return of Women to Local Governing Bodies. The events of her life are milestones in the movement.

Miss Twining is one of the old lights of London in a truly illuminating sense. She is the daughter of the late Richard Twining, head of the well-known firm in the Strand. She was born November 16, 1820, the year that George III. died, and has therefore lived in four reigns. The first sixteen years of her life were passed in her father's house, 34, Norfolk Street. Then the river ran past the end of the street, and there was a view across to the Surrey hills. She recalls the sound of the stage coach horn, blown in the early winter's morning at the top of Norfolk Street, when her brothers were returning to Rugby after the Christmas holidays. Then also the bell of the scarlet-coated postman summoned householders to bring out their letters, for which, if they were not franked, he took a shilling or ninepence for a quarto sheet. Those were the days of flint and tinder-boxes, when young ladies drove out in a yellow post-chaise, or in a glass coach on more ceremonious occasions. Miss Twining walked in the Temple Gardens when they had a rural aspect and a lime avenue, and as a special treat went to St. James's Park and got a drink of milk from the cows. She heard Sydney Smith preach in St. Paul's, Frederick Denison Maurice at Lincoln's Inn Chapel ; worshipped at the Temple before it was restored ; remembers the burning of the Houses of Parliament and the Royal Exchange and the beginning of the Thames Tunnel, and recalls the thrill of a first journey by rail in 1838, starting from Euston Square. As a girl she had delightful tours by post on the Continent, keenly noting all that she saw. Since 1829 Miss Twining has kept a pocket diary, and the "Recollections" of her useful and varied life were published in 1893. Her "Recollections of Workhouse Visiting and Management" had appeared in 1880.

As she grew to womanhood Miss Twining began to take an interest in the poor and sick, and at one time thought of becoming a nurse, and spent some time at the Ormond-street Hospital for Children. However, her energies were turned in the direction of nursing reform, and she has accomplished more than she would have had leisure to do had she been within the ranks of the profession. In 1847-48 she began to visit the poor in the old parish of St. Clement Danes in the Strand, and the sad case of a respectable old woman, one of her *protégées*, who was driven to enter the Strand Union, then in Cleveland Street, opened her eyes to the sufferings of the old and infirm paupers. Her first visit to a workhouse was paid to the Strand Union in 1853, to see this old woman.

The Strand district may be designated the cradle of nursing reforms in the metropolis. In its Union, Louisa Twining and Dr. Joseph Rogers began their work on behalf of the sick poor. The neighbouring King's College Hospital was the first to give facilities for a trained nursing staff; while in the squalid courts of the old Clare Market and other rookeries then adjacent to the Strand, the St. John's Sisters plied their ministrations amongst the sick.

Miss Twining's first visit to the Strand Union resulted in her effort to procure admission for lady visitors to the infirm and sick inmates. The master and matron were kindly disposed, but the higher authorities had decreed that "unpaid and voluntary efforts were not sanctioned by the Poor Law Board." Miss Twining courageously determined to interview the Central Board, and in a flutter of trepidation drove to Whitehall for the purpose.

Now, when the Prime Minister receives women suffragists with due ceremonial in Downing Street, and the Secretary of State for the Colonies places the library of the Colonial Office at the disposal of the annual gathering of the Colonial Nursing Association, it is not so easy to realize the intrepid enterprise of Miss Twining's visit to Whitehall. The attendant endeavoured to give her courage by saying, "You need not be afraid, ma'am; you will find them very nice gentlemen indeed." The Right Hon. Matthew Talbot Baines, the president of the Board, and Lord Courtenay, the secretary, received Miss Twining with courtesy, and promised that if she could obtain the sanction of one Board of Guardians to her proposal for lady workhouse visitors, they would not refuse permission. Alas! Bumbledom was not to be won over, and Miss Twining, roused by the appointment of a new master, the notorious Mr. Catch, to the Strand Union, redoubled her efforts to combat his tyranny, and braved the insolence of the gate-porters in trying to gain admission to her poor friends.

She also gained admission to the St. Giles' Union, which she found even worse than the Strand. The object of her visit was a poor old crossing-sweeper whom she had known for years plying his work in Bloomsbury Square. She found him in the basement ward, nearly dark, and with a stone floor; beds, sheets, and shirts were all equally grey with dirt. "To get in," Miss

Twining relates, " I had to wait with a crowd at the office door to obtain a ticket, visitors being allowed only for one hour once a week. The sick in the so-called infirmary, a miserable building, long since destroyed, were indeed a sad sight, with their wretched pauper nurses in black caps and workhouse dress. One poor young man there, who had lain on a miserable flock bed for fourteen years with spine complaint, was blind, and his case would have moved a heart of stone; yet no alleviation of food or comforts were ever granted him, his sole consolation being the visits of a good woman, an inmate, who had been a ratepayer, and attended upon him daily, reading to him to while away the dreary hours."

While pursuing her work of penetrating into the sick wards of the Metropolitan workhouses, Miss Twining began to rouse public opinion by her pen. In 1855 she published " A few words about the Inmates of our Union Workhouses," and in 1857 began a series of letters to the *Guardian*, afterwards printed as " Metropolitan Workhouses and their Inmates," and on November 25, 1858, appeared her letter to the *Times* on " Workhouse Nurses for the Sick," which was reprinted in 1861 as a pamphlet. It occupied three parts of a column in the *Times*, and, appearing when nursing was the subject of the day, drew considerable attention. Miss Twining referred to the efforts, following on Miss Nightingale's work in the Crimea, which were being made to improve hospital nurses, and asked what had been done about the large class of nurses who tended the destitute and helpless in workhouses, and proceeded to describe the existing state of things. One may smile to-day at the modesty of her demands. She did not venture to suggest that a staff of trained professional nurses should be employed, but thought that the pauper nurse's dress might be exchanged for a neat uniform, that she might be allowed hours for rest and recreation, have sufficient nourishing food and hot tea or coffee at night to enable her to do without stimulants, and ended by begging the Guardians to investigate the conditions of the workhouse wards for themselves.

Meantime, Miss Twining was very active in getting a petition signed in favour of Lord Raynham's motion in the House of Commons, asking for an inquiry into the management of workhouses. Mrs. Sidney Herbert, afterwards Lady Herbert, of Lea, and Mrs. Tait, wife of the future Archbishop, were among the ladies who signed. The appeal was not granted by Parliament, but the good leaven was working in the public mind.

An increasing number of ladies began to devote themselves to workhouse visiting and the amelioration of the lot of the infirm and sick. Prominent in the work was Miss Augusta Clifford, who rendered such generous service at the old Strand Union, Lady Alderson, the widow of the late Judge, and her daughter Miss Louisa. It was becoming desirable that an association of workers should be formed, and Miss Tucker, a visitor at Marylebone Workhouse, first put forward the proposition which resulted in the formation of the Workhouse Visiting Society.

This most important factor in pressing forward nursing and kindred reforms was founded in connection with the National Association for the promotion of Social Science which held its first meeting at Birmingham in 1857, at which Miss Twining read a paper on "The Condition of Workhouses." Miss Twining became the honorary secretary of the newly founded Workhouse Visiting Society. The president was the Rt. Hon. W. C. Cowper, and the committee included the Bishops of London, Oxford, Bath and Wells, Miss Burdett-Coutts, Mrs. Sidney Herbert, Monckton Milnes, M.P., and Roundell Palmer, Q.C. The Society was greatly aided by the important co-operation of H. B. Farnali, Esq., the Metropolitan Inspector of Workhouses. Among the ideas which it originated for brightening the dismal sick-wards was the taking of flowers to the workhouse every Sunday, a beautiful custom which spread to the civil hospitals and was the forerunner of the modern Flower Services.

The introduction of a better class of nurse into the workhouse wards was a special object of the Workhouse Visiting Society, and it pressed its views from time to time upon the authorities. The journal of the Society ventilated the abuses of the Poor Law system and throws instructive light on the then existing state of things. The journal ran from 1859 to 1865. In 1861, a first inquiry was made into the number of paid nurses—these were of course untrained—employed in London workhouses, and efforts were made to induce guardians to employ paid and responsible nurses to superintend the pauper nurses. A movement was also set on foot for the care of "destitute incurables," which had a far-reaching effect in bringing about a complete reform in the care of the sick in workhouses. The late Frances Power Cobbe, and Miss Elliot, of Bristol, were among the first to press forward the claims of these helpless ones. Among supporters of the movement were Miss Burdett-Coutts (now the Baroness), Lord Shaftesbury and the Bishop of London, and Mrs. Tait.

In May, 1865, a deputation of the Workhouse Visiting Society waited upon Mr. Villiers, President of the Poor Law Board, with a petition and statement as to the general condition of the sick in workhouse infirmaries. Meetings of influential people, including Dr. Sieveking and other medical men, had met at the house of the late Mrs. Gladstone, to promote the petition which specified amongst its objects "the employment of trained and competent nurses." In 1866, Miss Louisa Twining's vigorous pen was again at work, and her letters on workhouse management to the *John Bull* newspaper created considerable attention. And so in various ways public opinion was being roused, and the way paved for Mr. Gathorne Hardy's Bill of 1867, which revolutionized the Poor Law Unions of the metropolis, and laid the foundations of the separate and efficiently staffed infirmaries which now exist, and are the training schools for nurses in the Poor Law Service.

The provisions of this Bill were largely due to the recommendations of Dr. Joseph Rogers, who calls for special notice amongst the reformers of the period. Dr. Rogers was appointed medical officer to the Strand Union in 1856, and began a strenuous struggle with the authorities on behalf of the sick poor. Bumbledom regarded him as an "odious reformer," and was nearly petrified with astonishment when he advocated that a proper infirmary should be built for the sick poor, and staffed with qualified nurses. At the Strand he ran the gauntlet of some of the worst guardians and officials which the old Poor Law system harboured, and suffered accordingly in his profession. Dr. Rogers was a most important ally of Miss Twining and her friends in their efforts to introduce a better class of nurse into the workhouse wards. The story of his struggle against medical abuses is an important chapter in the history of workhouse nursing, and is related in his " Reminiscences," edited by his brother, Professor Thorold Rogers.

A few facts and incidents may be quoted as showing the ideas then prevalent regarding the care and treatment of the sick in workhouses. The female insane ward of the Strand Union was immediately below the lying-in ward, the unfortunate inmates of the latter having the "comforting" sound of the noisy lunatics. Immediately outside the male wards of the house the able-bodied were engaged all day in carpet beating. The noise was so great that it deprived the sick of all chance of sleep, and the dust so thick as to make it out of the question to open the windows until the day's work was done. In spite of medical protest the guardians persisted for ten years in having the carpet-beating carried on, as it brought in a considerable income. There were no paid nurses at the Strand Union for the first nine years that Dr. Rogers was there, such nursing as there was being performed by more or less infirm paupers. Those were the days when the notorious Mr. Catch was master. In 1865 the guardians, moved by the evidence of Miss Twining before the Select Committee, appointed a superintendent nurse, a young and respectable woman, but with no pretension to training.

Dr. Rogers had also given evidence before the Select Committee of the House of Commons in 1861, particularly as to the supply of drugs and medical comforts in workhouse infirmaries, and his views were adopted by the committee and pressed upon the department. What he advocated was the germ of the modern workhouse infirmary. Matters, however, were not brought to a crisis until 1865, when two scandalous cases of neglect in Metropolitan Unions led to great public indignation. The *Lancet* took up the cudgels and instituted, in 1866, a commission of inquiry into the condition of London workhouses and hospitals. Dr. Anstie reported on the condition of the Strand Union in its true colours. In the midst of the tumult caused by the exposures the Workhouse Infirmaries Association came into being, the prime movers being Dr. Rogers, Dr. Anstie, Mr. Ernest Hart, and Mr. John Storr, who generously offered one hundred pounds to float the association. Its efforts, like those of the Workhouse Visiting Society, started some seven years previously, were directed towards securing more efficient treatment of the sick and the medical inspection of workhouse infirmaries. While prison infirmaries and military hospitals were medically inspected, pauper hospitals were not.

We must now for a time leave the London movement and follow the channel of history which culminated in the introduction of trained nursing into the Brownlow Hill Infirmary at Liverpool, in 1865. Again the city on the Mersey takes a first place in nursing reform. Mr. William Rathbone was the originator of the scheme, which directly followed his pioneer work on behalf of district nursing. He was much struck by the horror with which the sick poor regarded the workhouse infirmary, and came to the conclusion that there must be something radically wrong with that institution. The Brownlow Hill was one of the largest in the kingdom, and in common with all other infirmaries had not a single trained nurse. Miss Eleanor Rathbone thus describes its condition at the time when her father began his investigations. "The twelve hundred sick persons in every stage of nearly every illness under the sun, a large portion of them incurable, or very old, and entirely helpless, were nursed—if it could be called nursing—by pauper women, selected from the adult wards of the workhouse. Able-bodied women were not employed unless there was something mentally or morally wrong with them, and in a seaport town like Liverpool they were a particularly vicious class. Their work was superintended by a very small number of paid but untrained parish officers, who were in the habit, it was said, of wearing kid gloves in the wards to protect their hands. At night a policeman patrolled some of the wards to keep order, while others, in which the inmates were too sick or infirm to make disturbance, were locked up, and left unvisited all night."

Mr. John Cropper, chairman of the Select Vestry, was anxious to see reforms instituted, but feared that the vestry would not face the expense of introducing trained nursing. A conference was arranged between Mr. Cropper, Mr. Rathbone, the Governor, Mr. Carr, and the Poor Law Inspector, Mr. Cane, not in an "upper room," but in the basement of the workhouse, and there, in dark and dingy surroundings, the secret reformers discussed their scheme. They had first to convince the vestry that their plan was an economical one.

At this time St. Thomas's Hospital was the Mecca of most pilgrims in search of information on trained nursing, and thither a deputation from the Liverpool Vestry repaired. To the Senior Honorary Physician at St. Thomas's, Mr. Hagger, the Liverpool Vestry Clerk, put this practical question:—"If you had to cure the sick by contract at so much a head, and had to choose between unpaid pauper nurses allotted to you gratis, or paying yourself for skilled nurses, which would you choose?" "To pay for skilled nurses, certainly," was the reply. It was, however, a private individual in the person of Mr. Rathbone, and not the vestry, who made the desperate plunge, and financed the first trial of trained nursing in a workhouse infirmary. Mr. Rathbone consulted with Miss Nightingale, who arranged that a nursing staff should be sent from St. Thomas's Hospital.

On May 16, 1865, the experiment was begun in the male wards of the Liverpool Infirmary, which were placed under the charge of Miss Agnes Jones, as superintendent, who had a staff of twelve nurses from St. Thomas's, eighteen probationers, and fifty-four old pauper women. At the end of the first year the pauper "nurses" were sent back to the workhouse as unredeemable drunkards. At the end of the second year the authorities were so favourable to the new system that the vestry decided to extend it throughout the infirmary, and to charge the expense on the rates, refusing further contribution from the unknown promoter, and invited him, through the chairman, Mr. Cropper, to help to develop it. Mr. William Rathbone now stood revealed. He became a member of the Select Vestry, and continued to serve until his death in 1902. In this as in his other reforms, Mr. Rathbone had acted on the principle of Dorothea Dix, who reformed the lunatic asylums in the States by presenting a plan to the people whose duty it was to put things straight.

Miss Agnes Jones, as the first trained superintendent of a Poor Law Infirmary, takes rank as the pioneer of workhouse nursing. She was young, attractive, and reared in affluence, but craved for a vocation. " In the winter of 1854," she wrote, " I had those first earnest longings for work, and had for months so little to satisfy them ; how I wished I were competent to join the Nightingale band when they started for the Crimea! I listened to the animadversions of many, but I almost worshipped her who braved all, and I felt she must succeed." Agnes Jones followed the example of her chief, and became a pupil at Kaiserswerth. She was amongst the first probationers at the Nightingale school of St. Thomas's, and her devoted life, and exceptional gifts, commended her to Miss Nightingale, when she was asked to choose a superintendent for the Liverpool Infirmary. There Agnes Jones laboured for three years, with unremitting zeal. She died in February, 1868, from typhus fever, contracted in the wards of the infirmary. Her system, weakened by the arduous and anxious nature of her work, could not resist disease. However, she had lived to see her pioneer work accomplished, and the nurses trained in her school were able to carry on the system, which began to spread to other infirmaries. Miss Nightingale contributed a beautiful tribute to her memory, entitled, "Una and the Lion," which subsequently formed the introduction to "The Memorials of Agnes Jones," by her sister. "She died, as she had lived," wrote Miss Nightingale, "at her post in one of the largest workhouse infirmaries in this kingdom—the first in which trained nursing has been introduced. When her whole life and image rise before me, so far from thinking the story of Una and her lion a myth, I say here is Una in real flesh and blood—Una and her paupers far more untamable than lions. In less than three years, she had reduced one of the most disorderly hospital populations in the world to something like Christian discipline, and had converted a vestry to the conviction of the economy as well as humanity of nursing pauper sick by trained nurses."

The object lesson of trained workhouse nursing, exhibited at the Liverpool Infirmary, helped to quicken the movement in the Metropolis. Abuses were brought into a stronger light by the famous *Lancet* Commission of 1866. Mr. Ernest Hart, of St. Mary's Hospital, published in the following year a condensed account of the investigations, in the *Fortnightly Review*. Shortly afterwards a public meeting was held in Willis's Rooms, presided over by Lord Carnarvon, and attended by numbers of influential people. The first resolution was moved by the Archbishop of York, Dr. Thomson, and seconded by Mr. Thomas Hughes, M.P. A deputation was appointed to wait on Mr. Villiers, president of the Poor Law Board, who admitted that "a case had been made out," and promised reforms. A change of Government took place at this juncture and matters were left in abeyance.

In 1867, Mr. Gathorne Hardy (Lord Cranbrook), who succeeded Mr. Villiers as president of the Poor Law Board, introduced the Metropolitan Poor Law Bill, the keystone of the present metropolitan infirmary system. The reports on the Metropolitan Infirmaries of Mr. Farnall and Dr. Edward Smith (returns to an order of the House of Commons) greatly helped to bring this about. The abuses which the Workhouse Visiting Society had proclaimed for fifteen years were at length recognized. The *Times* denounced the existing system as "a national disgrace." The Bill provided for the classification and separate treatment of the sick, by the establishment of workhouse infirmaries and dispensaries, and the supply of all medicines and medical appliances at the charge of guardians, and recommended the employment of paid and qualified nurses. In course of time, imbeciles and lunatics were placed in separate establishments, and special hospitals built for fever and small-pox cases. The Metropolitan Unions seemed to vie with each other in the erection of infirmaries, and with the new buildings came a new order of nurse. Unfortunately, the Act was not general, and the old abuses continued to flourish in country workhouses.

In 1870, at the new Highgate Infirmary, occupied by several of the London Unions, an experiment in trained nursing was made, when the council of the Nightingale Fund supplied the entire staff of trained nurses, and it was hoped that a permanent nursing school had been established for the supply of workhouse infirmary nurses.

It was carried out with complete success, until the lamented death of the matron, Miss Hill. The plan was then interrupted.

The first probationers in the Poor Law Service appear to have been appointed under orders of the Board, issued in 1873 and onwards, to managers of the metropolitan sick asylum districts, authorizing those bodies, in accordance with section 29 of the Metropolitan Poor Act of 1867, to use their "asylums for the sick poor" as training schools for nurses. The progress was slow, and the continued employment of pauper and untrained paid assistant nurses kept back educated women from entering the Poor Law Nursing Service.

The vigilant reformers who had done pioneer work in the past still continued their efforts to raise the tone of nursing, and in 1879 the Workhouse Nursing Association was started, on the initiative of Constance, Marchioness of Lothian, Lady Henry Scott, afterwards Lady Montagu, and Miss Louisa Twining. The inaugural meeting was held at the house of the Marchioness of Lothian, July 25, 1879, when the following resolutions were passed :—

1. That the present state of nursing in the majority of workhouse infirmaries and sick asylums is capable of improvement.
2. That it is desirable to promote the employment of paid and efficiently trained nurses in all workhouse infirmaries and sick asylums.
3. That the appointment of a hospital-trained lady superintendent to be at the head of each staff of trained nurses is essential to the efficiency of the system.
4. That an association be formed to carry out these objects, to be called an Association for Promoting Trained Nursing in Workhouse Infirmaries and Sick Asylums in co-operation with the Local Government Board and Poor Law Guardians.

Princess Mary Adelaide, Duchess of Teck, became president of the association; an influential committee was formed, which included the names of Dr. Acland, Sir William Bowman, Dr. Sieveking, Dr. Symes Thompson, together with many ladies well-known in the philanthropic world. Miss Louisa Twining undertook the duties of honorary secretary, which she continued to discharge with much ability and enthusiasm for many years.

One of the earliest actions taken by the Association throws a light on the Poor Law nursing of the time. There was an election of a nurse for a Norfolk workhouse infirmary. The only candidate was the cook of one of the guardians, who thought she would like a change from domestic service. She would probably have been elected had not the vigilance of the honorary secretary of the Association secured the introduction of a trained nurse from the Liverpool Infirmary. In 1881 the Association started to train nurses for workhouse infirmaries, who were called, after the president, the "Mary Adelaide" Nurses. This branch of work was discontinued after 1897. No less than eight hundred nurses had been trained.

So far had the movement progressed by 1886 that Dr. Joseph Rogers was thus able to review the changes which he had witnessed in the course of thirty years. "The change which occurred," he writes, "was enormous. Then [1856] there was hardly a paid nurse in any workhouse in London, the duties being performed by more or less infirm, drunken, and generally profligate inmates of the house. It was a miracle to find an honest one among them; they were a chance medley of Sairey Gamps and Betsey Prigs, who were elected at the will of master and matron, and who obeyed the orders of the medical officer just as much as, and no more than, their fancy led them. The scenes of untold misery which might have been witnessed by the guardians of the poor will never be fully exposed until the grave record of all things is opened to universal gaze. Fortunately, a change has come over the spirit of these things; in the present day the sick poor are housed in buildings which were never dreamed of twenty years ago; pauper nursing is now entirely a thing of the past."*

* The last statement requires qualification.

Still, much remained to be done, and in 1892, in response to the request of the Workhouse Nursing Association, a departmental committee of the Local Government Board was appointed to inquire into the question of workhouse nursing, and a mass of important evidence was given by experts. Two years later, Mr. Ernest Hart, editor of the *British Medical Journal*, a publication which has long been allied with humanitarian reforms, instituted an investigation into the condition of the English and Welsh workhouse infirmaries, and invited Miss Catherine Wood to undertake the work.

Miss Catherine Wood is a well-known figure in the nursing world to-day, and is a woman of strong personality and great ability. She began work in 1863 at the Children's Hospital, Great Ormond Street, at the time when its founder, Dr. Charles West, was introducing educated women as nurses. Miss Wood was co-founder with Mrs. Howard Marsh (then Miss Jane Spenser Percival) of the Alexandra Hospital for Hip-Joint Disease in Queen's Square. She was one of the founders of the British Nurses' Association in 1887, and acted as its honorary secretary until 1890. In 1889 Miss Wood started the Nurses' Hostel, the first of its kind, which now has commodious quarters in Francis Street. Miss Wood has been honorary secretary since 1878 of the Guild of St. Barnabas for nurses, which was founded by Miss Antrobus, and at the present time (1906) is undertaking a tour of the branches in the Colonies.

Miss Wood had gained experience for the task entrusted to her by the *British Medical Journal* by her work on the Committee of the Workhouse Infirmary Nursing Association. The report of her investigations into the nursing and care of the sick in the English and Welsh workhouses resulted in a request from the Irish Medical Association that she would make a similar investigation into the condition of the sick under the Poor Law in Ireland. Her report of these visits was also published in the *Journal*. These investigations played an important part in turning attention to the unsatisfactory condition of nursing in country Unions.

In 1894 the Countess of Meath, with the object of improving the class of workhouse infirmary nurses, started the Meath Workhouse Nursing Association, which continues to do useful work. Upwards of two hundred and thirty-four probationers have been accepted by the committee, and the majority placed as assistant-nurses in provincial workhouses. At present there are about one hundred and thirty holding Poor Law appointments. Princess Christian is patron of the Association, Dr. J. A. Shaw Mackenzie honorary medical officer, and Sir William Broadbent, M.D., one of the vice-presidents. Miss Mary E. Johnson is honorary treasurer, and Miss Annie Lee secretary. Lady Meath has long been associated with workhouse reforms, and was the founder of the Brabazon employment scheme, which affords occupation to the sick, bedridden, crippled, and infirm inmates, and is often the means of helping them to earn a living when they leave the House.

In Ireland, Gertrude, Countess of Pembroke, started, in 1897, the Workhouse Infirmary Nursing Association, to meet the difficulty of supplying Boards of Guardians with trained nurses, and to make strenuous effort to better the condition of the sick poor in workhouses in conjunction with the Irish Workhouses' Association. Both Protestant and Roman Catholic are employed as "Pembroke nurses." The secretary is Miss Armstrong, 42, Waterloo Road, Dublin.

The Local Government Board issued an important Nursing Order in 1896, by which it was directed that where three or more nurses are employed in one infirmary, one shall be appointed superintendent nurse, and be responsible, under the master and matron, for the management of the wards, and nurses, and patients. Under a further Nursing Order in 1897, pauper nurses were abolished, and the appointment of inexperienced assistant-nurses forbidden. The number of probationers has greatly increased since these Orders gave a better status to infirmary nu

The last important stage in the history of Poor Law nursing came with the publication, in 1902, of the Report of the Departmental Committee appointed ten years previously. The conclusions and recommendations are to the effect that the supply of nurses for the Poor Law Service should be encouraged by increased facilities for training, and better pay and conditions of work, and that the appointment of untrained persons as assistant nurses should no longer be sanctioned, and the appointment of trained matrons encouraged in the smaller infirmaries, where they might act as superintendents of nurses. Further suggestions are made for dealing with the difficulty which has arisen since the Nursing Order of 1897—appointing superintendent nurses—in order to more clearly define the duties and status of master, matron, and superintendent nurse respectively, and so avoid the conflict of jurisdiction occasioned by the grafting of the modern-trained superintendent nurse on to a system which still gave to the master and matron the control over the wards as laid down in 1847. The committee's proposition for the establishment of " minor " and " major " training-schools, and of " qualified " nurses and " trained " nurses caused considerable adverse criticism.

No action has yet been taken on this Report. The appointment in December, 1904, of a Royal Commission on the Poor Laws further raised the question, and the Workhouse Nursing Association appealed to the Local Government Board, that the care of the sick should receive adequate attention, and that at least one woman with a wide practical knowledge of the subject should be appointed on the commission. Miss Octavia Hill and Mrs. Sydney Webb * were appointed. The Workhouse Nursing Association, which had worked so vigorously for twenty-six years, unanimously agreed, on the motion

* And Mrs. Bernard Bosanquet.

of Lady Wantage, seconded by Lady Belhaven and Stenton, at the executive committee held on February 6, 1906, " That it is advisable to continue the work of the Association while questions connected with the sick Poor Law institutions are still in such an undecided and unsatisfactory condition." Her Royal Highness Princess Christian of Schleswig-Holstein is president of the Association, and those honoured workers in the cause, the Hon. Mrs. J. G. Talbot and Miss Louisa Twining, are vice-presidents. Miss Wilson is secretary. A great loss to the cause of Poor Law nursing recently has been sustained by the death of Lord Montagu of Beaulieu, who with Lady Montagu were among the founders of the Workhouse Nursing Association in 1879.

Training for the Poor Law Nursing Service is obtained at the schools in connection with the Metropolitan infirmaries, and with those in the large towns throughout the kingdom. The age at which probationers are received averages from twenty-one to thirty-five. The training is usually for three years, and a certificate is granted at the end of the course. The regulations are similar to those in civil hospitals. Training in infectious diseases is given at the special hospitals under the Metropolitan Asylums Board. Poor Law nurses can, if they wish, come under the Officer's Superannuation Act of 1896. Owing to the strong representations made, a further Act was passed in 1897, to enable nurses to " contract out " of the provisions of the superannuation fund if they so wish.

The Marylebone Infirmary was one of the first to start a training-school for nurses. The training home was opened by Her Royal Highness Princess Christian, in 1884, after which probationers were received. Mr. J. R. Lunn, medical superintendent of the infirmary since 1881, has from the first had the oversight of the training-school, and gives lectures to the nurses. The home sister has a class for practical work, and the matron, Miss Ramsden, sets questions before the examination to test the knowledge of the probationers. Miss Ramsden fills a very important post with much tact and distinction, and has a high ideal for infirmary nurses. She has an average of twenty-eight probationers in training. The nurses' home and matron's quarters compare favourably with those of large general hospitals. Mr. Henry Bonham Carter is an old friend of the Marylebone Infirmary, and was the means of first introducing trained nurses. A staff from St. Thomas's Hospital under Miss Vincent did admirable pioneer work. The probationers at Marylebone have hitherto received a gratuity from the Nightingale Fund.

The Kensington Infirmary, another of the model Poor Law institutions, has an old-established training school with an average of forty-nine probationers. There is a special maternity department where eight probationers are annually trained. Fee, ten pounds. Kensington has been well to the front in workhouse reforms. It was the first to have a lady guardian, and the first to introduce the Brabazon employment scheme. Dr. Potter is medical superintendent, and Miss Malim matron of the infirmary. Mr. and Mrs. Brimblecombe are the master and matron of the workhouse, which is extremely well managed.

One comes away from visiting such beautifully arranged and ordered infirmaries as Marylebone and Kensington, feeling that the most cherished ideals of the early reformers in workhouse nursing have been reached. In these, and indeed in all the large London and provincial infirmaries—one may specially mention the Charlton Union, Manchester, a model institution—the system works for the most part without friction; but in the small country Unions much remains to be done before the nursing is put upon a satisfactory footing. Women inspectors are greatly needed in the country workhouses, where trained nurses are in the invidious position of having the infirmary wards and the state of the sick examined by gentlemen who are without medical training.

The appointment of workhouse matrons who are trained nurses would be beneficial in the smaller unions, where to-day friction between the master and matron and the trained superintendent of nurses is of such common occurrence. To quote Miss Louisa Twining's terse summing up of the position, "What class of persons would ever consent to work under those who had no knowledge of their trade?" The report of the Royal Commission on the Poor Law and some action on the part of the Local Government Board are now awaited.

CHAPTER XV

NURSING IN ASYLUMS FOR THE INSANE

The old system—Dr. Browne's description of an asylum as it was—Treatment of the insane in ancient times—St. Vincent de Paul and Madame le Gras—Pinel's system in Paris—William Tuke founds the Retreat, York—Dr. John Conolly institutes new *régime* at Hanwell—St. Luke's Asylum—Legislation, 1815-45—Affliction of George III.—Lunacy Act, 1845—Commissioners and the attendants—Mrs. Jameson on asylum nurses—The work of Dorothea Dix in United States and Scotland—The Royal Crichton Institution, Dumfries—Dr. Browne institutes lectures for nurses—Sir James Crichton Browne tries to raise the status of nurses—First systematic attempt at training—Medico-Psychological Association Examining Board—Its course for certificate—Dr. Hyslop on the asylum nurse—Bethlem Royal Hospital—A contrast, past and present—A nurse thirty-five years ago—Claybury Asylum—Dr. Robert Jones—Nursing staff at Claybury—Rules and regulations—Berry Wood Asylum, Northampton—Dr. Harding—Dr. Robertson's "Ideals" at Larbert—Organization—Dr. Shuttleworth and the Asylum Workers' Association—Increased demand for mental nurses.

THE old system of nursing in asylums for the insane forms a blacker record even than the neglect of the sick and infirm in workhouse infirmaries. The "female keeper"—she rarely received the gracious name of nurse—was up to the forties, and indeed later, a woman of the very lowest type, uneducated, coarse, and brutal. Her only idea of nursing was terrifying the patient, and in extenuation of her diabolical practices it must be remembered that she worked in accordance with the accepted methods of dealing with the insane.

The unfortunate patient was, with curious inconsistency, treated as a criminal for being out of his senses. If refractory, he was flogged, put in chains, confined in a loathsome cell, or even put into a cage like a wild beast.

Little more than a century ago the good citizens of London were admitted at a penny a head to the old Royal Hospital of Bethlem to see the antics of the caged lunatics. While such was the attitude of asylum authorities and of the public towards the poor people deprived of the light of reason, it is not surprising that the male and female attendants on the insane were heartless and cruel. They were but a part of an inhuman system.

Classification was never thought of. There was no regulation of diet, baths, out-door exercise, or the provision of occupation or amusement. Moral treatment was unheard of, and the only methods used for bringing a lunatic to his senses (?) were bolts, bars, chains, whips, and cages. Diabolical devices were resorted to by keepers to keep their patients in subjection, and deaths from violence were frequent. It was put in evidence before the Parliamentary Commission, that at a private asylum a nurse or female keeper locked a harmless maniac down on her crib with wrist-locks and leg-locks, and horsewhipped her, the blood following the strokes. This was in 1812. When the Parliamentary Commissioners visited Fonthill Asylum, in Wiltshire, the cells were so foul that they could not enter them. One reads of a criminal lunatic, who had killed a man, being confined in a vault and fed like a wild animal for the period of twenty years. This in our own land in the year 1834. In evidence before the Parliamentary Commission, published in 1815, the case is given of a lunatic man who had been chained naked, lying on straw in a workhouse cell for fifty years! The morality of asylums was on a par with the cruelties practised. The male keepers not infrequently held keys which admitted to the sleeping-rooms of the female patients, and some women were put to sleep in the part of the house appropriated to men.

The late Dr. W. A. F. Browne, Commissioner in Lunacy for Scotland, and the father of the distinguished mental specialist, Sir James Crichton Browne, the Lord Chancellor's visitor in Lunacy, thus describes asylums as formerly regulated.* "The building was gloomy, placed in some low confined situation, without windows to the front, every chink barred and grated—a perfect gaol. As you enter, the crack of bolts and the clash of chains are scarcely distinguishable amid the wild chorus of shrieks and sobs which issue from every apartment. The passages are narrow, dark, damp, exhale a noxious effluvia, and are provided with a door at every two or three yards. Your conductor has the head and visage of Charib, carries fit accompaniment—a whip and a bunch of keys, and speaks in harsh monosyllables. The first common room you examine measures twelve feet long by seven feet wide, with a window which does not open, and is perhaps for females. Ten of them, with no other covering than a rag round the waist, are chained to the wall, loathsome and hideous, but, when addressed, evidently retaining some of the intelligence, and much of the feeling, which in other days ennobled their nature. In shame or sorrow, one of them perhaps utters a cry ; a blow which brings the blood from the temple, the tear from the eye, an additional chain, a gag, an indecent or contemptuous expression produces silence. And if you ask where these creatures sleep, you are led to a kennel eight feet square, with an unglazed air-hole eight inches in diameter ; in this, you are told, five women sleep . . . there is no bedding but wet decayed straw, and the stench is so insupportable that you turn away, and hasten from the scene. Each of the sombre colours of this picture is a fact. And those facts are but a fraction of the evils which have been brought home to asylums as they were."

Though things were at this terrible pass at the beginning of the last century, the treatment of the insane in ancient times was, in some instances, more humane, if mingled with superstition. Egypt had an enlightened method of treatment. The Temples of Saturn were, in many respects, asylums conducted on humane lines. The

* "What Asylums were and ought to be," by W. A. F. Browne, surgeon.

people who flocked to the shrines were treated as suffering from disease, and a healthy *régime* was prescribed. They walked in the beautiful gardens around the temple, rowed on the Nile, took excursions under pretence of pilgrimages, and had dances, concerts, and comic entertainments. These created pleasing impressions on the mind, which, united to faith in the deity, often brought about a cure. The priests, of course, claimed a miraculous intervention.

The influence of music was recognized amongst the ancients, as witness David being called to play before Saul. The Greek Hippocrates, the father of medicine, treated the insane by bleeding and purging, and Galen advocated classification. In the middle ages the insane were treated as people possessed of evil spirits, and sorcery and witchcraft were used to exorcise them. At the village of Gheel, near Antwerp, there was an ancient retreat for lunatics. The patients were employed in the gardens and fields, they had all kinds of out-door exercises and pastimes, and were boarded in the homes of the peasants, and allowed perfect liberty. The cure was not, however, attributed to these natural causes, but to the intercession of St. Dymphna, the patients being required to pass under the tomb of the saint. Dr. Robert Jones, resident physician at Claybury, read a most instructive and interesting paper on the history of the treatment of the insane at the Medico-Psychological Association in July, 1906. Dr. Jones took a national interest in the fact that the earliest reliable account of the treatment of the insane came from Gerald the Welshman (Gerald de Cambriensis).

In the seventeenth century an attempt to deal with the insane on humane principles was made by St. Vincent de Paul, inspired by Madame le Gras, his coadjutor in the organization of his sisters of charity. In the closing years of her life, Madame le Gras, having accomplished so much on behalf of the sick poor and the galle slaves, yearned to do something to alleviate the condition of the

R

inmates of the asylums. She laid the matter before St. Vincent, with the result that, in 1645, they took under their beneficent care the asylum, *Petites Maisons*, sending sisters of charity to nurse the inmates.

The beginning of the change in the treatment of the insane dates from 1792, when Pinel was appointed physician to Bicêtre, Paris. There he began to experiment with his theory, that the insane could be treated without mechanical restraint. His first experiment was on a furious lunatic who had been in chains for forty years. He was an English captain, and no one knew his history. Pinel entered the cell unattended, and calmly said—

"Captain, I will order your chains to be taken off and give you liberty to walk in the court, if you will promise to behave well, and hurt no one."

"Yes, I promise you," said the madman; "but you are only laughing at me."

"I will give you liberty," returned Pinel, "if you will put on this waistcoat."

After the chains were removed, the poor man, with difficulty maintaining his balance, staggered to the door, and, looking up at the sky, exclaimed, "How beautiful!" He behaved rationally, and during the two years that he remained at Bicêtre had no return of paroxysm. Later, Pinel was appointed medical superintendent of the vast establishment of Salpêtrière, which embraced an establishment for the insane, and there continued his humane methods. His ideas spread to other countries, and by degrees a total revolution took place in the treatment of the insane, which necessitated a different type of nurse and attendant.

In our own country, the first asylum to follow Pinel's system was the Retreat at York, founded in 1792 by William Tuke, a citizen of York. A woman, who was a member of the Society of Friends, having died in the old York Asylum under suspicious circumstances, the matter was investigated by the Society, with the result that William Tuke and other friends decided to build a new asylum to be managed on humane and open lines. Secrecy was the bane of the old system. When a name for the institution was under discussion a lady in the founder's family said, " Why not call it a Retreat ? " And so the famous institution was beautifully named, and we feel sure that those Quaker ladies had something to say in the choice of the nurses for the Retreat. That asylum long led the van of reform and remains true to its old traditions.

Other early reformers were Dr. Charlesworth, who experimented at the Lincolnshire Asylum in 1821 with the new system ; and Dr. Gardner Hill was, during the same period, engaged in similar work in a private asylum in London. But the most epoch-making reform was the work of Dr. John Conolly, at the Middlesex County Asylum, Hanwell. A most interesting account of this work is given in the "Life" of Conolly, by Sir James Clark, M.D.

Dr. Conolly was born in Lincolnshire in 1794, and in 1839 became resident physician at Hanwell. Although this was a new asylum the old methods were practised. Conolly found " each ward provided with a closet full of restraining apparatus, and every attendant used them at will." There were six hundred instruments in all, half of which were handcuffs and leglocks. At the end of ten years of humane management, Conolly reported that no hand or foot had been fastened, no instrument or mechanical restraint used, no patient placed in the coercive chair, or fastened to the bedstead by night. The result was increased tranquillity and diminished danger. The shackles which Conolly cut off the patients are to-day preserved at Hanwell, as relics of a barbarous age.

The great Asylum of St. Luke's, which was established by voluntary effort in 1751, to relieve Bethlem, stands well in the matter of instruction. Pupils attended this hospital in 1853. Dr. Ballie, a physician of that hospital, is said to have been the first to give lectures in London on mental diseases. The Parliamentary Commissioners did not discover many abuses at St. Luke's. It started the modern training of its attendants in 1892.

Legislation and inspection in regard to the conduct of asylums were active between 1815-45. The mental affliction of George III. had created national interest in the treatment of the insane. That unhappy monarch had not been exempt from harsh treatment. It is related that the aged king was knocked down by his keeper "as flat as a flounder." The Parliamentary Commission appointed in 1815 to inquire into the condition of the insane discovered an appalling state of things. The neglect and cruelty already described were found to prevail in most of the asylums. In 1828 an Act was passed, appointing official inspectors. Before 1828 only twelve of the fifty-two counties of England had public establishments for the insane, and until 1808 there was only one asylum in Ireland. All pauper lunatics requiring restraint were sent to prison with the felons, and most cruelly used. Lunatics were also found confined in loathsome cells in workhouses. Mr. Gordon Ashley and the late Lord Shaftesbury were the leading actors in bringing about legislation. In 1845 came the passing of the Lunacy Act, truly the Magna Charta of the insane.

An important result of the investigations by the newly appointed Lunacy Commissioners was the dismissal of large numbers of the old attendants and nurses. Nothing, however, appears to have been done towards instituting a system of training. The Commissioners in their 11th Report, 1855, recommended the appointment of head attendants of a superior class, to be responsible for the conduct of the other attendants. An experiment was also tried of placing educated ladies in some of the asylums as " companions to female patients of the upper classes."

In 1854, Mrs. Jameson drew attention, in her " Sisters of Charity," to the need of good feminine influence for insane men as well as insane women. "As to the use of trained women in lunatic asylums," she writes, "I will say no more at present, but throw it out as a suggestion to be dealt with by physiologists, and intrusted to *time*." To-day, the most advanced reformers in asylum nursing are proving the wisdom of Mrs. Jameson's advocacy of women nurses for insane sick men.

Mrs. Jameson had been stirred to interest herself in the nursing of the insane by the work accomplished in America by that remarkable woman Dorothea Dix, who travelled all over the United States, inquiring into the state of the asylums. She initiated a system of reform in which a more careful selection of nurses was a prominent feature, and was the means of founding some nineteen new asylums, and of enlarging others. The influence of Miss Dix was felt also in this country, more particularly in Scotland. She discovered a shocking state of things in some of the Scottish asylums. Her visits of inspection roused much opposition, and it was suspected that she would return to London and make revelations. A gentleman from Edinburgh tried to circumvent her, but Miss Dix, by taking the night express to London, outran him, and laid her statement before the Home Office. Her facts were so startling that a Royal Commission was appointed for Scotland.

There had been, however, at the beginning of the century, some stirring in the matter of reform at the asylums of Dundee, Aberdeen, and Perth, where the lunatics were employed in useful work. That far-seeing reformer Dr. W. A. F. Browne, medical superintendent at Montrose Royal Lunatic Asylum, and one-time President of the Royal Medical Society, Edinburgh, whose writings have already been referred to, delivered a course of lectures in 1840, which were published in a volume, entitled " What asylums were and ought to be." The book is now out of print, but it contains suggestions which have long since been carried out. Dr. Browne dwells specially on the need for a different class of attendants in asylums. He thought it was necessary to " cure the keepers " before attempting to cure the patients. Dr. Browne was able to carry his theories into practice when he became medical superintendent at the Royal Crichton Institution, Dumfries, the founding of which marks an epoch in the movement in Scotland.

Up to 1839 there was no provision for the insane south of Edinburgh and Glasgow, except six squalid stone cells attached to the Dumfries Infirmary. Dr. Crichton, of Friar's Carse, Dumfries, had bequeathed to his widow £120,000 for charitable purposes. Mrs. Crichton determined to devote it to the founding of an institution for the insane, on humane and advanced principles. This enlightened lady directed that a Bible should be placed as the foundation of the building instead of a stone, to signify that it was to be conducted on the principles of Christian philanthropy as well as of science. Dr. W. A. F. Browne was appointed medical superintendent of the Crichton Institution, and there put in practice the most enlightened methods of treatment, after visiting the best conducted institutions in Paris and elsewhere. The institution, founded in 1839, is situated in beautiful grounds outside the town of Dumfries, and a few miles inland from the Solway. Freedom, employment, and recreation have from the first been the keynotes of the asylum, which receives patients of various classes. The treatment initiated by Dr. Browne has been successively carried forward on modern lines by the late Dr. Gilchrist and the present medical superintendent, Dr. Rutherford. Lectures to the nurses have for many years been a feature of the institution, and it is now insisted upon that all charge attendants hold the certificate of proficiency of the Medico-Psychological Association.

An extract from the annual report of the Crichton Institution for the year 1854 states that Dr. Browne had arranged a course of lectures for the attendants and nurses. "Since the diminution and discontinuance of physical restraint, and the introduction of education and amusement as remedies," runs the entry, "these officers are called upon for greater intelligence, higher motives, and a clearer comprehension of what that human nature, which in its morbid phases they have to guide and govern, really is. Instruction of some kind is obviously necessary. To these persons is in great measure intrusted the moral treatment of the insane. They pass the whole day with their charges, while the visits of the medical officers are necessarily brief and at intervals. The instruction offered will embrace a full, if somewhat popular, discussion of insanity in the different forms, intelligible by the shrewd and sensible, if somewhat illiterate class of persons, employed as attendants and nurses, with practical demonstrations of methods of treatment employed." These were the first lectures given to mental nurses in the British Isles or, I believe, in the world.

Education did not spread rapidly amongst asylum nurses, for when Dr. Browne's distinguished son, Sir James Crichton Browne, had charge of an asylum in 1865, there were nurses in the wards who could not read the directions on the medicine bottles, and had to get the lunatics to help them. Sir James had one hundred and fifty nurses under his charge, drawn from the lower domestic class, and when he raised the wages of the under-nurses from twelve pounds to fourteen pounds per annum, the ladies of the district laid a complaint before the committee of the asylum, saying that their kitchenmaids were being taken away to be made into nurses. Sir James Crichton Browne's continued efforts for improving the education and status of asylum nurses are well known.

The first systematic attempt to train asylum nurses began within the Council of the Medico-Psychological Association, 11, Chandos Street. Amongst those who took special interest in the work were Sir James Crichton Browne, Dr. Yellowlees, Dr. Cluston, Dr. Savage, Dr. Hays Newington, Dr. Spence, and Dr. Robert Jones, honorary secretary of the society for the past ten years.* Lectures and demonstrations were started, and by degrees the present system of training and examination established.

* Dr. Robert Jones has been elected President of the Society, 1906-7.

This began about twenty years ago ; now there is not an asylum in the three kingdoms which does not go in for special courses of training.

The Medico-Psychological Association remains the examining body for mental nursing, and some 7250 men and women have obtained its certificate. The course which was originally for two years has now been raised to three years' work, and instruction in an asylum or hospital for the insane, including the trial probationary period of three months. The system required by the association consists of—

(*a*) Systematic lectures and demonstrations by the medical staff at the various institutions. At least twelve lectures, each of one hour's duration, must be given in each year of training ; and no attendant will be admitted to examination who has not attended at least nine lectures in each year.

(*b*) Clinical instruction in the wards by the medical staff.

(*c*) Exercises under the head and charge attendants in the practice of nursing and attendance on the insane.

(*d*) Study of the handbook of nursing issued by the Association. Other books may be used in addition.

(*e*) Periodical examinations, the nature and frequency of which are left to the discretion of the superintendent, but one examination at least is held in each year. The scope of training required by the Association is such as will impart a knowledge, (1) of the main outlines of bodily structure and function, sufficient to enable attendants to understand the principles of nursing, and of "first-aid," especially with regard to the accidents and injuries most likely to occur among the insane ; (2) of the general features and varieties of mental disorder ; (3) of the ordinary requirements of sick nursing, and especially of the requirements of nursing and attending on the insane.

Twice a year, in May and November, examinations for the granting of certificates to successful candidates are held at every institution in which there are candidates. The examinations are partly written, partly *viva voce* and practical. The papers are set and examined by examiners in nursing appointed by the Medico-Psychological Association. A certificate is given at the successful completion of the three years' course. The examination is the same, though conducted separately, for male and female nurses. The names of all persons who have received a certificate are placed upon a register kept by the registrar of the Association, Dr. Miller, Hatton Asylum, W. Warwick.

The training of an asylum nurse is of a twofold character, for not only has she to study the nursing of bodily disease in the hospital or infirmary wards attached to asylums, but the special treatment also for dealing with the mind diseased. To nurse a mad person afflicted with some other disease, such as fever or pneumonia, presents a more difficult task than nursing a sane patient similarly afflicted. That it takes a person of superior skill and intelligence to make an asylum nurse has been very slowly recognized. She must be tactful and patient to a degree which is angelic, for she is permitted no weapon but moral suasion in the control of a refractory patient or for the protection of her own person. To quote Dr. Theodore B. Hyslop, the distinguished Superintendent of Bethlem, " Asylum nurses need qualifications over and above those of general nurses. When one remembers that they are constantly the butt, not only of malicious sayings by the insane, but actually of their fists and feet, that they have to endure all this without complaint, and to display constant amiability, that when struck by patients they must make themselves as soft as possible to avoid injuring the toes or knuckles of the aggressors! lest there should be an inquiry, one feels that, instead of asylum nurses being blameworthy, they deserve credit for their pluck, endurance, and Christian fortitude. I remember one case in which the nurse deserved the Victoria Cross, and consider that the qualifications of asylum nurses far exceed anything required from general nurses."

Bethlem Royal Hospital, the noble institution over which Dr. Hyslop reigns, forms an object lesson of the change which has been made in the treatment of the insane, and in the education of the attendants. Bethlem is the oldest hospital for the insane in Great Britain, and I believe in the world. It was originally founded in 1247, by Simon FitzMary, as a priory in Bishopsgate for Brethren and Sisters of the Order of St. Mary of Bethlem. It was seized by the crown in 1375, under the pretext that it was a foreign priory. When Bethlem or "Bedlam," as it came to be called, was first used as an asylum for the insane is not definitely known. In 1547, Henry VIII. granted it by Royal Charter to the citizens of London, and at that time it housed a small number of insane persons. The portrait of Henry VIII. hangs in the committee room of the hospital. The institution was removed from Bishopsgate to Moorfields in 1750, and to its present fine open position in St. George's Fields in 1812. The wits of the town expended their fun on the fine building, and said that the authorities must " be mad to build so costly a college for such a crackbrained society." Even at that time the bedroom windows were unglazed, and the other windows placed high so that the patients could not see out. Successive additions and improvements have been made, to bring the ancient hospital to its present state of perfection, but I noticed that in some of the single rooms the old high windows remain. It stands on a part of the site of the old Dog and Duck, and the quaint sign of the old inn is preserved in an outer wall of the asylum.

Bethlem has a notorious past. Within the walls of the old hospital the most diabolical practices reigned. There is probably no device for the mechanical restraint and torture of the insane which has not been put into practice at Bethlem. In Tuke's " History of the Insane " * occurs a picture of a ward in the hospital, in 1745, which

* "History of the Insane in the British Isles," by Daniel Hack Tuke, M.D., F.R.C.P.

shows a half-naked lunatic held down on the floor by
three keepers, while a fourth manacles his limbs. Up to
the year 1770 Bethlem was one of the sights of London.
People were admitted at a penny a head to see the antics
of the unhappy lunatics, who were encouraged to eat
filth and to disport themselves indecently in order to
amuse the low and vicious. Fine ladies, it would seem,
resorted there also, according to the picture drawn by
Hogarth, when he finally ends the progress of his Rake
within the walls of Bethlem. In olden times it was the
custom to periodically turn out a number of the more
harmless lunatics, who roamed the country begging, and
were known as " Tom-o-Bedlams." Shakespeare describes
the practice in *King Lear*—

> "The country gives me proof and precedent
> Of Bedlam beggars, who, with roaring voices,
> Stick in their numb'd and mortify'd bare arms,
> Pins, wooden pricks, nails, sprigs of rosemary."

I am afraid Bethlem hugged its malpractices. It
strenuously opposed the work of the Parliamentary Commissioners in 1815-35. Not until 1853 was the old
Royal Hospital placed under inspections, like other institutions. Since then, a new order of things has been
introduced, culminating in the present admirable administration.

Dr. Theodore Bulkeley Hyslop, C.M., M.R.C.P.,
L.M., the physician superintendent of Bethlem, and also
of Bridewell, is, it need not be stated, one of the first
authorities in the kingdom on the treatment of the insane.
He is lecturer on psychological medicine at St. Mary's
Hospital, and senior examiner of the Medico-Psychological
Association. Dr. Hyslop sets high ideals for the asylum
nurse, and uses his influence to further in every way the
education and status of attendants on the insane. As well
as being the author of a text-book on mental physiology,
and various articles on the subject, Dr. Hyslop is both a
musician and an artist. He has exhibited in the Royal
Academy, and his paintings adorn the recreation room at

Bethlem. His orchestral compositions have been played at the promenade concerts, and he is a playing member of several orchestras. Nothing gives Dr. Hyslop greater pleasure than to use his musical gifts for the pleasure and amusement of those in whom the light of reason has failed.

Bethlem as it was, and Bethlem to-day, what a contrast! No chains, no cells, no strait-jackets. In the lower ward, one sees the acute cases just received being reduced to obedience and trust by the kindly cheery manner of the nurse. "I won't go to bed," says a distraught woman with threatening look. Nurse smiles, persuades the lady that she looks "so tired," and almost by magic that refractory patient's arm is linked in that of the nurse, and she passes to her room subdued as a little child, glad to be taken care of. Conquests are not all so easy as that. The nurse must be able to assert and maintain authority, but kindness rules. In the beautiful Alexandra ward, with its flowers, and plants, and singing birds, and pretty objects of all kinds, one sees the patients, who will soon be ready to go to the convalescent home at Witley, for the completion of their cure, chatting, and reading, doing needlework for Dr. Barnardo's Homes, or playing the piano, while the sister and her staff treat them more like paying guests than asylum patients. The nurses complain that they lose their patients as soon as they become companionable and interesting, while the hospital nurse is able from the first to establish at least a conversational footing with those under her care.

Bethlem receives for free treatment patients who are from the educated classes, chiefly reduced gentlepeople, and there are also some who pay, but the nurses are not allowed to know who pays, so that all receive equal attention. Only cases of recent insanity are received, and if not cured within a year they are transferred to one of the London County asylums.

In the recreation room, concerts and dances for the patients are held throughout the winter, and the grounds of Bethlem, wonderfully pleasant and spacious for a London hospital, afford a delightful place in summer for tennis and other games. It is a most useful qualification for an asylum nurse to be able to play and sing. Dr. Hyslop is a great believer in the beneficial effect of music on the insane. The chaplain conducts services for the patients in the asylum chapel.

I was much interested when going over Bethlem to meet a nurse who had been connected with the institution for thirty-five years. In the old days she did single-handed the work performed now by six nurses. As night sister, she went alone all round the hospital, from top floor to basement, carrying a little lamp to light her through the gloomy passages. She was liable at any moment to meet the wild spring of some lunatic, as she opened the doors of the various sleeping rooms. She parted with a good many handfuls of hair in those days. Things came to a climax one night, when she was called to the assistance of a nurse who was being nearly strangled by a lunatic on the floor of one of the corridors. This led to a much-needed reform, which provided that two nurses should go the rounds together at night. Now, two night sisters go round the wards together, and every half-hour peg their clock, which registers the time in the office of the medical department. In the observation wards there are five other nurses who peg their clocks every quarter of an hour, and if anything happens, the medical superintendent is able to tell where each nurse was at the time of the occurrence.

At the beginning of last century every "female keeper" at Bethlem had sixty patients under her care, all suffering from different degrees and kinds of insanity. To-day the staff in the hospital, where there is an average of 250 patients, consists of fifty nurses of all grades. At the head of the female nursing department, working under the Medical Superintendent, Dr. Hyslop, is the matron, Miss Meikle. There are six sisters, one to each ward, each having under her six charge nurses and four

under nurses, who are being trained. There are also lady
probationers, who receive no salary, and are taught the
treatment of the insane to fit them for being companions
to the feeble-minded. They are not certificated as trained
nurses. The age at which nurse probationers are received
is from eighteen to thirty. The salary is a little higher
than the average in general hospitals.

Leaving Bethlem, our oldest hospital for the insane,
which has emerged through all the terrors and revolting
practices of the old *régime* into the light of modern treatment, we will journey to Claybury, one of the ten London
county asylums, and one of the largest institutions for the
insane in the world. There are about 2400 inmates.
Dr. Robert Jones, the distinguished head, must con-
gratulate himself that Claybury has " no past." He
began his work in 1893, with a new model institution
beautifully situated on high ground above the village of
Woodford Bridge, Essex, and from its elevated site overlooking a finely wooded country. The grounds, which
cover 269 acres, are most tastefully laid out. There
are walks and drives, shrubberies, and vegetable and fruit
gardens within the domain, and plentiful provision for
tennis, cricket, and other out-door games. Immediately
surrounding the building are a succession of airing courts
or gardens, each appropriated to one class of patient. In
summer the flowers are luxuriant, and in winter the
gardens are still bright and beautiful with evergreens.
Dr. Jones takes great pride in the floral culture of the
estate. Turn where you will at Claybury, there is something beautiful for the eye to rest upon. In summer one
sees even the acute patients enjoying picnic teas upon the
grass.

In-doors every portion of the huge building is light,
bright, and airy ; I do not think there is a dark room or
a dark corner to be discovered. All the windows have
pleasant, cheerful views. Almost every ward has a separate day- and dining-room for the patients, and these are
arranged in a manner which destroys the idea of a public

institution. In one large dining-room, flooded with sunshine, I saw some thirty or more women patients seated in parties of five or seven at round tables prettily set out for afternoon tea. A couple of nurses passing to and fro, chatting and joking, maintained perfect order. The affection with which the patients regard their nurses is very striking. To nurse they tell the sorrows of their distraught brains, fully persuaded that she is their great and particular friend. If, as sometimes happens, a patient shows an aversion to some nurse or attendant, he or she is removed to another ward. It is not an unusual thing for a nurse herself to take out for a holiday some lonely patient who has no friends to visit her.

There is a handsome chapel, as big as a large parish church, attached to the institution, a palatial recreation-room for balls, concerts, and theatricals, and a library and reading-room. The dormitories are models of simplicity and cleanliness. The infirmary wards are equal to those of a good general hospital, and have low windows, which enable the patients to look from their beds over the surrounding country. The only thing which reminds you of the special character of the patients are the protected fireplaces. There are no iron bars to the windows. There is a small maternity ward, very sad in many respects, and yet it has its bright side, for sometimes the joy of motherhood calls back the wandering intellect. There is an up-to-date operation theatre, and at a little distance from the main building an isolation block for infectious diseases.

Dr. Robert Jones is one of the most advanced advocates for the non-restraint treatment. Not even the strait-jacket has ever been used at Claybury. If a patient arrives in one from a workhouse infirmary it is promptly removed. The padded room is used for the unmanageable cases. Dr. Jones is against the single-room system, even for acute cases, and prefers to place them in dormitories under observation.

The nursing staff, who are well accommodated with

quarters, consists of 159 nurses on the female side to 1400 patients, and 131 attendants on the male side to 1000 patients. At the head of the staff, under the resident physician, is the matron, Miss Cottis, who was appointed on the staff at the opening of the institution. She has been connected with asylum work for twenty-three years, and worked her way through the various grades of that branch of nursing. When she began, trained nursing had not been introduced into asylums, but later Miss Cottis passed the examination of the Medico-Psychological Association for her certificate. Before coming to Claybury she had been ten years at the Wandsworth Asylum. She has a valuable and skilful coadjutor in the assistant matron, Miss Eaton Smith, who takes rank as an " officer."

Candidates are received on three months' probation, and if satisfactory engaged for three years' training and service. They are encouraged to work for the certificate of the Medico-Psychological Association. It is desirable that they be not less than five feet five inches in height, proportionately well-built and healthy, of fair education, excellent character, and good-tempered, with some knowledge of music and singing. It is not forgotten at Claybury that David was sent for to play before Saul. The attendants are divided into two grades. The second-class begin at £18 a year, rising £1 a year to £24 ; the first-class begin at £25, rising £1 a year to £33. The female night attendants receive £25, rising £1 a year to £33. Board, lodging, uniform, and laundry free in all cases. A gratuity of 10s. per quarter is given for good conduct. Attendants in the choir receive an annual gratuity. The hours on duty are from 6 a.m. to 8 p.m., after which a day attendant has the privilege of going out until 10 p.m. The night attendant is encouraged to take off-duty time in the afternoon. Each attendant has one day off in every seven, and twenty-one days' annual leave.. Although the hours are long, an asylum nurse has a good deal of variety in her work. Her duties take her constantl into the open air, and she is much engaged in games andypastimes with the patients.

The Berry Wood Asylum, Northampton, of which Dr. Harding is medical superintendent, is to the front in pioneer reforms. From its establishment in 1838 it has adopted the non-mechanical restraint system. As early as 1890, Dr. Harding instituted a three years' course of training for nurses, with examinations, and was the first to do so in connection with mental nursing. The education is very thorough, and includes fever nursing. The textbooks used are, first year, St. John's Ambulance Handbook; second year, Miss Eva Lückes' "General Nursing;" third year, Dr. Harding's "Mental Nursing." Each fortnight, nurses write answers to questions on the subjects of the lectures, which are corrected by the lecturer. At the end of each course of lectures, three examinations are held, written, oral, and practical, and the student must pass in all three before going on to the next year's work. In addition, a lecture is given every week in a ward or the sick-room on some subject illustrated by a patient. Bandaging and dressing of wounds, moving and lifting of patients, etc., are practised at every course of lectures. The nurse's ward work and general conduct must be satisfactory before she can be admitted to examination. On passing the third year's examination, a nurse receives the Berry Wood Nursing Certificate and a silver medal. If any nurse is first in all examinations for the three years, she gets a special or extra medal.

Worcester, Prestwich, and Dorset asylums, also the Retreat, York, have followed the example of Northampton, and grant their own certificates. In most other asylums e certificate of the Medico-Psychological Association is tbken.

The most recent development in mental nursing is in the direction of making an asylum more like a general hospital. In the old days an asylum was practically a prison both in construction and in administration. Now insanity is regarded as a disease, and treated in the medical spirit. Some years ago Sir James Crichton Browne proposed the building of a new asylum in London on purely hospital lines. For the past five years Dr. Robertson, medical superintendent at the Stirling District Asylum, Larbert, has been developing the nursing in that admirable institution on hospital lines. The matron on the female side is a hospital-trained nurse, and on the male side there is also a hospital-trained matron in place of the usual head male attendant. Dr. Robertson has also created a new officer in the assistant matron (hospital-trained), of whom there are five at Larbert. It is their duty to supervise the nurses in the wards. There is also a hospital-trained night superintendent, who inspects the hospital four times each night. She receives a salary of £52 a year, and ranks as a superior officer. The night nursing is arranged on novel lines. The patients are classified in the dormitories, as in the dayrooms. To six hundred and ninety patients there is a staff of twenty night nurses, who give as effective care and supervision by night as by day. Incarceration in single rooms, even for the noisy and violent, is not used at all in this asylum. The door of every single room is left standing open at night, a plan which, as Dr. Robertson admits, seemed as Utopian as the abolition of restraint in Conolly's day at Hanwell.

The special feature of Dr. Robertson's plan is the employment of women in the male sick and infirm wards by night as well as by day. Mrs. Jameson, writing in 1854, advocated the employment of women nurses amongst the male asylum patients, and after fifty years Dr. Robertson is proving the wisdom of her suggestion. Out of forty-two persons engaged by night and by day at Larbert, in the care and supervision of male patients, nineteen, or practically half, are women, and three are hospital trained. All the aged and infirm male lunatics are nursed by women in a special infirmary ward. The result is that bed sores are abolished, the imbecile and feeble folk are more carefully and patiently tended, and

the male patients prove more amenable. There have
been no scandals to report, nor any assault. Male
attendants are employed for some offices, such as bathing
and dressing and undressing the male patients. Much
credit is due to Miss Wise, the matron, for the manner
in which she has administered the asylum under these
novel conditions.

Dr. Robertson has written of his " Ideals for the Care
of the Insane," in the *Journal of Medical Science*, April,
1902, and foremost amongst these is the employment of
women nurses in the male wards, and " the extent to
which they may be employed," he writes, " and their
usefulness have exceeded all expectations. . . . I consider
the qualifications of mind and heart and of body needed
for an asylum nurse infinitely greater than for a hospital
nurse, just as disease of the mind is more complex than
disease of the body, and when acute includes the latter."

We have now reached the period at which mental
nursing had become an important branch of the profession, and organization became inevitable. Miss Honor
Morten first suggested the idea of starting an Association
to improve the status of asylum workers, and found a
sympathetic supporter in Miss Laura Evans, the matron
of Berry Wood Asylum. They laid their scheme before
Dr. Harding, and under his auspices, as honorary secretary,
the Asylum Workers' Association was started in 1896.
The first president was the late Sir Henry Ward Richardson. He was succeeded by Sir James Crichton Browne,
who for five years was an indefatigable president, and
now acts as chairman of the Association. The president
is Sir James Batty Tuke, M.D. Dr. Walmsley succeeded
Dr. Harding as honorary secretary, and was instrumental
in getting two thousand people to join. For the past ten
years Dr. Shuttleworth, who has recently removed from
Ancaster House, Richmond Hill, to Sheen, has acted
as honorary secretary of the Association and has developed its organ, the *Asylum News*. Dr. Shuttleworth is a
specialist on mental disease in children, and was formerly

Superintendent of the Royal Albert Asylum for Defective Children, Lancaster. Mrs. Chapman is honorary treasurer, Mr. W. J. Hill, honorary auditor; and Mr. J. B. W. Wilson, assistant secretary.

The objects of the Association are to raise the status of asylum nurses and attendants, and to promote their general welfare. Grants are made to enable members in ill health to obtain rest and change at Homes of Rest in various resorts. Long and meritorious nursing service in asylums is rewarded by a yearly grant of two gold and two silver medals. The subscription is eighteen pence a year, which includes a copy of the *Asylum News*. The Association numbers upwards of three thousand nurses and attendants, not by any means a large proportion of the vast army of asylum workers. In the event of State registration, the Association propose that asylum nurses should be placed on a separate section of the register. The demand for mental nurses is steadily increasing, as, unhappily, the number of the insane is growing larger. The first Report of the Commissioners in Lunacy, issued in 1844, gives the number of registered lunatics at 16,821. The Report for 1906 shows the number, in England and Wales, to have risen to 121,979. The asylum nurses and attendants number about 20,000; 7555 have passed the Medico-Psychological examination, and of these 4006 are women. The male attendants are trained as sick nurses at the National Hospital for the Paralyzed and Epileptic, Queen's Square, Bloomsbury.

CHAPTER XVI

PRIVATE NURSING

The best paying and most criticized branch of the profession—Dissatisfied patients—Private nurse expected to be a paragon of perfection—Some ground for complaint—Nursing plays an increasingly important part in recovery of patient—Private nurse and district nurse compared—Need of special training for private nurses—First attempts to organize private nurses—Mildmay Institution—The Royal Scottish Nursing Institution—Miss M'Alpin's Home, Glasgow—Abuses of Nursing Homes—Princess Christian's Nursing Home at Windsor—Beginning of the co-operative movement in nursing—Miss Firth formed the London Association in 1873—Her devoted life—Progress of her Association—Its rules—The Nurses' Co-operation—The Registered Nurses' Society—Large proportion of nurses take up private work—Three principal classes—Daily private nursing—Marylebone Daily Visiting Nursing Association—The Ada Lewis nurses—The bitter cry of the middle classes.

THOUGH private nursing has become the most lucrative and is generally regarded as the most attractive, it is certainly the most criticized, branch of the profession. People are apt to grow irritable under the idea that they are called upon to pay for being ill, and consequently the nurse shares with the family doctor the general grumble when bills have to be met.

The active old lady seized with influenza, who is persuaded by her friends to have a trained nurse, cannot reconcile herself to the luxury. She thinks that two guineas a week, very generous board, including wine, and two shillings and sixpence per week for laundry, "a preposterous charge" for the privilege of having her temperature taken, her back rubbed, and being washed between blankets by a three years' certificated lady in immaculate uniform. She broods in bed over the days of her youth, when " good faithful Mary " nursed everybody in the family when they were ill, and sat up at nights without a grumble. *She* did not keep a man and a horse constantly going to the country town for unnecessary things, *she* did not want servants to wait on her, and *she* was grateful for proper wages. And so the invalid extols the old and denounces the new. When the day for nurse's departure comes, the convalescent sings her *Te Deum* over the tea-cups : " My dear, I was never so thankful in all my life as when I saw that woman go out of the house. Why, she objected to my measuring the brandy with my own tea-spoon ! "

If the same old lady had watched nurse pull an idolized son through typhoid fever, she would have sung a *Te Deum* in a different strain. It is people suffering from small ailments who are usually so impatient at the demands of the trained nurse. During the first epidemics of influenza, when, if a member of the family sneezed, a nurse was telephoned for, the profession reaped an aftermath of adverse criticism. In many cases skilled nursing was not needed, yet the usual fee must be paid, and chagrin at the unnecessary outlay was heaped upon the nurse's innocent head.

The rebound from the discomforts endured at the hands of the Gamp class has led to an unreasonable expectation with regard to the modern nurse. People are so astonished if she is not an absolute paragon of perfection. The general cry of patients and their friends is for a nurse with a sweet sympathetic face, a melodious voice, noiseless manner, and pacific demeanour. She must be a beautiful reader, and able to play and sing if desired. She must be willing to take advice from older people, not intrude her own opinions, be conciliatory to the servants, do without off time and sleep if circumstances require it. Also, she must show marked aversion to male society. Of course she is expected to nurse her patient well, but take the advice of the family as to what he should eat. If her religious and political opinions coincide with those of her employers for the time being, it is greatly in her favour.

Still, though the modern private nurse is, I think, in many respects a victim to unreasonable expectations on the part of the community, it cannot be denied that there is some ground for the strictures levelled at her. To be a private nurse is a severe test of character. A woman who is one month pampered and petted in the mansion of the rich, and in the next is called to nurse amidst the small economies of a struggling professional man's home, is apt to lose balance of judgment and treat her poorer patients to the imperious airs, impossible demands, and unsympathetic attitude of which one hears so much. The constant change from place to place, family to family, and sometimes country to country, is apt to induce an unsettled disposition, and the desire to get the best for themselves out of everybody breeds intolerable selfishness in some nurses. Superintendents of nursing institutions sadly bear testimony to the deterioration of character which they observe in some private nurses, who evidently have not been fitted to withstand the tests or the temptations of the life.

One finds it difficult, however, to take seriously the people who affirm that Sairey Gamp was on the whole a more satisfactory person than the modern trained nurse. The treatment of disease has absolutely changed since those "good old times;" nursing now plays such an important part in the recovery of the patient that doctors seem each year to demand greater efficiency on the part of the nurse. Can one imagine Sir Frederick Treves performing an operation with Sairey Gamp or Betsey Prig at his side?

One cannot put back the hands of the clock, or stem the progress of medical science, and the nurse in her highest function is the co-operator with the doctor. If anything goes wrong with the patient, the nurse has usually to take the blame. The private nurse does not require less, but more training. The majority of

complaints made against private nurses are in relation
to character and behaviour, and rarely have to do with
technical skill, and one feels that complaints would be
considerably lessened if all nurses intending to take up
private work went through a special training on similar
lines to those laid down for Queen's Nurses. The
brilliantly certificated graduate of a great hospital training-
school has much to learn and unlearn before she can
successfully nurse people in their own homes. Like her
sister, the district nurse, she has, if in a lesser degree, to
learn to do without. A patient's home cannot be made
into an up-to-date hospital, and the successful nurse must
stoop to make-shifts. To worry anxious relatives to
supply her patient with countless things which they can
ill afford to buy is a thoughtless and mistaken policy. It
is inexplicable to the lay mind that, while highly trained
women of education and refinement will do as district
nurses the most menial offices for the poor, and tax
their ingenuity to the utmost to improvise appliances to
save outlay, the private nurse is so often lacking in the
accommodating spirit when in the home of the paying
patient of limited means.

The district nurse has to learn tactful management,
and get her wishes carried out by the gentle arts of suggestion and persuasion. The open window, the daily
ablutions, and the turning out of germ preserves have to
be effected by diplomacy. If she entered the poorest
one-roomed tenement with the air of a dictator, she would
be ordered out even though the patient died. The
lessons in dealing with the foibles of human nature, and
the art of sympathetic management which the Queen's
Nurse learns during her probationary period in her
district training-home, are a necessary equipment for the
nurse who enters the homes of paying patients. She is
apt to forget that she is not dealing with the recipients of
charity in a public hospital governed by set rules, but with
people who are her employers and expect to be masters
in their own homes. The family doctor maintains his

dignity, self-respect, and popularity by managing his patients. The present is, however, a transition period, and when the private nurse has been longer in an assured professional position, she, like the family doctor, will have learned the value of the *suaviter in modo* attitude.

The matrons and superintendents of the best private nursing institutions and associations recognize the need for special training for private nursing for the nurse who has just quitted her hospital training-school, and do their best to exercise an influence in this direction. Complaints from patients are investigated, and if sufficient cause is shown the nurse is removed from the register of her association, society, or hospital institute. But, alas! only too frequently she gravitates to a third-rate association, to some fraud on the public in the shape of a Nursing Home, or sets up in " practice " for herself, and there is nothing to prevent her remaining a terror and a danger to the community so long as she can impose on credulous people who do not demand her record.

The first attempts to train and organize nurses for private families began, as we have already seen, with the starting of Mrs. Fry's Institution of Nursing Sisters in 1840, and the foundation of St. John's House in 1847. These were followed by the All Saints' Sisterhood and other religious communities, which came into being on the wave of the Tractarian movement, and had for their objects the care of the sick poor, and the supplying of nurses to private families and hospitals.

In 1869 the Mildmay Nursing Home was founded as a branch of the religious and philanthropic work started by the late Mrs. Pennefather, and remains one of the oldest established nursing institutions in London. From the beginning the nurses went into private families, and one district nurse was kept for work amongst the poor in the parish of St. Jude's, Mildmay Park. The nurses were trained in the large hospitals by the Mildmay institution, and were expected to remain on the staff for three years. A pension scheme was started to provide for their future. Now, however, only nurses who are engaged on that understanding are eligible for a pension. Nurses now receive a salary of forty pounds per year and a commission of three per cent. on their earnings. All the surplus revenue of the nursing branch is devoted to the benefit of the nursing staff. Nurses are cared for when ill, and provided with medical attendance. The institution is federated to the Royal Pension Fund for Nurses. Mildmay has a staff of fifty fully trained and certificated nurses, who live in the nurses' house at 10, Newington Green, N., which is one of the most interesting old houses in London. It dates from the reign of Henry VIII., and has some good oak carving. It has always been the aim of Mildmay to get nurses with a high ideal of their calling, and who are actuated by a love of their work. The institution, though imbued with a religious spirit, is unsectarian, and has no rigid rules, except that it is thought best for the nurses to be total abstainers. The superintendent of the Nurses' House is Miss Annie Carter, and it is under the direction of Mrs. Tottenham, who is the head of the women's work at Mildmay. There is a mission hospital and dispensary at Austin Street, Bethnal Green, where probationers are received for three years' training.

The nursing world received its second great period of quickening at the outbreak of the Franco-German War, and the result is seen not only in a greater interest in military nursing, but in the foundation of three important associations for private nurses—the Royal Scottish Nursing Institution, 1872, the London Association of Nurses, 1873, and Miss M'Alpin's Training Home for Nurses, Glasgow, 1874.

The Royal Scottish is the pioneer of nursing institutions in Scotland, and is the oldest and largest in Edinburgh. It was started in 1872, under the patronage of the Duke of Buccleuch, with four nurses. Now [1906] it has one hundred and fifty on the staff, including fifteen probationers, and has further advanced its usefulness by the opening, December 5, 1904, of an admirably equipped surgical and medical Nursing Home at 20, Torphichen Street. The parent Home is at 69, Queen Street. Queen Victoria granted the designation of "Royal" to the institution in 1877, when the Duchess of Edinburgh became patroness.

The marked success of the institution is mainly due to the untiring energy and great organizing ability of Miss Dundas, the first honorary secretary, who worked for a period of upwards of thirty years with unflagging zeal, until enfeebled health compelled her to relinquish the duties. Lady Warrender, the first president, and an influential committee of ladies, ably supported Miss Dundas in her efforts. Upon the death of Lady Warrender in 1875, Miss Dundas became president of the institution, without, however, relinquishing her work as honorary secretary.

Another name much honoured in the profession, and very dear to Royal Scottish nurses, is that of Miss Harland, who was appointed matron of the institution in 1875, and devoted herself to the work for nineteen years.

The "Royal Scottish" is the only Nurses' Home in Edinburgh which is not run on co-operative lines. It has a pension fund for its nurses, which was started soon after the establishment of the Home. A nurse is entitled to fifteen pounds a year after fifteen years' service, twenty pounds after twenty years' service, and twenty-five pounds after twenty-five years' service. A new regulation was made some six years ago to meet the views of younger nurses who felt that fifteen years was a long time to wait for the pension. Now, a nurse may go on the pension fund or take a bonus. The bonus is paid at the end of each year, and varies with the profits, which are counted according to the number of weeks which the nurse works. The highest bonus has been about twelve pounds. There is no special age for retirement, but the pension nurses who desire to do so may take their pension. They are, however, prohibited from nursing within a ten-mile radius of the Home. Many of the nurses also belong to the Royal National Pension Fund. The Royal Scottish nurses have a three years' training at one of the large hospitals in England or Scotland. The salaries are from thirty pounds to forty pounds per year. Miss King, R.R.C., the present matron, was appointed in 1897. She was an army sister for ten years, and went through two campaigns in Egypt. Miss King has received the Royal Red Cross, the Egyptian War medal, and the Khedive's Star in bronze.

Mrs. Kirke, who succeeded Miss Dundas as honorary secretary, has indefatigably worked with her husband, Colonel Kirke, late C.K.E., Sc. Dist., to establish the Surgical and Medical Nursing Home, recently started in connection with the institution, on a sound commercial basis. The Home has a splendidly equipped operating theatre. The patients' rooms are very bright and attractive, and owe much to Mrs. Kirke's taste and ingenious devices for comfort. The aim is to benefit gentle-people at moderate fees. The matron is Miss Louisa Burton, a thoroughly skilled medical and surgical nurse, who was formerly in charge of Professor Clarke's surgical ward in the Royal Infirmary, Glasgow.

Some years ago the Royal Scottish extended its borders and started a branch at Carlisle. This was, however, removed in 1895 to Dumfries, the pleasant border town sacred to the memories of Bruce, Burns, Scott, and Carlyle, where there is a nicely appointed Home in Castle Street, with twenty nurses constantly employed. The matron is Miss Sutherland.

Amongst Scottish nursing pioneers no name is more honoured than that of Miss M'Alpin, a lady of independent means, who founded, in 1874, the Glasgow Training Home for Nurses, 250, Renfrew Street, the first of the kind established in Scotland. For thirty-two years Miss M'Alpin has given her services as honorary lady superintendent of the Home.

Miss M'Alpin's attention was first drawn to the need of trained private nursing by an experience of serious illness in her own family, when only a nurse of the "Gamp" order was available. Encouraged by some medical men of her acquaintance, Miss M'Alpin made a beginning in a modest house in St. George's Road, Glasgow, with one nurse and one patient. She had determined that the venture should be on a business footing, and resolved that she would not start the Home until the expenses were paid, and a thousand pounds in hand. Her friends told her she was mad. Miss M'Alpin is a woman of religious faith and striking personality, and was not to be daunted. The Home was opened free of debt, and with a thousand pounds in hand, on February 9, 1874, and from that time until the present it has never been in debt.

For a fortnight Miss M'Alpin waited before she could get a nurse, the occupation being regarded, even at that comparatively recent period, as very inferior. At length a lady friend called with the tidings that she had found a nurse, and next day another lady brought a patient, and so the work was started, and since then neither patients nor nurses have ever been lacking. From this small beginning the Nursing Home has grown until it now requires the services of more than one hundred nurses, and about one thousand cases annually pass through the books. The object of the institution was to supply trained women of high character as nurses for the sick, and to employ them either in the Home or in private families.

The idea was a benevolent one, and originated with the desire to enable people of moderate means to obtain trained nursing, either in the Home, as in surgical cases, or in their own residences, and the scheme has not been developed for the purpose of making profits. Any accumulation of funds, arising either from profitable business or from the subscription list, has been devoted to the purchase and extension of buildings, and to the increase and betterment of the staff. The institution is managed by an influential Board of Directors. Miss M'Alpin's services as superintendent are honorary, and for twenty-seven years her sister worked with her as honorary secretary. The names of these ladies are honoured in the religious and philanthropic world of Glasgow for their unselfish efforts to ameliorate the condition of the sick and distressed. Miss M'Alpin has taken a keen interest in the progress of hospital and district nursing, and is a much appreciated visitor in the wards of the Royal Infirmary.

Miss M'Alpin trains her own nurses, and will not take any who have been elsewhere. She is not in favour of the hospital system for nurses who are to engage in private work. Probationers are received between the ages of twenty-five and thirty for a month's trial, and if satisfactory they enter the service of the institution for three and a half years and undergo a course of training. Lectures are given twice a week by the visiting medical staff, and practical work is taught in the Home. The nurses have to pass stiff examinations in technical studies and practical work. No premium is required, but nurses give their time for the first six months, and receive board, lodging, uniform, and laundry free. The salaries are from fourteen pounds to twenty pounds, rising to thirty pounds per annum, if the nurse re-engages on the expiration of her term. Wages and bonuses are assured, whatever decrease takes place in earnings, and the nurses of the Home have first claim for residence in the convalescent home at Busby, founded by the late Dr. Samuel Johnstone Moore. A new block has recently been built to the Home, and provides excellent rooms for patients, and a well-equipped operating theatre.

Since Miss M'Alpin founded her Nursing Home for private patients, such institutions have spread to all parts of the kingdom; some are excellent, and others irredeemably bad. There is no occasion to dwell on the scandals which from time to time crop up in connection with nursing and surgical Homes. In some fees are extortionate and nurses inferior, but when well managed and staffed, Nursing Homes are a great convenience to the community. Princess Christian's admirably equipped Nursing Home at Windsor is a model of its kind.

For the first thirty years of the movement, the private nursing institutions were conducted on the lines of employing nurses at a stated salary, while the entire profits arising from the fees of patients became the property of the institution. A step in advance for securing better remuneration for the private nurse was made in 1873, when Miss Maria Firth formed the London Association of Nurses, 123, New Bond Street. It is claimed that this is the first organization which secured to nurses a proper remuneration for their work. Miss Firth may therefore be regarded as the pioneer of the principle of payment since developed in the Nurses' Co-operative Associations.

Miss Firth was a woman of a singularly unselfish and devoted life, and with ideas greatly in advance of her time. She practised medicine before women could hold diplomas, and was remarkably successful. Most of her patients were unable to pay her, but the joy of restoring some poor woman to health and enabling her to resume her work as bread-winner was its own reward. She held what were considered at the time very advanced views with regard to women's work and remuneration, and it was her strong sense of justice which induced her to establish the Association of Nurses.

She was led to nursing work when a comparatively young woman by an incident which occurred while on a visit to a relative. A member of the family was taken seriously ill, and Miss Firth volunteered to nurse him. The case was a very serious one, and the physician in attendance was so struck by Miss Firth's competence as a nurse, that he said to her, "I do not know what your occupation in life is, but I am sure God intended you for a nurse." She acted upon the suggestion, and went for training in midwifery to Queen Charlotte's Hospital, and, after a little experience in private nursing, became matron of the Lying-in-Hospital, Endell Street. It was then in a wretched condition, the building old, the conditions insanitary, and so many of the patients died from puerperal fever that the women almost regarded it as a death warrant to be brought there. With the consent of the Governor, Miss Firth set to work to reform the hospital, and, single-handed, gathered the money to rebuild some of the wards, and completely renovated the others. The death rate from being the highest became one of the lowest in such institutions. In recognition of her service she was made a Life Governor of the hospital. Miss Firth remained at Endell Street until her health broke down, and she was obliged to take a long rest. Later she became lady superintendent of Mrs. Ranyard's Bible-women Nurses.

In the course of her work Miss Firth was moved with the desire to improve the condition of nurses, whom she felt did not receive adequate remuneration from the institutions and hospitals which they served. While it was the fashion of the day to denounce the nurse for her lack of education and training, Miss Firth saw the other side of the question, and felt that good conditions and remuneration for the workers was an important factor in raising the standard of nursing. In a booklet, "The Hospital Nurse," printed for private circulation, Miss Firth gives some of the experiences of the then hospital nurse. "No, I don't complain of the pay itself (from ten pounds to twenty pounds per year), though it was hard-earned," said one, "but I didn't like hospital work all the same; an' I don't think nurses get a fair chance there. I know when I was night-nurse I'd to come on at 11 p.m., an' stay till 4 p.m. on the following day. I'd to give the patients their meals an' medicines, cook my own food an' some of the patients', an' do all the dressings; an', ma'am, I think it was too much for one woman to do properly. As to my meals, I could hardly

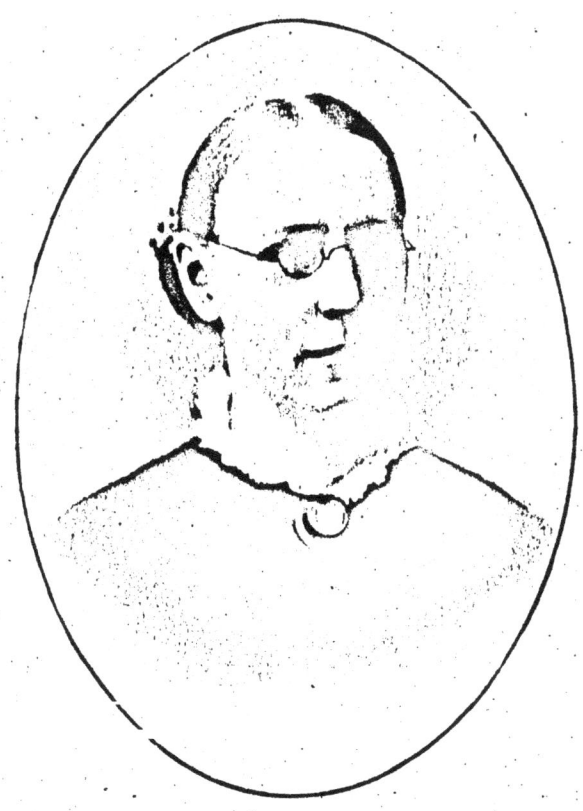

Miss MARIA FIRTH.

Founder and First Superintendent of the London Association of Nurses.

[To face p. 272.

get time to take 'em at all. It was generally a chop or steak, because that took quickest to cook; but, bless you, m'm, it as often as not got charred up to a cinder, an' then as cold as ice twice over afore I'd time to eat it; an' then only by a mouthful at a time. As to vegetables, they was out of the question; an' the tea stood on the hob all day simmerin' and stewin', till it was more like boiled cabbage-leaves than anything else." Such were the conditions of a nurse's life in the good old times!

Miss Firth began her experiment for the amelioration of the nurse's lot in her own home in London, where she received seven or eight nurses. She found them private work, and allowed them to take the whole of their earnings subject to a small commission for office expenses and advertisement. The numbers grew rapidly. Great care was taken in the selection of the nurses, and in suiting the nurse to the special patient. Miss Firth had the faculty in a very marked degree of creating an *esprit de corps* amongst her workers, and they regarded her with peculiar love and veneration. She was nevertheless a strict disciplinarian, and instantly dismissed from the Association a woman who gave way to intemperance. The culprit was not lost sight of, and every means was used to help her to recover herself. Miss Firth had a faith in men and women which sometimes led her to be deceived, but more frequently led to the redemption of the fallen one. "Do good unto all men, despairing of no one," was the motto upon which she acted.

The following testimony to Miss Firth's beautiful character is borne by her niece, Miss Moorhouse, for so many years the Principal of Greenhill House School, Stourbridge: "A nature so absolutely free from selfishness I never knew. She seemed to have a heart big enough to cradle all the human race. She literally 'went about doing good.' She said to me once, when I remonstrated with her on working far beyond her strength, 'When any one asks me for help I feel it is the voice of God speaking, and I must obey if it is at all possible to do what is asked.' No one knows the number of women who were helped up, and set on their feet, and enabled to earn a living by her. Her self-devotion to the ser- e of the sick and suffering had no bounds. To her the service of humanity was the service of God." Miss Firth died in February, 1882.

The Association which she founded has made great strides since it removed to 123, Bond Street, in 1887. It met a great public need at a time when there was very limited provision for the supply of private nurses, and for many years it was the only nursing institution which secured to the workers their earnings. It is superintended and managed by ladies intimately connected with Miss Firth's family, who make it their aim to carry out the ideals of the founder. Miss Briggs, the acting superintendent of the Association, has been connected with it for twenty years. She was trained under Miss Firth, and is ably assisted by her sister and Miss Firth's niece, Miss Sipman.

A three years' course of hospital training and satisfactory references as to character are indispensable qualifications for membership. Nurses taking mental cases only must have had three years' training in an asylum containing not less than fifty beds, or a year's training in a general hospital in addition to two years' training in an asylum. Nurses taking maternity cases only must hold a monthly or midwifery certificate from a lying-in hospital, and also have had a year's training in a general hospital. During the first year a salary of thirty-five pounds or more is given, and the nurse when not at work resides in one of the Homes belonging to the Association, of which there are four. At the end of the year of probation—in which the previously trained hospital nurse is receiving her special training for private nursing—the nurse is placed upon the staff, and instead of a salary receives her earnings, less a percentage, which varies with the amount of the fees. Between cases the nurse boards at a very moderate fee in one of the residential Homes of the Association. One Home is reserved for nurses who have been in attendance on infectious cases, another is specially reserved for the monthly nurses, who usually devote themselves entirely to this branch of work. The London Association now employs about two hundred and fifty nurses. The staff is varied as much as possible, so that all cases can be suitably supplied. The fees are moderate, and range from one and a half to three guineas a week. Miss Firth's nurses have held high places of trust. One was attached to the royal nursery of Russia, another was for several years with the late Lord Tennyson, and several have served with the Army Nursing Service, and one of the number, Sister Emma Durham, has received the Royal Red Cross.

The first nurses' association to take the name of "co-operative" was founded in London in 1891, some eight years after Miss Firth's pioneer association. It was called the Nurse's Co-operation, and provided not only that the members should take their earnings less a percentage, but that the society should be managed on co-operative lines. It claims to be the oldest and largest association of the kind in existence. The headquarters are at 8, New Cavendish Street, Portland Place. It owes its existence chiefly to Miss Mary Belcher (now Mrs. Belcher Houghton), who originated the proposal that private nurses should be enabled to co-operate for their mutual advantage. Miss Honor Morten gave assistance in formulating a workable scheme, which was taken up by Sir Henry, then Mr., Burdett, and other gentlemen. Financial aid was given by Mr. Cheston and Mr. Slaughter, who advanced £100 and £200 respectively. Four nurses came forward with loans. Miss Belcher lent £75, Miss Ward £50, Miss Napper £25, and Miss R. Napper £50. They were protected from risk by their loan of £200 being underwritten by the late Mr. Burns. They received an interest of 4 per cent. until November, 1892, when the capital was repaid. Mr. Cheston and Mr. Slaughter made their advances free gifts to the co-operation. The society thus founded in 1891 was registered in 1894, the Memorandum and Articles of Association being signed, May 13th, by Henry C. Burdett, Herbert P. Hawkins, Mary M. Belcher, Charles Cheston, solicitor, and W. Capel Slaughter, solicitor. The signatures were witnessed by Miss Honor Morten.

The articles provide that ten representatives of the nurses of the society shall be on the committee of management. These are elected annually in general meeting to fill vacancies created by compulsory retirement in rotation or otherwise. The committee of management consists of seventeen persons, seven being elected from members of the co-operation, two of whom retire annually, but are eligible for re-election.

Members of the co-operation are elected by the committee of management, after being proposed by two or more members, who certify in writing that the candidate is a fit person to be a member. The terms of membership are an annual subscription of one guinea, or compounding of the same by a payment of five guineas.

Candidates must not be over thirty-five years of age. A nurse is not admitted to the general staff unless she has had three years' experience of nursing, and holds a certificate from a recognized training-school attached to a general hospital with over a hundred beds. Recent experience in private nursing is also necessary. Nurses for mental cases only must hold the certificate of the Medico-Psychological Society. Nurses taking maternity cases only must hold a recognized monthly or midwifery certificate, and have had two consecutive years' training in a general hospital.

Nurses receive their own earnings, less 5 per cent. in the case of nurses who joined the co-operation by the end of 1898; $7\frac{1}{2}$ per cent. being paid by the rest of the nurses. It is proposed to add nurses who joined the co-operation during the year 1899, to the list of those paying percentage at the lower rate.

The patroness of the Nurses' Co-operation is Her Royal Highness Princess Louise, Duchess of Argyll, the president is Alice Countess of Strafford there is a list of distinguished vice-presidents. Mrs. Lucas succeeded Miss Roberts as lady superintendent in 1904, the home sister is Miss Baker, and the secretary Miss H. F. Gethen. There are now about four hundred and ninety-one nurses on the general staff, and some twenty-three asylum-trained nurses for mental cases only. There is a Nurses' Home and Club at 8, New Cavendish Street, and the members of the Co-operation have opportunities for meeting each other at the monthly "At Homes."

Another co-operation of private nurses was founded in 1894 under the title of The Registered Nurses' Society, and has its offices at 431, Oxford Street, W. It claims to be the "first co-operation of chartered nurses," and was founded by Mrs. Bedford Fenwick, late matron of St. Bartholomew's Hospital. The objects of the Society are to secure work for fully trained nurses, together with a just remuneration for their services, and to promote the advancement of their calling. Members receive their own earnings, less $7\frac{1}{2}$ per cent. for office expenses, and are encouraged in self-government, six of them always serving upon the executive committee, and retiring in rotation after a term of two years.*

It is estimated that two-thirds of the nurses now take up private work after the completion of their training. Hospital matrons complain that they are constantly losing good nurses who are attracted by the freer life and better chances for making money which private nursing offers. Most of the large hospitals have started private nursing institutions. The pioneer of such institutions was founded in connection with the London Hospital on the suggestion of Miss Lückes, and the youngest is that of St. George's Hospital, opened 1906.

Private nursing is divided into three principal classes—

* The Society of Chartered Nurses was founded on co-operative lines by Mr. T. Mark Hovell in 1896.

the institution nurse, who works for a given salary from the institution where she is trained or to which she attaches herself; the independent nurse, living in her own home and forming a private connection of clients, generally through the recommendation of local medical men ; and the co-operation nurse, who receives her fees minus a percentage paid to her association. The introduction of the co-operative system has given a great impetus to private nursing, and upon that line it seems destined to progress.

At present the middle classes, in respect to trained nursing, are left practically out in the cold. The sick poor are freely provided with skilled nursing in their own homes, or in the hospitals, and the rich can dictate their own terms, but the people of limited means are stranded between the expensive private nurse or doing without a nurse altogether. No reasonable person would wish to have the services of a highly skilled nurse at a less fee than is commensurate with her value and the expense of her training, but means may be arrived at by which the patient is suited at a low fee, and the nurse properly compensated.

The scheme for daily private nursing, which has been growing in practice since 1889, is a step in the right direction. A nurse working independently can make from two pounds to five pounds per week, by paying daily visits to a *clientèle* of patients, requiring partial attention, or several nurses may work a district by co-operating together. Nursing institutions and associations are now finding it desirable to meet public requirements by arranging daily nursing.

An admirable experiment was started in May, 1902, by the Marylebone Daily Visiting Nursing Association, founded by Mrs. Stephen Spring Rice and Miss Ellen Desart, to meet the requirements of those unable to afford or to house a resident nurse. The scheme was floated by a strong committee, and subscriptions solicited for three years. The Association employs a fully trained certified nurse, at a salary of one hundred pounds a year. The

fees for her daily visits are received by the Association.
Since 1905 it has been self-supporting.

The Ada Lewis Nurses' Institute was started in October,
1905, by that well-known philanthropist, Mrs. Ada Lewis
Hill, with the object of providing daily visiting trained
nurses for people of limited means. The duties of the nurse
are confined to washing and dressing the patient, making
the bed, dressing wounds, or applying surgical or medical
treatment, or any nursing required for the immediate
comfort of the patient. The institute is at 62, Oxford
Terrace, Hyde Park, and the nurses visit cases within a
two-mile radius. The minimum fee is five shillings, and
the maximum fee ten shillings per week. The services of
the nurses are much appreciated by residents in small
flats, in private lodgings or boarding-houses, where the
lot of the invalid is often so lonely and sad. Mrs. Lewis
Hill takes the full financial responsibility of the work,
and hopes in the future to further develop the scheme by
starting branch Homes in various London districts. The
work is benevolent, and great care has to be exercised
that only the necessitous are supplied with nurses at
these low fees. An old lady who applied to the institute
soon after it was founded, and who appeared to be a most
distressing case of genteel poverty, was found after her
death to have hoarded a considerable sum of money.
The Ada Lewis nurses wear purple bonnets and cloaks.
The lady superintendent is Miss M. Rye, the daughter
of the late Mr. Rye, F.R.C.S., of St. Bartholomew's
Hospital. She was trained at the Glasgow Royal
Infirmary. Only fully trained and certified nurses are
employed.*

The difficulty of placing trained private nursing within
reach of middle-class people, at moderate fees, but without
the suggestion of charity, might be met by a great central
organization, with branches throughout the kingdom, to
provide daily nurses for paying patients, on similar lines

* Mrs. Lewis Hill died October 13, 1906, and the future of the Institute is unsettled.

to the Queen's Jubilee Institute, or it might be conducted on the co-operative principle. Such an organization might have its own surgical Nursing Homes.

Private nursing must be viewed from the broad national standpoint, and the bitter cry of the middle-classes, that they shall not be left in a worse position in time of sickness than the class below them, is one which the twentieth century has to face. The people who help to support hospitals, and who pay rates for infirmaries and asylums, where the indigent poor have the best medical skill and nursing free, and the doctors and nurses obtain their training, have a decided grievance in the present position of things. The *viâ media* between paying high fees for home nursing or accepting the aid of charitable institutions has yet to be worked out.

CHAPTER XVII

DISTRICT NURSING: ITS RISE AND PROGRESS

District nursing specially commends itself to public favour—Stirring of public opinion in the fifties—Mrs. Ranyard's Bible-women—She starts a nursing branch—Its position to-day—Article on deaconesses in 1860—William Rathbone, M.P., of Liverpool—Founds district nursing—Develops quickly in Liverpool—District nursing in London—The National and Metropolitan Association started 1874—Miss Florence Lees—Her tour of inspection—Report of the sub-committee on district nursing—Miss Nightingale's appeal for funds for a District Nurses' Home—Training of the Bloomsbury Square nurses—The "auld lichts" of the profession—Homes of the London poor—Miss Octavia Hill—The district nurses had to overcome the prejudice of the poor—Steady increase of the Metropolitan Association—Contemporary work in Scotland—The work of religious organizations—Parish nursing—The Alexandra nurses.

THERE is, perhaps, no branch of the profession which so universally commends itself to public favour as that of district nursing, or one which is so well organized and officially inspected. The care of the sick poor in their own homes appeals on the broad ground of common humanity, and has a more far-reaching influence than even the tending of the sick in hospitals, important as that is. The nurse with her bag, threading her lonely way through the crowded courts and alleys of our great cities, crossing the moors to Highland cottage or hut, trudging over the bogs to remote Irish cabins, or climbing the rough mountain roads of Wales, is a figure which commands something akin to veneration. She takes the new-born babe in her arms and gives it the skilled care which ensures it a good start in life, she comforts the dying, tends the chronic cases and the bed-ridden and infirm, and is often the first to note the sign of infectious disease. But she carries more with her than bandages and dressings and technical knowledge. Into the squalid slum she brings an educative and refining presence; teaches by gentle suggestion the laws of health and hygiene, puts heart into the overburdened mother, helps the husband to regain self-respect, brightens the lives of little children, and gives even to the meanest one-roomed tenement the semblance of a home. Though her work may be a form of charity, it engenders the spirit of self-help. To quote the words of Charles Booth, "Of all the forms that charity takes, there is hardly one that is so directly successful as district nursing. It is almost true to say that wherever a nurse enters, the standard of life is raised." And Archdeacon Wilberforce, recently speaking at the Mansion House, said, "Women are to be found at the root of every movement for the benefit of mankind, but the district nurse exercises the most civilizing, humanizing influence of all."

It is difficult to exactly place district nursing in history. It is as old in spirit, if not in organization, as Christian charity. Phœbe, a servant or deaconess of the church at Cenchrea, was commended by St. Paul to the Christians at Rome as one who had been a "succourer of many." The deaconesses of the early Christian Church are the prototypes of the modern district nurse.

To come to recent times, we have seen that the pioneer nursing institutions of Devonshire Square and St. John's House made the nursing of the sick poor in their own homes a branch of their work. It was, however, in the period immediately succeeding the Crimean War that there began to be a general searching of heart amongst philanthropic people regarding the sufferings of the poor in time of sickness, and a desire to formulate some system for their relief. Women were tentatively coming forward as social reformers, encouraged by the more far-seeing and liberal-minded men. Mrs. Jameson's admirable lectures on "Sisters of Charity" and

"Communion of Labour" aroused much attention in
1855-56, and inspired thoughtful women with a desire
to take part in the work of social service. "Practical
Letters to Ladies," by Rev. J. Ll. Davies, was an effort
in the same direction, particularly the Lecture on
"District Visiting." At this period, too, Miss Louisa
Twining was writing vigorous letters to the press on
the neglect of the sick in workhouses. There was,
in brief, an uncomfortable feeling taking root in the
public mind that the sick poor were in a sadly neglected
condition.

The Bible-women and Nurses' Mission, founded by
the late Mrs. Ranyard in 1857, was an important pioneer
effort to remedy the existing evils. The Bible-women
visited the homes of the London poor with the object of
selling Bibles by a system of weekly payments. It was a
part of their duty to try and raise the moral and physical
condition of the families visited by enabling them to buy
not only Bibles, but bedding, clothing, and necessaries for
sickness. In the course of their house-to-house visitation
the Bible-women heard of cases of sickness in need of
nursing, and to meet this need Mrs. Ranyard, in 1868,
started the nursing branch of the Mission. She aimed
from the first at bringing her nurses into touch with the
hospitals, and much good was accomplished by taking
nursing charge of out-patients. The system was one of
district nursing, and Mrs. Ranyard summed up her
ideal in the terse phrase : " Hospital Work outside all
Hospitals." Miss Agnes Jones and Miss Maria Firth
were workers in the early stages of this beneficent movement. Agnes Jones, after achieving at the Liverpool
Infirmary the first great reform in workhouse nursing,
was laid to rest on the day that Mrs. Ranyard initiated
her nursing branch. One of the earliest donors to the
nurse fund was Florence Nightingale, who, with her
contribution, sent the following message :—

" A small gift to the nurses, with Florence Nightingale's
deepest sympathy for this noble attempt to provide

nursing and cleanliness for the very poor, with gratitude to God and fervent prayer for its extension and progress."

The Bible-women nurses formed the first modern Association of any size for district work, and steadily increased in efficiency under the superintendence of Mrs. Ranyard and her successor, Mrs. Selfe Leonard. In June, 1906, this admirable institution celebrated its Jubilee, when Sir Frederick Treves gave the members an inspiring address. Sir Thomas Barlow is honorary consulting physician and a kind friend to the Society. At present the nurses number sixty-five, and are engaged under four superintendent nurses in the poorest districts of London. They are hospital-trained nurses, and work under doctors. Candidates are received for three years' training according to the rules issued at the offices, 2, Adelphi Terrace, Strand. Miss Andrews is the honorary secretary and general superintendent. The Society is dependent on voluntary contributions. In connection with it is the Training-Home for candidates, the Seaside Convalescent Home for patients, and the Home of Rest for members of the staff. The society is federated with the Royal National Pension Fund for Nurses.

An early account of Mrs. Ranyard's mission published in 1859 under the title, "The Missing Link, or Bible-women in the Homes of the London Poor," created considerable interest in the subject. This was followed in 1860, by an able and suggestive article on "Deaconesses of the Church of England" in the *Church Monthly Review*, in which the deaconesses of the Kaiserswerth Institution were described as a model for the kind of nurse-visitor required in this country. "It is beautiful," says the writer, " to see the accomplished parish deaconess visiting. She makes her round in the morning. She performs little offices for the sick, who do not require a nurse living in the house, but which the relations cannot do well ; she teaches the children little trades, knitting, making list shoes, etc., and all this with a cordiality and charm of manner which win sufficient confidence from the parents to induce them to *ask* to be taught to sweep, cook, and put the house in order ; . . . wherever she goes the cottage puts on a tidy appearance." The writer goes on to plead for the establishment of a central home in each parish as the headquarters of a district visiting society—a community of "extra parochial workers" to live in the midst of the poor and carry out a similar work to that of the Kaiserswerth Deaconesses. Through these various channels the leaven had been working until a master of organization initiated a scheme in 1860, which developed into the modern system.

To William Rathbone, M.P., of Liverpool, belongs the honour of being the founder of trained district nursing. The great city on the Mersey has a noble roll of men and women devoted to humanitarian work, and amongst these the name of Rathbone holds an honoured place. Greenbank, the family home on the outskirts of Liverpool, has for more than a century opened its hospitable doors to men and women of light and leading. Its walls have echoed to the voices of William Roscoe, Robert Owen, Dorothea Dix, to the friends of Abolition, and many others whose names are written on the page of history. William Rathbone, sixth of the name, was born to a noble heritage, and his fifty years of social service adds another chapter to the family record. He came of Quaker stock, and his grandmother, who had a notable reign as hostess at "Greenbank," is described as "an exquisite specimen of eighteenth-century Quaker womanhood." She was the admired friend and counsellor of many distinguished men. Her husband, however, was expelled from the Society of Friends for the publication of "A Narrative of Events that have recently taken place in Ireland among the Society called Quakers," and her son, the father of William Rathbone, having married a lady of Unitarian family, finally joined the Unitarian body. The Quaker connection is interesting in the case of Mr. Rathbone, as the Friends have been prominently associated with pioneer efforts on behalf of nursing both in this country and in America.

In a private memorandum, written in the closing years of his life, Mr. Rathbone thus modestly estimates his work: "If I were to venture to express what seems to me the lesson of my own life by an adapted proverb, I should say, 'Great are the uses of mediocrity!'" Though his personality was not one to dazzle the popular mind, few men have toiled more strenuously, conscientiously, and modestly for the public weal than William Rathbone. In Parliament and in civic affairs he laboured in the cause of education and social reform, but the movement with which his name is most intimately associated as a pioneer is that of nursing. In 1890, he published "The History and Progress of District Nursing," and to this record, the admirable memoir of William Rathbone by his daughter, Miss Eleanor Rathbone, adds some intimate touches of his connection with that work.

Private grief first drew him to an interest in the subject. In 1859, Mr. Rathbone was left a widower with five little children, the youngest of whom was an infant a few days old. His wife had been much comforted in her sufferings by the skill of a nurse, Mary Robinson, and the circumstances brought home to William Rathbone the cruel fate of the poor who lacked comforts, appliances, and skilled nursing in time of sickness, and he determined to try an experiment. He engaged Nurse Robinson for three months, and, furnishing her with necessary appliances and medical comforts, sent her to a certain district in Liverpool to nurse the sick poor. At the end of a month the nurse returned, and begged, with tears in her eyes, to be released from her engagement as she could not bear to witness so much misery. Mr. Rathbone encouraged her to persevere, with the result that when the three months was up, she declared her determination to devote herself wholly to the nursing of the poor, the good she had been able to do and the gratitude of her patients having led her to this resolve. Not only had lives been saved, patients considered chronic restored to health, but a moral and sanitary influence had been exercised in the homes. Husbands who had given way to drink from sheer hopelessness and misery, when the wife was laid low by sickness, returned to habits of sobriety, after nurse's care had made the home inviting.

Mr. Rathbone now sought to extend his operations, but was confronted with the usual difficulty—there were no suitable nurses to be found. This was in 1860-61, and as yet the Nightingale School at St. Thomas's and the St. John's House Nursing Institution at King's College were the only hospitals in London with training-schools, and they had no sisters or nurses to spare for Liverpool. Mr. Rathbone consulted Miss Nightingale, who, with characteristic common sense, suggested that Liverpool should start a training-school of its own. This was subsequently effected, as related in Chapter IX., by the founding of the "Liverpool Training-School and Home for Nurses," in 1862, one object of which was to provide nurses for poor patients in their own homes.

The organization of district nursing now quickly developed, and by 1865, six years from the time Nurse Robinson started on her lonely work, the whole of Liverpool had been divided into eighteen districts, each presided over by a lady or group of lady superintendents, and placed under the care of a paid nurse. A paid inspector superintended the nursing. So eager was Mr. Rathbone to see exactly how the system worked, that in the early stages of the movement he took the place, for a year, of an absent lady superintendent, overlooking arrangements and accounts, and even going once a week with the nurse to visit her patients. He was thus able to gauge the work from intimate knowledge.

In the organization of the districts, Mr. Rathbone was greatly aided by Mr. Charles Langton, who for thirty-five years made it his special care to find lady superintendents for the districts. So successful was Mr.

Langton in his choice that in 1898 there were no less than six ladies, Mrs. W. Rathbone, Mrs. C. Langton, Mrs. H. B. Gilmour, Mrs. Paget, Mrs. G. Holt, and Mrs. R. D. Holt, who had held the office of superintendent for thirty years. The work became something of a family heritage, in some cases being handed on from mother to daughter.

The chief difficulty connected with district nursing was to avoid pauperizing the people by indiscriminate charity, as with the compulsory attendance of children at school, the question of food inevitably came in. A half-starved child is not in a condition to profit by instruction; and yet to provide free meals lessens parental responsibility. In like manner, when the recovery of a patient largely depends on suitable nourishment and medical comforts which the home resources cannot supply, the nurse feels that in some way the need must be met. The superintendent of each district had at her command funds subscribed for such charitable purposes, and at first there was a danger of district nurses becoming little more than mere almoners. In one of the Liverpool districts the yearly amount p for relief and medical comforts was about two hundred pounds, including forty pounds for stimulants. One superintendent set the example of giving plenty of milk and very little stimulant, which was followed by many other ladies. By degrees, the doles became less, the nursing more efficient and the system was worked on more professional lines. In cases of extreme poverty, the aid of the parish authorities was called in or help solicited from charitable agencies. A nurse was to be a nurse, not a district visitor in the old sense of the term.

In 1868, the first District Nursing Association was founded in London, by the Honourable Mrs. Stuart Wortley and Mr. Robert Wigram, under the name of the East London Nursing Society, now affiliated to the Queen Victoria Jubilee Institute. The central office is 43, Rutland Street, E. In the same year was formed, as

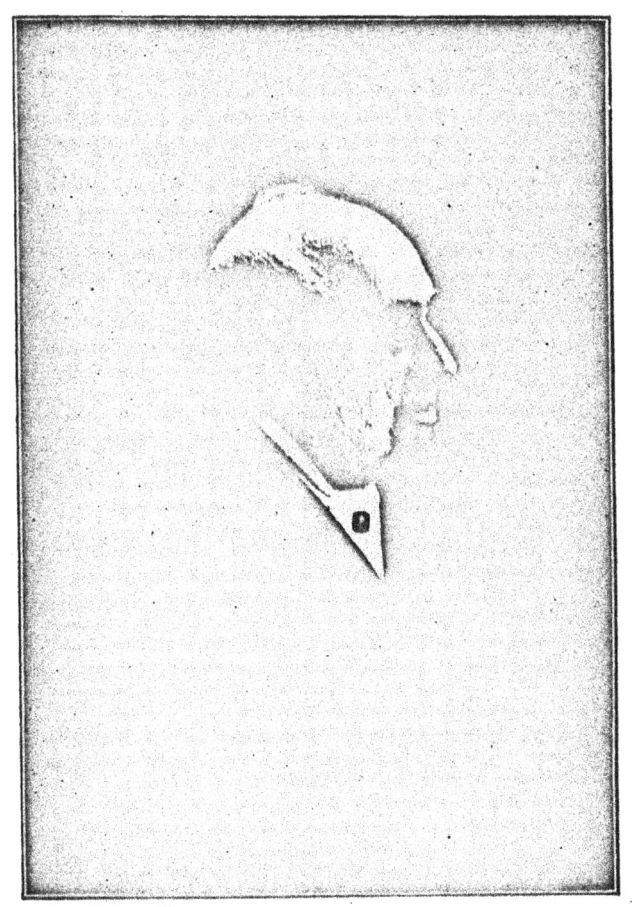

WILLIAM RATHBONE, ESQ., M.P.

The Originator of Trained District Nursing.

(*By permission of Miss Eleanor Rathbone, Author of "William Rathbone—A Memoir."*)

[*To face p.* 288.

we have seen, the Nursing Branch of the London Biblewomen and Nurses' Mission. These societies did useful pioneer work in London.

An important step in advance was made in 1874, when Sir Edmund Lechmere and others, connected with the English Branch of the Order of St. John of Jerusalem, met in London, to consider an organization for district nursing in the metropolis. The result was " The National Association for providing Trained Nurses for the Sick Poor." The late Duke of Westminister was an active supporter of the scheme, and consulted Mr. Rathbone, who, on account of parliamentary duties, lived in London for half the year. A sub-committee of inquiry was appointed, of which Mr. Rathbone became chairman, and Lady Strangford and Miss Florence Lees (now Mrs. Dacre Craven), honorary secretaries. Its members also included Dr. (afterwards Sir Henry) W. D. Acland, Bart., F.R.S., etc., Regius Professor at Oxford, Sir Rutherford Alcock, K.C.B., Mr. Henry Bonham Carter, Sir James Stansfeld, G.C.B., Dr. Sir Edward Sieveking, and others. The object of the committee of inquiry was to ascertain how far existing institutions throughout the country fulfilled the requirements of nursing the sick poor in their own homes, and teaching and introducing among them rules of health, cleanliness, order, and ventilation.

Miss Florence Lees was entrusted with the important task of making a tour of inspection. Miss Lees was one of the earliest Nightingale probationers at St. Thomas's Hospital, and, like her illustrious chief, had quitted a life of social ease to devote herself to nursing. She spent some time at Kaiserswerth, and visited hospitals abroad. She volunteered for service on the outbreak of the Franco-German War, and was placed in charge of the second fever station of the 10th Army Corps at Marangue, before Metz. When that was closed, Miss Lees accepted the Crown Princess of Germany's (the late Empress Frederick) invitation to superintend her

Lazarette for the wounded soldiers at Homburg, and was favoured with many marks of esteem from members of the Prussian royal family. In 1873, Miss Lees inspected the nursing in the principal hospitals in the United States and Canada, and immediately after her return from this tour entered upon work on behalf of district nursing.

One of the chief requisites for a nurse amongst the poor is that she shall nurse the home as well as the patient, or rather that she shall see that the home, be it only a top attic in a dingy court, is kept in " nursing order," and often she has to help in bringing about that reformation with her own hands. It was in this particular, quite as much as in lack of knowledge of the technique of nursing, that the early district nurses were lacking. Miss Lees visited all the leading centres of the work which had been established throughout the country, and was constantly confronted with the nurse whose dignity was touched if it was suggested that she should make a dirty room clean. The women then employed largely came from the same class as their patients, and the few months' training given them in hospital had inflated them with foolish importance. The lady superintendent of the district was untrained also, and more disposed to order comforts than to criticize the nursing, and was afraid of offending the dignity of the nurse by suggesting that she should do anything for her patient beyond dosing and feeding. " I never sweep patients' rooms, ma'am," was an answer often received by Miss Lees ; " nurses are not expected to do anything menial. Our visiting lady (the superintendent) pays a woman to come and clean up now and then." On another occasion it would be, " No, indeed, ma'am, I've no time to wash patients and comb their hair. I am here to nurse, and have a lot of patients to go round." The old district nurse considered that her duty lay in giving milk and beef-tea, and " doing dressings." It did not occur to her to examine the drainage or water-supply, to rout out dirty clothes and refuse from under beds, to disinfect and ventilate the patient's room, or instruct the family in these matters. A special fault was the large amount of relief given, while, says Miss Lees, "the pseudo-doctoring and surgery done by these women was appalling!" "She could cure it without a doctor," or "leave your finger to me, I'll save it," was talk characteristic of this order of nurse, and the "saving" sometimes ended in the finger producing blood-poisoning and causing death. Many of these nurses were little more than "Sairey Gamps" and "Betsey Prigs," with a thin veneer of training.

A turning-point in the history of district nursing came in June, 1875, when, after the investigation into the condition of the work, the sub-committee of inquiry issued a report, which defined the object of the newly formed National Association as being the organization of a system of training and supplying district nurses for the whole country. "We have seen," it runs, "through the eyes of a trained nurse [Miss Florence Lees] of the very highest grade, the actual working of the best organized district nursing systems in London and other towns." It was found that the metropolis had only two organizations, already referred to, which supplied trained nurses for the sick poor in their own homes, viz. the Bible and Domestic Female Mission, employing fifty-two Bible-women nurses, and the East London Nursing Society, which employed seven district nurses. London had in all about one hundred nurses engaged in district work, and of these one-third were untrained, and could do little save in the administration of nourishment, medical comforts, and general relief.

The existing system was found to be open to grave objections, which may be summarized as—

1. Too much relief, and too little nursing.

2. Too little control and direction, and consequent lapses into slovenliness and neglect, sometimes dangerous to the very lives of her patients, on the part of the nurse.

3. Too little communication between the nurse and the doctor.

4. Too little instruction given to the patient's friends and family in regard to the care of the sufferer, to ventilation, cleanliness, disinfecting, etc.

The recommendations of the sub-committee were, in brief, that the nurses should have systematic hospital training, based on Miss Nightingale's suggestions, to make them real aids to the doctors. They were to work under trained superintendents and devote themselves entirely to nursing, while the work of granting relief should be left to parish authorities, district visitors, and charitable agencies. Hitherto the district nurse had lived in private lodgings, and an important provision of the new organization was that in London and large towns Homes for the district nurses should be established and placed under the management of highly trained superintendents. These Homes were to be places of residence for the nurses engaged in the district, and of training for probationers in district nursing. The Association adopted the principles of the report. The sub-committee were thanked for their labours, and the liberality of Mr. Rathbone in defraying the expenses in connection with the inquiry was warmly acknowledged.

Florence Nightingale made a special plea in the *Times*, April 14, 1876, for funds to establish a central Home for district nurses in connection with the National Society, or, as it had been renamed, "The Metropolitan and National Association." She had been in close touch with the Committee throughout its work, and now pleaded with characteristic eloquence that the nurses who were to be factors in reforming the homes of the poor, should themselves be suitably housed. Her plea aroused special interest in the work, and eventually the Central Home and Training-School for Nurses was established at 23, Bloomsbury Square.

Miss Florence Lees, who had already done such valuable work on behalf of the National Association, was appointed Superintendent-General, and had special charge of the Home and the branches to be formed in connection

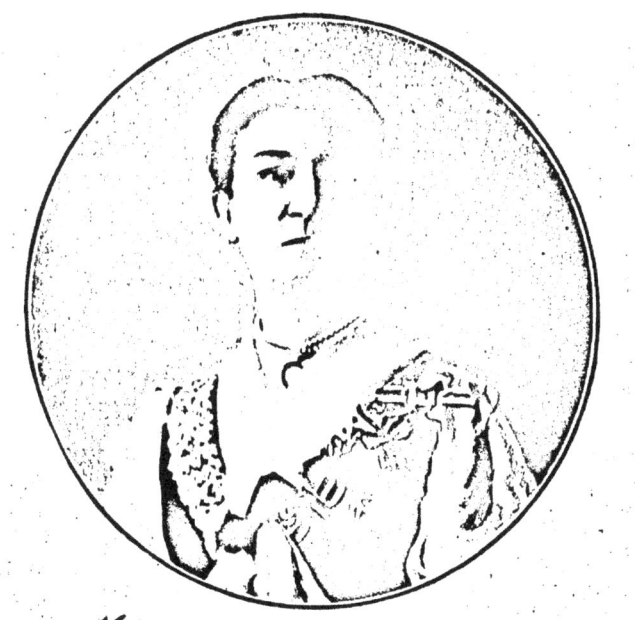

Florence S. Craven

Mrs. Dacre Craven.

(*Photograph by Barrauds.*)

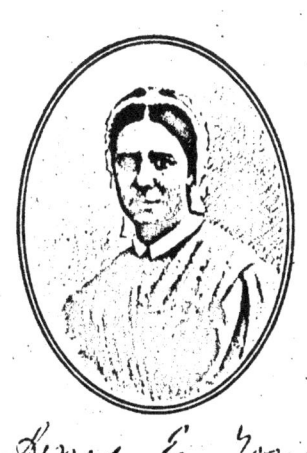

Agnes E. Jones.

with it. She was a strong advocate for making district nursing a profession for educated women, and gathered around her nurses of superior social position. When the Crown Princess of Germany (the Empress Frederick) visited the Home in Bloomsbury Square, Miss Lees was able to preface the individual introduction of her staff to the Princess by the remark that all were eligible for presentation at Court, and several had been presented. This feeling was a rebound from the want of breeding and education of the old class of district nurses. Moreover, it was highly necessary to attract to the work gentlewomen who should become trained superintendents and take the place of the lady bountifuls and amateur superintendents of the old system.

The new organization had to combat the idea that any respectable working-class woman is good enough to nurse the sick poor, and that a district nurse is not in need of such thorough training as a hospital nurse. To quote a medical man of the time, what was needed for the sick poor in their homes was, " a calm, steady discipline existing but unfelt; the patient, cool control which a stranger, if a trained nurse, is far more likely to exercise than a relation ; and the experience of illness to note changes and call for aid when really needed, as well as to recognize symptoms and correctly report them." While the hospital nurse is in constant touch with the doctor, the district nurse sees him but once in twenty-four hours, or even a much longer period, and should be able to give provisional treatment if necessary. A highly trained and superior woman was needed to be a real aid to the medical man, capable of teaching the laws of health, and of such nobility of character that she was willing to become a servant of the sick poor.

The nurses of the Association were required to pass (1) A month's trial in district work ; (2) a year's training in hospital nursing ; (3) six months' training in district nursing, combined with attendance at a special course of theoretical instruction given at the Central Home by qualified medical men, and tested by written and *viva voce* examination at the end of each course. The nurse was not permitted to give alms to her patients, but where help was a necessity it was her duty to report the case to the parish authorities or a charitable agency. She was not only to nurse the sick poor, but reform and recreate their homes—show the family how to clean, sweep, dust, air, disinfect, and teach habits of personal cleanliness. It was the golden rule of the Association that wherever a nurse entered, order and cleanliness should enter too.

The auld lichts of the " profession " sniffed the air in disdain at " them Bloomsbury nurses," to whom they probably added the epithet " bloomin' " not in a complimentary sense. " If I was you, I wouldn't send for the parish doctor," counselled one of the fraternity to a poor woman with a wound in her leg; " because the first thing he'll do will be to send for one of them district nurses from Bloomsbury Square, and if they come here you'll have to keep your room clean and open your winder, clear out the things from under your bed, and they'll turn the whole place topsy-turvey so as you won't know your own home ; and you'll feel just as if you was in a horspital. And then they'll never give you no grocery tickets, nor milk, nor nuthin' else." After this alarming picture, the poor woman thought it would be a deal more comfortable to have the ministrations of her mentor. However, the wound in the leg grew worse, the " nurse " decamped, and the neighbours sent for the doctor, who promptly brought in a dreaded Bloomsbury nurse. She fulfilled the worst of her predecessor's prophecies, but the patient recovered, and announced her resolve to keep her room the same as the nurse had done. To quote Miss Nightingale's terse summing up of the work of the district nurse, " Every room thus cleaned has always been kept so. This is her (the nurse's) glory. She found it a pig-stye ; she left it a tidy, airy room."

The homes of the London poor, even thirty years

ago, were deplorable from a sanitary point of view, as the experience of that noble philanthropist, Octavia Hill, shows. The spirit of inquiry into the subject of the better housing of the poor, which her work aroused, has borne fruit in these later times. Miss Hill has herself cleared out rookery after rookery, intrusted to her management by the Ecclesiastical Commissioners, and established in their place comfortable cottages and tenements where the poorest may live in order and cleanliness. County Council model dwellings have been springing up, and on all sides are evidences of improved conditions of living. Legislation, too, has been active with regard to sanitation and infectious diseases, and the modern district nurse is not confronted with the same horrors which met the pioneers of Bloomsbury Square.

On one occasion, Miss Lees was called to a miserable "home," consisting of a single room, where she found one child lying dead from scarlet fever on the window-sill, the little sufferer having asked to be carried there; another child dying in bed; and a third, suffering from the same disease, lying beside her. The young, ignorant mother was in a state of frenzied grief. She had carefully excluded all fresh air from the room by pasting up the windows; small wonder that the first victim begged to be laid on the window-sill to die. Miss Lees and her nurse took up the dirty strips of carpet, and wiped over the floor with a disinfectant. The begrimed curtains were removed, and the fresh air let in. They performed the last offices for the dead child, calmed and comforted the mother, and taught her how to keep the room ventilated and disinfected. It was arranged for one nurse to come three times a day, and another one at night. "If the district nurses had been called before," said the doctor, "they would have saved both children instead of only one," and the medical officer testified that the careful disinfection practised had prevented the fever spreading beyond the family attacked. As the work progressed, medical and sanitary officers in the poor districts of

Her Royal Highness Princess Christian is president of the Association, Henry Bonham Carter, Esq., is president of the council and of the executive committee, and the Rev. Dacre Craven is honorary secretary. Miss Hadden has ably discharged the duties of superintendent of the Central Home since 1899, and has had a valued assistant in Miss Kent. There are branch Associations at Holloway, Paddington, Battersea, Hampstead, Kensington, Newington and Walworth, Westminster, Chelsea, and Haggerston, which are managed and supported by independent committees. Many important district nurses' Homes have been established in recent years, but a special interest will always attach to the old Home in Bloomsbury Square, where the seeds of trained district nursing in the metropolis were sown.

In Scotland contemporaneous pioneer work in district nursing was done by Mrs. Mary Orrell Higginbotham, who, in 1875—the year after the National Association was founded in London—started the Glasgow Sick Poor and Private Nursing Association. Mrs. Higginbotham had, prior to that date, been working with one or two nurses amongst the Glasgow poor. The headquarters are at 209, West George Street, and the Nurses' Home at 218, Bath Street. The nursing staff consists of twenty-eight district nurses, twenty-one private nurses, and twelve probationers training in hospitals. The district nurses attended 2916 cases last year. The president is Lady Blythswood; the vice-president is Mrs. C. T. Higginbotham; the honorary treasurer, Lady Kelvin, and the honorary acting-secretary and treasurer, Miss Story. The Association is affiliated to the Queen Victoria Jubilee Institute.

It is impossible even to mention the many religious and private schemes which are at work all over the land to ameliorate the condition of the sick poor. There is scarcely a church or chapel in a crowded neighbourhood which does not do something to further district nursing, while great organizations like the Salvation Army, West

London Mission, and the Church Army employ nurses amongst the sick poor.

Parish nursing is being developed in country towns, and experiments are being made in village nursing and cottage nursing. Miss Broadwood started the Holt Ockley Nursing Association, 12, Buckingham Palace Road, which employs nurses of the village class, trained in midwifery and district nursing, to do the domestic work as well as the nursing. The cottage nurses work on similar lines, and receive systematic training in workhouse infirmaries or small hospitals for six months. Village nursing, as we have already seen, is organized by the Queen Victoria Jubilee Institute. It is a branch of work beset by many difficulties.

In concluding this account of district work mention should be made of that useful Order called "Alexandra Nurses," who practically are the district nurses for the Army and Navy. They were organized by Col. Gildea in connection with the Soldiers and Sailors Families' Association, and attend the families of our soldiers and sailors all over the world.

CHAPTER XVIII

THE QUEEN'S NURSES

Queen Victoria devotes the Women's Jubilee gift to founding an Institute for district nursing—Provisional committee formed 1888—The Institute incorporated—St. Katharine's Royal Hospital—The Institute removed to Victoria Street—Mr. William Rathbone's interest in the Institute—Affiliation of existing Homes and Associations—Organization of branches—Rules for Queen's Nurses—The council of the Institute—The Irish Training Homes—Lady Dudley's scheme for district nurses—The Training Home and work in Wales—Rural district nursing—The County Associations—School nursing—Present estimate of the work of the Queen's nurses—Funds of the Institute—Resignation of Miss Peter, general superintendent, and of Miss Wade, the superintendent for Scotland—A round with a Queen's Nurse—Her civilizing and refining influence—The Queen's Nurses' Journal—Council of superintendents—Proposal for a League of Queen's Nurses—Miss Amy Hughes. THE SCOTTISH BRANCH—Its formation—Miss Guthrie Wright, honorary secretary—Pioneer work of Miss Peter in Edinburgh—Progress of the work—The Nurse's Pension Fund—Miss Wade—Miss Cowper—Success of the Scottish Branch—Jubilee Day at the Central Home.

THE year 1887 marks an epoch in the history of district nursing. A most powerful impetus, which has converted the movement into a great national organization, was given when Queen Victoria decided to devote seventy thousand pounds of the Women's Jubilee Offering to the furtherance of this benevolent work. The Duke of Westminster, Sir James Paget, and Sir Rutherford Alcock were appointed trustees of the Fund, and for six months worked as an informal committee of inquiry, helped by the expert knowledge of Mr. William Rathbone, who, as his daughter relates, used to describe the committee as " the most efficient he had ever known, as it hardly ever met." In point of fact, he issued suggestions and memoranda to the trustees, who returned them with assents or comments, and there was no waste of time and words.

In June, 1888, a provisional committee was formed, which, in addition to the three trustees, included the following members : Lady Rosebery, Lord Lyttelton, Mr. Henry Bonham Carter, Mrs. Henry Grenfell, Mrs. Theodore Acland, the Rev. and Mrs. Dacre Craven, and Mr. W. S. Caine. Mr. Rathbone undertook the duties of honorary secretary. In the course of a year a plan was formulated, and it was decided to apply the interest of the Fund, amounting to about two thousand pounds per annum, to the founding of a Queen Victoria Jubilee Institute for the education of nurses to tend the sick poor in their own homes, and to promote the establishment of branches all over the kingdom.

The Institute was incorporated by Royal Charter, September, 1889, and was connected with St. Katharine's Royal Hospital, Regent's Park, which had been under the sole control and patronage of the Queens of England since its foundation by Matilda, Consort of Stephen, in 1148, by the Tower of London. I am indebted to the Master of St. Katharine's, the Rev. Arthur Peile, for an account of this most ancient and interesting institution. It is not a hospital in the usual sense of the word, but an ecclesiastical foundation for the promotion of things spiritual. The community from the first has consisted of a master, three brethren, and three sisters, and it was the duty of the sister to minister to the sick and infirm. Alms under certain conditions were distributed to the poor in and around the hospital precincts. Bedeswomen lived in the hospital and took part in the service and prayers for the foundress, and helped the sisters to minister to the sick poor. There were strict rules about the dress of the community, red and yellow being forbidden to be worn. The bedeswomen were to wear "a cloak and cap of grisette, and of no other colour." They were subject to punishment by the master, though not "by stripes." The community lived in their allotted houses in the cloisters surrounding the fine collegiate church of St. Katharine's, one of the most famous of the old London churches, and capable of holding two thousand persons. It is noteworthy that the sisters of the foundation have always held an equal rank and dignity with the brothers, and exercise the right of voting in the chapter. St. Katharine's is a relic of a time when communities of women had an ecclesiastical position in England, and remains a solitary survival of those ancient religious houses, as it escaped dissolution. Though spared by Henry VIII., his widow Catharine Parr altered its character somewhat by appointing a lay master in the person of her husband, Sir Thomas Seymour, 1547, and for three hundred years lay masters continued to rule over it, though the brothers were ecclesiastics. In 1825 the buildings and the beautiful old church of St. Katharine's were swept away from the old site by the Tower to make room for St. Katharine's Docks, and the community removed to a new home in Regent's Park. The organ and pulpit and some of the ancient carvings were saved from the old and put into the new church.

Queen Victoria, when called upon to exercise her prerogative in appointing a master to St. Katharine's, reverted to the original custom, and chose one in Holy Orders. She also, in 1878,[*] appointed a small number of nurses in connection with St. Katharine's to attend cases in which she was specially interested. They were the first "Queen's Nurses," wore Her Majesty's brassard upon the arm, received a grant from St. Katharine's, and met there once a year. When the Jubilee Institute was founded they ceased to exist. The Queen, however, desired to connect her new Order of nurses with the old institution, and appointed the master of St. Katharine's

[*] Mrs. Dacre Craven had presented a petition to Queen Victoria in 1877, asking that St. Katharine's might be restored to its original object, and be made a training-school for nurses of the sick poor.

for the time being p s of the Jubilee Institute, and placed a house and offices within the hospital precincts at Regent's Park as a home for the superintendent and her assistants. It is extremely interesting that the Queen's Nurses should thus be a link uniting the great modern organization with those early sisters of St. Katharine's who eight centuries ago went in and out amongst the sick poor around the precincts of their religious house by the Tower of London.

Changes have recently taken place. In 1903 the Jubilee Institute was removed to its present central and commodious quarters at 120, Victoria Street. The following year King Edward granted a Supplemental Charter by which Queen Alexandra was constituted patron of the Institute, and the official connection with St. Katharine's Hospital was terminated. The Rev. Arthur Peile, the present master, retains for his life the *ex officio* position as president of the Queen Victoria Jubilee Institute, to which he has devoted sixteen years of labour. The first superintendent of the Institute was Miss Rosalind Paget, who still serves upon the Council. She in turn has been succeeded by Miss Mansel, Miss Peter, and Miss Amy Hughes.

Mr. William Rathbone was appointed vice-president of the Institute, and retained the office until his lamented death in 1902. He derived no small satisfaction from the fact that the Metropolitan and National Association was adopted by the Provisional Committee of the Institute as the nucleus in London, and its scheme formed the model upon which the new organization was formed. He and Mr. Henry Bonham Carter rendered immense service in the early years of organization, and they found an invaluable Court of Appeal in Miss Nightingale. The old Home of the Metropolitan Association in Bloomsbury Square, was affiliated with the Institute, and became the Central Training Home, and still remains the chief educational centre for lectures. Liverpool, and the majority of the other district nursing Associations already established, also became affiliated to the Queen Victoria Jubilee Institute.

Not only did the Institute receive the great majority of existing Associations into affiliation, but primarily acted as an organizing centre for establishing a network of branches and training Homes all over the country. From the first the pivot of the scheme was inspection. Highly trained paid inspectors were appointed to periodically visit every affiliated Association, while nurses working singly in small districts are subject to extra inspection. The Institute exists to superintend the training of nurses, to give general advice and assistance in the carrying out of district nursing, and watches and safeguards the interests of its nurses.

Those engaged in the work enjoy the distinction of being Queen's Nurses, and wear a silver badge and brassard with Queen Victoria's monogram. The royal prestige is extended to the patients, whom it is customary to call the "Queen's Poor." Some of them accept the position in a literal sense, and in 1896, when Queen Victoria reviewed her nurses at Windsor, many sent messages regarding their particular ailments. "Tell the dear Queen," said one old woman, "that the pain in my head is not near so bad, and I takes my food better; and don't forget, nurse, to ask her opinion about them pills, as you said wasn't no good." The gentle art of prevarication must have been widely practised by district nurses on the day after that great event. Many suffering people to-day derive innocent satisfaction from the idea that the Queen knows all about their individual case. Slum language, however, is not always complimentary, and one has heard a Queen's Nurse dubbed "jubilee tramp" by an idle loafer trying to be witty.

The qualifications laid down for a Queen's Nurse were training at any approved general hospital for at least two years—now the time has been raised to three years — training in the special art of district nursing for not less than six months, including the nursing

south-western counties; Miss K. MacQueen, London area. Inspector for Wales, Miss F. W. Pritchard.* Superintendent of the Irish branch, Miss Lamont. Secretary, Miss A. Martin Leake.

The work in England, Wales, and Ireland is directly under the central council; but Scotland has a separate branch. The difficulty which arose in Ireland through conflicting religions was met by the wise suggestion of Mr. William Rathbone, that there should be two central training Homes in Ireland, one for Protestant, and the other for Roman Catholic nurses. The Protestant Home of St. Patrick's is situated at 101, St. Stephen's Green, Dublin. It had been doing good pioneer work amongst the sick poor for some years before the Jubilee Institute was founded. It was affiliated to the new organization, and became the central training Home for Ireland. The Report shows that two thousand one hundred and forty-two cases were nursed, and thirty-six thousand seven hundred and two visits paid by nurses from this centre last year, and the work is progressing most satisfactorily under the superintendence of Miss Lamont. The president is the Archbishop of Dublin; vice-president, Lord Ardilaun; patroness, Lady Ardilaun, vice-patronesses, the Countess of Meath, the Lady Plunket, the Hon. Mrs. Barton, and Mrs. Tottenham. The affairs of the Home are governed by an influential executive committee. The honorary secretary is Sir Edmund T. Bewdley, L.L.D.; honorary treasurer, Major D. C. Courtney; honorary physician, Sir John W. Moore, M.D., and the honorary surgeon, E. H. Bennett, Esq., M.D.

St. Lawrance's Catholic Home is situated at 34, Rutland Square West, Dublin, and was founded in 1892 for the Roman Catholic sick poor. The patron is the Archbishop of Dublin; the honorary treasurers, Charles

* Miss Pritchard has resigned and been appointed superintendent of the Brixton Branch, and Miss Ellinor Smith has been appointed Inspector for Wales.

Martin, Esq., and Charles Kennedy, Esq.; the honorary secretaries, L. A. Teeling, Esq., and H. J. Monahan, Esq.; the honorary physician, Joseph M. Redmond, Esq.; and the lady superintendent, Miss Julia Horan.

The work shows a steady increase, and has been conducted in a manner which won high encomium from the Queen Victoria Jubilee Institute inspector. A permanent staff of three nurses is kept in the Home, and a number of probationers are always in training for district work in the country. The report 1904-05 shows the number of new cases attended as one thousand eight hundred and sixty-one, and the number of visits paid thirty-four thousand five hundred and twenty-six. The figures bear strong testimony to the need there is for district nurses amongst the poor of Dublin. A Queen's Nurse is supported in the west by the Manchester West of Ireland Fund, and one by the *Irish Homestead* newspaper.

A very important extension of district nursing in Ireland was effected in April, 1903, when Lady Dudley, wife of the then Lord Lieutenant, established a scheme for providing district nurses in the poorest parts of Ireland by means of a fund raised outside the districts where the nurses work. In outlying districts around her country home in Connemara, Lady Dudley had seen much of the poverty of the people in these neglected wilds, and her appeal came from a full heart. It met with a generous response. The Queen Victoria Jubilee Institute voted a sum of one hundred and eighty pounds per annum to form the nucleus of a special fund to be raised by private contribution, and undertook to supervise the nurses through their Dublin branch. Queen Alexandra headed the subscription list with fifty pounds, and many well-known Irish ladies collected subscriptions in their respective counties. The 17th of August, 1903, saw the establishment of the two first nurses under the scheme: Nurse McCoy, at her little thatched cottage at Geesala, County Mayo, on the verge of a desolate bog,

with two thousand scattered inhabitants; and Nurse
Cusack at Bealadangan, County Galway, one of the most
poverty-stricken wilds in Ireland. If the district nurse
finds her ingenuity taxed in carrying out her work in
the poor homes of towns and villages, her difficulties in
the rough stone cabins which form typical patients'
dwellings in Ireland can be readily imagined. Instruction
on hygiene, cookery, and cleanliness must have an amusing effect on an ancient Biddy who likes her pig for
company. Still the Irish peasant is warm-hearted and
good-tempered, and nurse is a much-appreciated person
if she is tactful.

The applications coming in from congested districts
prove the great need there was for this scheme. Amongst
typical cases cited by Lady Dudley is Knocknalower, a
bleak moorland district of seventy thousand acres, where
there is scarcely a dwelling of any kind except the wretched
cabins of the five thousand small landholders, and so
utterly poverty-stricken that it is difficult to find a doctor
who will remain, no less than ten appointed having
resigned during five years. In many parts the people
have to journey a whole day across the bogs to get
medical relief. Already twelve nurses have been established in such needy districts, each centre having a permanent endowment of one hundred pounds a year out
of funds subscribed. Generous as the response has been
to Lady Dudley's appeal, the cry for help from these
forsaken regions demands continuous gifts in money,
clothing, and comforts. The clergy and medical officers
alike write gratefully of the work of the nurses. The
scheme is affiliated to the Queen Victoria Jubilee Institute,
and each nurse is subject to its inspection. The Catholic
nurses are trained at St. Lawrence's Home, and the Protestant ones at St. Patrick's Home, Dublin. They wear
Lady Dudley's special badge—a heart with a shamrock
leaf in the centre, surrounded by the words " By love serve
one another." At Lady Dudley's wish, Lady Aberdeen,
as wife of the Lord Lieutenant, has succeeded her as head

of the organization. The secretary is Miss Dorothea Keyes.

In Wales a central training Home, in affiliation with the Queen Victoria Jubilee Institute, was established at Cardiff, and nurses have gradually been introduced throughout the principality. Miss Morgan has been superintendent of the Cardiff Home since 1900. In many of the rural districts it is found necessary to employ Welsh-speaking nurses—particularly in the north. There is also a small Home at Bangor, with a superintendent and four nurses, and another at Barry, with a superintendent and four nurses. There is a special maternity training home at St. Andrew's Crescent, Cardiff. Miss Ellinor Smith is the inspector for Wales.

The nurses, working singly in the country districts of Wales, have, as in Ireland, to face great difficulties. There are long distances to walk over the hills where railways do not exist; bicycles are useless, and there are no funds to provide a pony and trap. Journeys have often to be made at night through pitch darkness when nurse is suddenly called to a case. Two nurses in the South Wales district have been provided with a pony and trap each, which they harness themselves and drive fearlessly off on their errands of mercy. Owing to the wide distances which separate her patients, the nurse's work is much retarded when she has no such convenience. Bicycles are usually a part of a country nurse's outfit, but do not meet the difficulty in rough hilly country. The long distances, too, which some nurses daily cycle, have brought about cases of serious breakdown in health.

The work in Wales is spreading rapidly, and is greatly aided by Lady Victoria Lambton in the south, and Lady Penrhyn in the north. The nurses have to gently combat some of the old customs dear to the hearts of the poor. The old-fashioned box-bed, for example, fitted against the wall is a trial to a conscientious nurse, who desires to surround her patient with fresh air, while the making of these beds, with a very sick and helpless patient in them, is something of a feat. The Welsh miners are very appreciative of having a nurse always ready in cases of accident, and in some districts the miners themselves subscribe a nurse's fund. Not long ago, the men engaged at some steel works, among whom rheumatism is very prevalent, subscribed for a Scott's electric bath, which has been erected in a little red-tiled cottage, and has a nurse in charge.

Rural district nursing is now chiefly carried out by the various county nursing associations, a large proportion of which are affiliated to the Queen Victoria Jubilee Institute. The work was originally started in 1888 by the Rural Nursing Association, the aim of which was to provide nurses and midwives for the country poor. It was affiliated to the Institute in 1891, and in 1896 entirely amalgamated with it. The Plaistow Maternity, Charity, and District Nurses' Home is affiliated also to the Institute as a training Home for village nurses.

As district nursing extended from urban to rural places, it was found desirable to form county nursing associations, to meet the needs of villages and hamlets unable to support a nurse. Miss Amy Hughes, as superintendent of county nursing associations, proved a most successful organizer, and since her appointment as General Superintendent of the Institute, a special inspection for the county associations has been established. The county associations work under a special agreement, and are affiliated to the Institute. Many county associations, started independently, have also entered into affiliation. Each association has a county superintendent, who is responsible to the county committee for the maintenance of a high standard of the nursing work. In addition to Queen's Nurses, subject to the institute rules for training, the county associations employ village nurses, certified as midwives, who have had a year's training.

"School Nursing" is another important development in which Queen's Nurses have been the pioneers. The School Nurses' Society in London and the Liverpool and other Queen's Nurses' Associations have undertaken work amongst the children of the Board Schools in the poorest districts. There is a distinct movement amongst local education authorities to provide nurses for their elementary schools, and it is probable that some arrangement will be made for the employment of Queen's Nurses.

The scope of the Jubilee Institute is ever widening, and the number of Queen's Nurses steadily increases. The number on the roll January, 1906, stands thus—

England	777
Scotland	271
Ireland	104
Wales	108
Total	1260

The number of nursing associations in affiliation with the Institute is 694, thus distributed—

England	365
Scotland	174
Ireland	80
Wales	75
Total	694

There are sixteen county nursing associations affiliated—

England	12
Scotland	3
Wales	1
Total	16

These associations employ three hundred and two village nurses in addition to forty-nine Queen's Nurses.

While there are district nursing associations who prefer to work under their own organization, and some ladies who maintain district nurses under their own charge, the general tendency is towards making the Jubilee Institute an all-embracing national organization.

The funds have been augmented by the generosity of a few friends, who placed eleven thousand pounds at the disposal of the Council. The Queen's Commemoration Fund raised forty-eight thousand pounds, and of this nineteen thousand pounds raised in Ireland was invested for the work in that country, and eleven thousand pounds collected in Scotland was returned to the Scottish Council. By the Queen's Memorial Fund in 1901, eighty-four thousand pounds was raised in England, Wales, and Ireland, and twelve thousand pounds in Scotland. The Council have now at their disposal an income of eight thousand two hundred pounds a year, but the sum is insufficient by two thousand pounds to meet the needs of such a vast work.

Queen Alexandra recently made an appeal to meet the deficit. A ladies' committee was appointed to raise a Commemoration Fund. The Countess Cadogan consented to act as president of the committee. The response was very gratifying to the Queen, a sum of two thousand pounds having been raised. A further plan has been sanctioned by Her Majesty, namely, that two hundred ladies should be asked to guarantee ten pounds each per annum for helping forward the ever-extending work of the Queen Victoria Jubilee Institute.

The Queen's interest in the needs of the poor is well known. One of her first acts after the King's accession was the reception of Queen's Nurses at Marlborough House in July, 1901. No less than seven hundred and seventy were able to be present. The King, as he looked on the rows of nurses covering the lawn, asked how the patients were faring, and the president assured His Majesty that the patients had shown the utmost anxiety for the nurses to attend. The Queen gave a further proof of her deep interest in the Institute by a gift of a thousand pounds in 1903, to facilitate the removal to the present offices.

In 1905 Miss Peter resigned the position of General Superintendent, which she had held for thirteen years. The Council placed on record their high appreciation of her services to the Institute, and the Queen received Miss Peter in private audience and thanked her for her devotion to the work of the Queen's Nurses. The Council selected Miss Amy Hughes to succeed Miss Peter. The Council also received with great regret the resignation of Miss Wade, the superintendent for Scotland. The Institute has also lost the valuable services of Mrs. Theodore Acland, the honorary secretary. She has been succeeded by Mrs. George Byron.

Although the public which generously supports the work of district nursing, understands the kind of attention given to the sick, it does not so readily realize the nurse's work as a civilizing and refining agent. The following instances of this influence came under my notice when accompanying a Queen's Nurse in a London district. A little girl was dying with a lingering disease. The children in the street below were playing noisy games, and the suffering child could get no peace. As nurse came along to make her morning visit, she stopped and told the children that their games disturbed her little patient, and asked them to play away from that part of the street. The suffering child lingered long ere the end came, but nurse's injunction was never forgotten even by the most high-spirited of the boys. On the day of the funeral a deputation of the children came to the house carrying a wreath of flowers, which, on their own initiative, they had subscribed their halfpence to buy. It was a touching tribute to the better feelings aroused by nurse's little appeal.

In a house with a smart exterior, there was a case of the most distressing kind. When nurse was summoned, she found the husband in the last stage of consumption, three children, the eldest two and a half, and the youngest ten days old, all suffering with tuberculosis, the wounds being in a most shockingly neglected

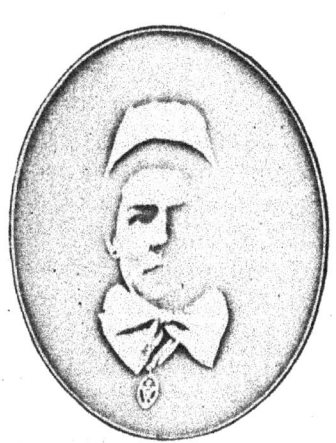

MISS AMY HUGHES,

General Superintendent, Queen Victoria Jubilee Institute for Nurses.

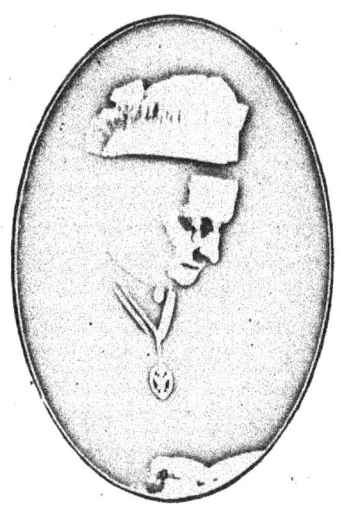

MISS PAULINE PETER.

General Superintendent, Queen Victoria Jubilee Institute, 1892-1905.

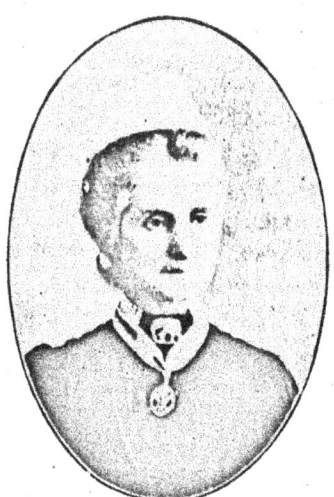

MISS COWPER.

Superintendent, Scottish District Training Home, Q.V.J.I., Edinburgh.

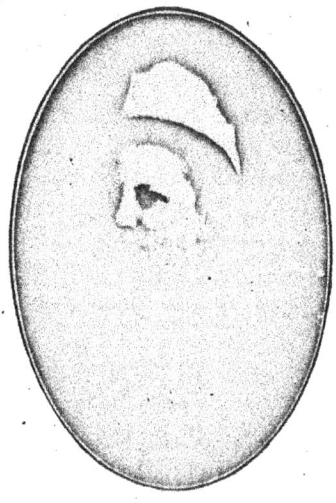

MISS WADE.

Superintendent, Scottish District Training Home, Q.V.J.I., Edinburgh, 1893-1905.

[*To face p.* 312.

condition. The young mother of twenty-four had been keeping a boarding-house, but had lost her people by reason of ill-health and incapacity to attend to them. Now she found herself with no boarders, an expensive house on her hands, no money, no friends near, and her husband and children in the condition described. In a desperate moment, dazed by circumstances and weakened by her recent confinement, she was preparing to poison herself and children. The entry of nurse saved the situation. She calmed and comforted the distraught woman, tended the husband, bathed the children, and dressed their wounds, put the room, where they were all huddled together, in order, procured food through a charitable agency, and stayed the extreme misery of the household. The husband eventually died, and nurse turned her attention to helping the wife to recover her position. She was a respectable and fairly educated woman, capable of clerical work, and was advised to take a situation, dispose of the house which she could not maintain, while the second child, who was the greatest sufferer, was placed in a hospital, and the two others, after good nursing had improved their condition, were sent to a *crêche* near the mother's place of business. Nurse had made the case known to a kindly man, who extricated the poor woman from her financial difficulty by the advance of a loan, under a proper business arrangement, and so by timely advice and help, tragedy was averted, diseased children given a chance of recovery, and a most deserving woman saved from going under into the abyss of the hopeless.

The third case is more trivial, but illustrates the influence of the district nurse from another point of view. We entered the house of a patient suffering from pneumonia. It was the usual one-roomed home in which most of the London poor live. When nurse went to get water to wash her patient she found the sink stopped up. Inquires resulted in the admission that, as three week's rent were owing, the tenant was afraid to approach the landlord to have the sink put right. Nurse, however, knowing that her patient was a respectable man, temporarily behind in his rent through illness, brought a little pressure to bear in the right quarter, and the sanitary condition of the home was secured. While the sink was under discussion, a young girl, needing a light on the staircase, lighted a piece of paper in the fire, and rushed off with it flaring. Nurse looked so horrified that the patient laid down the law to his wife and family as impressively as his feebleness would allow, and we fancy that something was done towards saving that building from future destruction by fire. Similar incidents occur daily in districts all over the kingdom, and when we consider them in the aggregate, the importance of the influence exercised by a district nurse apart from the actual care of the sick will be realized. The ideal district nurse, in addition to the best professional training, must have the elements of character which enable her to be the tactful counsellor, the cheery friend, the trusted confidante ; in a word, she must be at once the servant and the teacher of the poor. At her best, she is the most perfectly bred woman one can meet, for she has made delicate consideration for the feelings of others a fine art.

The Queen's Nurses are one of the most important bodies of skilled workers in the world, and their beneficent influence in the homes of the people it is impossible to overestimate. The *Queen's Nurses' Journal* is the organ of the Association. The superintendents of the Institute meet together in council to discuss questions of interest, and for mutual help. There is now a scheme for forming a league of Queen's Nurses.

In recognition of the valuable services rendered by the General Superintendent, Miss Amy Hughes, the gold badge of the Institute was, with the sanction of the Queen, recently bestowed upon her. Miss Hughes began her nursing career at St. Thomas's Hospital in 1884, and amongst the appointments which she has held are those of superintendent of the Central Home, Bloomsbury, 1895; superintendent of nurses in the Bolton Union Workhouse, 1896; superintendent of the Nurses' Co-operation, 1897; superintendent of County Associations affiliated to the Queen Victoria Jubilee Institute, 1901; and in 1905 she was appointed General Superintendent of the Queen's Jubilee Institute. Miss Hughes has visited the United States and Canada and seen the district nursing in those countries.

The Scottish Branch

When the Queen Victoria Jubilee Institute was founded, provision was made for a separate Scottish branch working under its own council and executive committee. Queen Victoria entrusted to the Countess of Rosebery the formation of the Provisional Scottish Committee, which received an endowment of four hundred pounds per annum as its share of the Jubilee gift. Lady Rosebery remained president of the Queen's Nurses in Scotland until her lamented death in 1891, when Queen Victoria appointed Her Royal Highness Princess Louise, Duchess of Argyll, to be president. The vice-presidents are the Duchess of Buccleuch, the Lady Blythswood, the Lord Justice-General, and A. H. F. Barbour, Esq., M.D., F.R.C.P.E. Dr. Joseph Bell is chairman of the Executive Committee, and his constant interest in the nurses and care of them when ill is much appreciated. Miss Butter is convener of the House Committee, and J. S. Pitman, Esq., W.S., convener of the Finance Committee. The late Miss Flora Stevenson, chairman of the Edinburgh School Board, and her sister, Miss Louisa Stevenson, who is upon the Council, have taken a deep interest in the work.

Miss Guthrie Wright has been honorary secretary of the Scottish branch since its initiation, and its steady progress, and especially its good financial position, are greatly due to her untiring efforts. She was honorary secretary for the Queen Victoria Commemoration Fund in 1897, and for the Queen Victoria Memorial Endowment Fund, for the benefit of the institution. She is an indefatigable collector for the general funds, and there is a little pleasantry to the effect that Miss Guthrie Wright had never realized how many people had their front door steps washed at the same hour until she began her early morning collecting pilgrimages round the Edinburgh squares. She is a member of the Council of the Queen Victoria Jubilee Institute as representative for Scotland.

Miss Peter was the first superintendent of the Queen's Nurses in Scotland, and started work in a temporary Home in North Charlotte Street, Edinburgh, in April, 1889, with three nurses. She had many difficulties to overcome in her pioneer work. The national prejudice in Scotland was strong against permitting a stranger to enter the home even though on an errand of mercy. At the end of two years, however, the work was on a secure basis, and the Scottish District Training Home established in excellent quarters at 29, Castle Street, midway between old and new Edinburgh, and under the shelter of the old grey Castle rock.

From their picturesquely situated Home the nurses, by devious short cuts, quickly reach their patients in the crowded courts and alleys of the Cowgate, Grassmarket, Lawnmarket, and the towering tenements of the old High Street. One fancies that there must be a touch of romance in nursing amid such historic surroundings. The poor room in which the suffering one lies was, may be, an apartment of a lordly mansion in the days when the houses of the nobility lined the lower High Street, and Holyrood Palace kept a gay court.

The extent of the work done by the Queen's Nurses amongst the Edinburgh poor may be gauged by the following comparison : In a recent year Edinburgh Infirmary nursed 5592 cases from among the inhabitants of Edinburgh and Leith, and during the same period the number of sick poor attended in their own homes by the district nurses amounted to nearly an equal number, being 5173. The Edinburgh Home has an average of 410 cases per month.

The Jubilee grant is augmented by private subscription. The appeal of the Duchess of Buccleuch resulted in an addition of twelve thousand pounds to the capital funds. An anonymous gift of one thousand pounds was received in 1903, and the Edinburgh Parish Council increased its grant. There is, however, an ever-present need for more funds to meet the increasing demand for district nurses in the capital, and for the extension of the work in the country districts.

The Council is very thoughtful for its nurses, and a pension fund has been founded to increase the provision which nurses may make for themselves. There are two pensions of ten pounds each, viz. the Florence Nightingale Pension and the Lady Rosebery Pension, and to be eligible for these, Queen's Nurses must (1) have served twelve years in that capacity, and of that time not less than six years in Scotland; (2) they must satisfy the Council, or a committee appointed by the Council, that they have made satisfactory and systematic effort to make provision for themselves, unless prevented by approved family claims, or by ill-health; (3) they must have attained the age of fifty years.

Miss Wade succeeded Miss Peter as superintendent of the Central Home and inspector of Queen's Nurses in Scotland in 1892, and for twelve years devoted herself most assiduously and successfully to the work. She was followed in 1905 by Miss Cowper, who had been assistant-inspector. All three superintendents graduated in nursing at the Edinburgh Royal Infirmary.

The Scottish branch may indeed be proud of its progeny. Its district nursing associations now form a network all over the country, and number upwards of 174. The roll of the Queen's Nurses in Scotland numbers 271. Besides the central Home in Edinburgh, which has 52 nurses and probationers, training Homes have been established in Glasgow, Dundee, Aberdeen, and Paisley. An interesting reunion takes place in Edinburgh on Jubilee Day, June 20th, when Queen's Nurses from many parts of Scotland meet at the Central Home. Miss Nightingale has always taken special interest in the Scottish nurses, and often sends them greeting on Jubilee Day.

CHAPTER XIX

MIDWIFERY AND MONTHLY NURSING

Midwifery closely allied with nursing—Mrs. Gamp—In early times forbidden to men—After the Reformation, midwives licensed by bishops—Ignorance and cruelty—"The Woman's Booke"—The Chamberlen forceps revolutionize the practice—Warfare between midwives and the "he-practisers"—Distinguished midwives try to educate their sister practitioners—The Society of Apothecaries' action—The Female Medical Society—Miss Nightingale's scheme—Dr. Farre shows high mortality statistics—London Obstetrical Society appoints a commission—Public opinion roused—Dr. Humphrey's articles—Efforts to bring about legislation—The Midwives' Institute founded—Its incorporation—Its objects—It drafts a Midwives' Registration Bill—Various agencies at work—Passing of the Midwives Act, 1902—Its provisions—The Association for Promoting the Training and Supply of Midwives—The Rural Midwives' Association—Enrolment of midwives under the Act—Training for midwives and monthly nurses—The Rotunda Hospital, Dublin—Rise of other lying-in hospitals—Queen Charlotte's Hospital, Marylebone.

ALTHOUGH midwifery is not a branch of nursing, it is so closely allied with the profession that some account of its history seems to be in point. In the old days of untrained nursing, women who acted as midwives often undertook monthly nursing, and the care of sick people also. Most country villages had some ancient dame, who was by turns a midwife in the homes of the poor, and a sick-nurse in the houses of better-off people. "Mrs. Gamp" is the immortal illustration of this class of woman, and though she set up the sign of "midwife" at her lodgings in Holborn, "Sairey" counted herself, in the highest walk of her art, a "monthly nurse." To-day the distinction is more clearly defined. The midwife is a licensed practitioner acting independent of the doctor, while the monthly nurse attends the birth under a medical practitioner, and takes charge of the mother and infant. Both may or may not be trained nurses, but the midwife is compelled to be certified as such, and is now required to pass the examination of the Central Midwives' Board.

In olden times the practice of midwifery was forbidden to men, and midwives were protected by strong corporations. In those days medicine and surgery were under ecclesiastical rule, and the Church deemed the practice of midwifery as most fitting for women. When, in the reign of Henry VIII., the organization of medicine and surgery began, and the control of medical science passed from the Church to the State, midwifery was still left in the hands of women.

After the Reformation, midwives were required to be licensed by the bishops, and the first license was drawn up by Bishop Bonner. I am afraid the bishops did not go into the matter of training and qualification. Judging from an old licence before me, they required the woman to swear that she would not be a party to smuggling supposititious infants into the bed ; that she would not kill, injure, or maim the babe ; and that if called upon to christen it, as midwives frequently were in cases of emergency, she would religiously perform the ceremony in the name of the Father, the Son, and the Holy Ghost, and abstain from unholy incantations. The licensing by bishops continued in full force until 1642, when midwives began to be licensed at Chirurgeons' Hall, after being examined by six skilful midwives and as many chirurgeons. Then, in 1662, came another change, and the midwives took oath at Doctors' Commons, paid their fee, and obtained their licence, apparently without any test of their qualification. The licensing by bishops still continued in some districts until modern times.

The old midwives were generally low and vicious, ignorant and superstitious, and more or less barbaric and cruel. They put their faith in quackery and nostrums, had a supreme disregard of the method of nature, and devised various revolting practices. Attention has recently been drawn to the barbarous birth customs amongst the Philippinos, but prior to the nineteenth century, things were not much better in our own land, so far as many of the old midwives were concerned, and even up to recent years, extraordinary practices were in vogue in remote parts of Wales.

In the middle of the sixteenth century English-women began to complain that midwives were without education for their work, and an attempt to provide instruction was made by the publication of "The Woman's Booke," by Andrew Boorde, a translation from the Latin of Rhodion's "Birth of Mankynde." It suggests that the "licensing" bishops should, with the consent of the doctor, examine and instruct the midwife; "it is necessary to give instruction to midwives, and a guarantee of their skill to the public," runs the recommendation. In 1616, Dr. Peter Chamberlen petitioned James I. "that some order may be settled by the State for the instruction and civil government of midwives." A movement in this direction was then going forward on the Continent.

The invention by Peter Chamberlen and his distinguished son of the obstetric forceps changed the situation, and eventually destroyed the supremacy of the midwife. At first, as we have seen, men were forbidden to practise midwifery; then came a period in which they despised it, and left it to women, but the Chamberlen forceps created professional interest, medical practitioners had the monopoly of their use, and gradually the female midwife became a secondary person.

She was not dethroned without a struggle. War to the knife followed between the old midwives and the doctors, whom they contemptuously dubbed the "he-practisers." A compromise seems to have been effected in the case of royal and distinguished ladies, by which the midwife took charge of the case while the doctor was in readiness if needed. In such manner was the birth of Queen Victoria ushered in, the Duchess of Kent being attended by a famous German midwife, dubbed "Doctor Charlotte," and the male practitioner was not required. One reads of some of the most celebrated midwives, who, when they were obliged to summon the doctor, compelled him to crawl into the chamber on his hands and knees so that the patient might not be disconcerted by seeing him enter the room. Queen Victoria was the first royal mother to dispense with the midwife, and be attended by an accoucheur and a monthly nurse.

The middle of the eighteenth century saw the rise of lying-in hospitals, which followed each other in quick succession, and to these we refer later. From that time efforts to train and educate midwives and monthly nurses became continuous. It is to the credit of some of the most distinguished midwives that they tried to educate their sister practitioners. Mrs. Jane Sharp published a book on the subject, and Mrs. Sarah Stone of Piccadilly, at the beginning of the eighteenth century, wrote, "In my humble opinion it is necessary that midwives should employ three years at least with some ingenious woman in practising this art. For if seven years must be served to learn a trade, I think three years as little as possible to be instructed in an art where life depends." Mrs. Stephen, midwife to Queen Charlotte, gave lectures to her sister practitioners.

The Society of Apothecaries in 1813 tried to persuade Parliament to pass enactments for the examination and control of midwives, but the House of Commons would not allow the mention of female midwives. The London Obstetrical Society, founded in 1859, took up the question, and the Female Medical Society, started in 1864, had for one of its objects the employment of educated women in midwifery. Miss Nightingale interested herself in the matter, and at this period elaborated a scheme for the instruction of midwives. She suggested the building of a lying-in institution on an open, healthy site, and to have a staff, consisting of matron, midwives, and thirty pupils, with a visiting medical officer to give scientific and practical instruction to the pupils. Unfortunately, Miss Nightingale's wise plan for a separate hospital was not carried out, and the first attempt to found a modern school of midwifery was made at King's College, where, as already related in the account of that hospital, lying-in wards were started with the view to the training of midwives and monthly nurses, a grant from the Nightingale Fund being devoted to the purpose. Owing to the proximity of these special wards to the general wards, the result was such a high rate of mortality amongst the women that after a few years the experiment was abandoned.

Dr. Farre, of King's College, who had charge of the Nightingale wards, had laboured earnestly in the cause of reform. That distinguished physician began to call public attention to the high rate of mortality amongst mothers and infants. He showed, from the Reports of the Registrar-General's department, that fifty to ninety per cent. of births in England and Wales were attended by midwives, and that there was a total absence of training amongst these women, and the result was an alarming rate of mortality. In 1869, a commission was appointed by the Obstetrical Society to investigate the cause of infant mortality. The returns induced the Society to arrange a course of instruction for midwives, and to grant a diploma to those who successfully passed examination. Candidates must have been six months in a lying-in hospital or have attended twenty-five cases. For twenty-three years the Obstetrical Society remained the examining body for midwives.

The lying-in hospitals, in which at one time the mortality had been so great that it seemed like a death warrant to enter one, had, under improved antiseptics, greatly reduced their death rate. But all over the country ignorant midwives were practising, who regarded Lister and antiseptics—if they ever heard of them—with characteristic scorn. The publication of Dr. Aveling's "English Midwives" in 1872, a book to which I am greatly indebted, vividly brought the matter before the public. Then came some exposures in the *Times*, the subject was freely discussed, and the long battle, which ended in the Act of 1902, was fairly begun. Dr. Humphreys, L.R.C.P., M.R.C.S., in the course of a series of papers in the *Nursing Times*, in the spring of 1906, has succinctly traced the steps in the progress towards legislation. In 1872, the General Medical Council appointed a committee to deliberate on the subject of the examination and regulations of midwives in connection with the question of the medical employment of women. The British Medical Association and the Obstetrical Society joined in a friendly discussion regarding legislation, and various proposals were made.

In 1881 the Midwives' Institute, 12, Buckingham Street, Strand, was founded by Miss Louisa Hubbard and the late Mrs. Henry Smith, for the purpose of raising the efficiency and improving the status of midwives, and proved an important factor in pressing forward parliamentary legislation. Miss Wilson, now the president, and Miss Rosalind Paget, the honorary treasurer, have indefatigably worked from the beginning to promote the objects of the Institute. It was incorporated in 1889, and the following ladies signed the articles of association —Miss Louisa Hubbard, Mrs. Henry Smith, Mrs. Scharlieb, M.D., Miss Freeman, formerly matron of the British Lying-in Hospital, Miss Wilson, Miss Rosalind Paget, and Miss Fynes-Clinton, now organizing secretary. Valued friends of the Institute, who helped it through the years of toil and stress, were Sir John Williams, M.D., Mr. Thomas Bryant, F.R.C.S., one time president of the College of Surgeons, Dr. Humphreys, L.R.C.P., M.R.C.S., and the late Mr. William Rathbone, M.P., Mr. H. Fell Pease, Dr. Bristow, and Sir Frederick Fitz-Wygram.

The objects of the Midwives' Institute are : (1) To raise the efficiency and improve the status of midwives ; (2) To establish a register for members, and to establish a centre of information for the public ; (3) To provide a good medical lending library and club-room for friendly meetings ; (4) To arrange courses of medical lectures, and to afford opportunities for discussion on subjects connected with the profession. Associated with the Institute is the Trained Nurses' Club. Special information of interest to members is published each month in *Nursing Notes*. The Institute is an admirable educational and social centre for midwives and monthly nurses, also masseuses, and acts as a medium between its members and the public. The subscription is five shillings a year, with two shillings and sixpence entrance fee.

The year that it was incorporated (1889), the Institute drafted a Midwives' Registration Bill, which was introduced into the House of Commons in 1890, passed the second reading, and was referred to a Select Committee ; but was finally blocked and withdrawn. In 1892 the whole subject was referred to a Select Committee. Some years of agitation followed. A Society was formed amongst medical men for promoting the registration of midwives, and another for enlisting the interest of lay women in the subject. Public and private meetings were organized, statistics were obtained to prove the great mortality incident upon the attendances of untrained midwives, and the need of registration as a safeguard against incompetency. There was in some quarters strong medical opposition, and the passing of bills introduced was hindered by obstructive methods. There is no occasion to follow the strife occasioned by the proposal to register midwives. The agitation at length bore fruit in the Registration of Midwives Act, 1902. The Act is administered by the Central Midwives' Board, 6, Suffolk Street, S.W., from which all information can be obtained.

A three years' grace was given to the old untrained midwife, who was permitted to be certified under the Act provided that she had been in *bonâ fide* practice as a midwife for a year previous to July 31, 1902, and bore a good character. Since March 31, 1905, midwives have been required to pass the examination of the Central Midwives' Board before they could be enrolled. The names of certified midwives are entered upon the midwives' roll. The fee for enrolment is ten shillings. The Act does not apply to Scotland or Ireland. The Board's examinations are held three times a year in London, and at the provincial centres of Bristol, Manchester, and Newcastle-on-Tyne simultaneously.

The organizing and regulating of a profession which had sunk out of recognition, and chiefly fallen into the hands of a particularly ignorant and untrained class of women, are a heavy piece of work, and at present much confusion reigns in the provinces. In every county large numbers of women are retiring from practice now that training for their work has become compulsory, and the number left is inadequate for the needs of the mothers.

The Association for Promoting the Training and Supply of Midwives, Dacre House, Dean Farrar Street, Westminster, secretary, Miss Gill; and The Rural Midwives' Association, 47, Victoria Street, secretary, Mrs. Browne, are doing excellent work in promoting the training and supply of midwives to take the places of the great army of the untrained who, happily for the lives of mothers and infants, are now passing—though slowly in some districts—into oblivion.

The full provisions of the Act will not come into force until April, 1910. After that year no woman may practise (*i.e.* habitually and for gain attend women in child-birth otherwise than under the direction of a qualified medical practitioner), unless certified as the Act provides.

The Midwives Board held its first examination under the Act in June, 1905, and up to the present (1906) some 23,942 midwives have been enrolled. The Midwives' Institute supplies candidates with advice and information, and provides a course of instruction to prepare for the C.M.B. certificate. The recognized training for midwives is three months in a maternity hospital or the lying-in wards of a workhouse infirmary. Fees for tuition, board, and lodging, from £10 to £26 for the thirteen weeks. The registration fee is £1 1s. For monthly nursing, the training is for six or twelve weeks. The fees for tuition, board, and lodging vary from £7 7s., for a six weeks' course, to £15 15s., for a twelve weeks' course. A registration fee of £1 1s. is usually paid on making application.

We must retrace our steps somewhat to give the history of the earliest training-schools.

The Rotunda Hospital, Dublin, takes front rank as the pioneer training-school for midwives and monthly nurses. It was the *first* lying-in hospital established in the British dominions. As early as 1755 it fixed the length of training for female pupils at six months, and in 1786 began to grant certificates of proficiency, while in 1788 a bye-law was passed requiring all pupils to pass an examination. A special prestige also attaches to the hospital because of its School of Midwifery for medical students, which is the largest and oldest chartered school of midwifery, not only in Great Britain, but, with one exception, in the world, and attracts students not only from the United Kingdom and Ireland, but from remote British colonies, and from America, France, and other countries.

This world-famous institution owes its origin to Dr. Bartholomew Mosse, son of the Rev. Thomas Mosse, rector of Maryborough, Queen's County. Having received "a genteel education," as an old manuscript memoir runs, he was sent to Dublin to study medicine. In 1733 he was licensed as a surgeon, and practised surgery and midwifery with great success. He travelled through Europe, studying in various hospitals, and on his return home resolved to start a free lying-in hospital in Dublin. He had been moved by compassion for the poor women of the city, who had no place for themselves and their new-born infants but garrets open to the wind, or damp cellars subject to floods. He took a large house staff in connection with the hospital, and nurses are sent out after six months' training. The Rotunda School has been formally approved by the Central Midwives' Board as an institution for the training of midwives under the rules of that Board. Already (1906) four hundred and twenty-seven nurses trained in the Rotunda have been placed on the roll of registered midwives kept by the Central Midwives' Board, London, under the second section of the Midwives Act, 1902. The master of the hospital, elected for the usual term of seven years in November, 1903, is Dr. E. Hastings Tweedy, F.R.C.P.I.; the assistant physicians are Dr. Gibbon Fitzgibbon and Dr. A. Norman Holmes, and the lady superintendent is Miss Lucy Ramsden. An additional wing is in course of erection for the accommodation of the nursing staff.

For four years after its foundation the Rotunda remained the only lying-in hospital and school of midwifery in the kingdom. In 1749 London followed suit, and founded the British Lying-in Hospital in Brownlow Street, Long Acre, which was rebuilt a hundred years later in its present position, Endell Street, St. Giles. Next followed the City of London Lying-in Hospital in 1750; the General Lying-in Hospital, Bayswater, 1752 (to be known later as Queen Charlotte's), and the Westminster Lying-in Hospital (ultimately removed to York Road, Lambeth), in 1765. All of these old institutions have to-day recognized training-schools, but Queen Charlotte's is the largest, and stands foremost in point of history. It, like the Rotunda, has a school for medical pupils as well as for midwives.

Queen Charlotte's Hospital was originally founded in Bayswater, in 1752. Mr. Thomas Ryan, formerly secretary to the hospital, has published a detailed history of the institution, in which he patiently unravels the mystery of its early site. Suffice it to say that it was removed to its present position in the Marylebone Road about 1813. It had the good fortune to secure the warm interest of His Royal Highness the Duke of Sussex, at whose request Queen Charlotte consented to become its patron in 1809. The name was then changed from the General Lying-in Hospital to the Queen Charlotte's Lying-in Hospital, and the institution was renovated and reconstituted. At this period it was opened as a training-school for resident male pupils. Hitherto London students had been obliged to go to the Rotunda, Dublin, for practical training in this branch of medical science. Queen Charlotte was anxious that the training of midwives should be arranged for, but curiously enough the hospital was only opened to women in the event of there being no male pupils in the hospital. The old rule runs : "Women desirous of being instructed in the practice of midwifery, may be admitted to the hospital on the recommendation of the physician or surgeon in ordinary, on the same terms as the male pupils, provided there shall be no male pupils then residing in the house."

The home of the hospital in Marylebone from 1813 to 1856 was the old Manor House of Lisson Green, and judging from an old picture which hangs in the Board-room, and which was rescued from a lumber cellar by the late matron, Miss Davies, the hospital then stood detached amongst rural surroundings, very different to its present busy environment. One may imagine Queen Charlotte coming in her sedan chair to visit her favourite charity. No less than five portraits of this excellent Queen hang round the Board-room. In 1856 the present hospital was built on the site of the old Manor House.

An interesting branch of training was started in 1868, namely, the training of women to act as midwives for the army. It was resolved that " The governors of this hospital, in endeavouring to benefit the army of this country, are willing, on receiving a recommendation from the commanding officer of a regiment or depôt, to receive, as they can accommodate them, pupils for learning midwifery at half the sum usually charged, and to board the pupils during the time of tuition."

In 1872 the administration of the hospital had fallen

into an unsatisfactory state, and changes were effected during the succeeding years to bring it into line with the modern system. A revised code of rules was made in 1874, by which a resident medical officer was appointed. The finishing touch to the new arrangements was made in 1879, when a housekeeper was appointed, leaving to the matron the charge, under the medical officer, of the patients and the nursing department. From this period, 1874, dates the modern training-school for medical pupils, midwives, and monthly nurses. The advance in the number of midwives and nurses trained was rapid. A trained matron was not however appointed until 1894, when Miss M. F. McCard came and continued in the post for ten years. In 1899 the well-appointed Nurses' Home in the Marylebone Road, opposite the hospital, was built. New wards have recently been added to the hospital, the total number of beds being now sixty-nine. Last year one thousand five hundred and sixty in-patients were received. They usually remain for fourteen days. The total number of new out-patients attended and nursed in their own homes was one thousand nine hundred and sixty-nine; the total number of attendances on out-patients nineteen thousand six hundred and ninety. At the Convalescent Home one hundred and fifty patients were received. The enormous increase in the charity compels the committee to appeal earnestly for increased support. Her Majesty the Queen is patron.

The following are the regulations for the training of pupil midwives and monthly nurses. The course of training for pupil midwives is specially adapted for those candidates who wish to present themselves for the examinations of the certificate of the Central Midwives' Board, and for those who wish to qualify for appointments as midwives under the Local Government Board, and other similar appointments. The course is for five months, and the fee, which includes board and lodging (not washing), is thirty-five pounds. Nurses who hold a certificate of three years' training from a recognized training school may enter under the same regulations for a course of four months' training in midwifery and monthly nursing at the reduced fee of twenty-eight pounds.

Pupil monthly nurses are received for sixteen weeks' training, the fee being twenty-four pounds, which includes board and lodging. Certificates are granted by the hospital to midwives and to monthly nurses on the passing of an examination. The number of pupils varies from sixty to seventy. Miss Bröchner, a Swedish lady, has recently, 1906, been appointed matron of the hospital. She was trained at St. Bartholomew's. Miss Bröchner has made a speciality of midwifery work, and holds the London Obstetrical Society and the Central Midwives' Board certificates. Under her superintendence this old pioneer school of Queen Charlotte's Hospital will doubtless be kept in the forefront of progress.

CHAPTER XX

MASSAGE

Definition of massage—Revival of an ancient practice—The ideal masseuse—The rise of modern massage—The Society of Trained Masseuses founded 1895—List of the Founders—Objects of the Society—Conditions of membership—Fees—Examinations—Where instruction can be obtained—Fees and length of training.

THE history of massage to most of us begins from the days of childhood, when after a tumble we were told "to rub the place and make it well." There was nothing scientific about the matter, but the homely adage often proved efficacious.

To-day massage is defined as "a scientific method of curing disease by systematic manipulations," and is useful in paralysis, neuralgia, rheumatism, joint diseases, and various other complaints. It is also resorted to for promoting beauty of form and improving the complexion, and for the latter is a more healthful method than the use of cosmetics. Face massage belongs to the province of the beauty specialist.

Massage is a modern revival of a very ancient practice, recommended by the fathers of medicine some thousands of years before the Christian era. It was used by the Indians and by the Chinese, and has long been in use in the Sandwich Islands under the name of *lomi-lomi*, and in Tonga it is called *toogi-toogi*. The word massage is from the Greek *masso*, to work with the hands, to knead dough.

It is a distinct employment, and not necessarily followed only by those who are trained nurses; many nurses, however, add a course in massage to their general training. Never has the trite saying, that a "nurse is born, not made," proved truer than in the case of the masseuse; if she has not the physical as well as the moral fitness for this branch of work, no training can make her successful. She needs exceptionally good physique and good health, intelligence, refinement, the ability to ensure confidence, and a bright though calm and placid manner. Hers should be the hand of Diana, full of energy and power, yet withal soft, smooth, fleshy, and dry. The masseuse, like the private nurse, has a great responsibility in her hands, and needs to be a woman of high character and discretion, one who knows the professional value of the silent tongue. Only the other day a distinguished physician told me of a masseuse whose services were invaluable to his patient, but her gossiping habit had caused estrangements in the family of her patient, and he was compelled to dispense with her skilful services.

It is about twenty years ago that massage began to be talked about in this country as a fashionable remedy. Dr. Thomas Dowse and his colleague Dr. Herbert Tibbits gave lectures on massage and electricity, and demonstrations at the Hospital for Diseases of the Nervous System, in Welbeck Street, with the intention of creating a class of masseurs and masseuses. Lady Janetta Manners wrote an article on massage in the *Nineteenth Century*, December, 1887, drawing attention to its efficacy and tracing its early history. Crowds at this period, too, were being drawn to Amsterdam by Dr. Metzyer, who used massage on the late Empress of Austria with great success.

Numbers of irresponsible people, however, began to practise the new remedy, and brought it into ill-odour. To afford status and protection to *bonâ fide* professional workers, the Society of Trained Masseuses was founded by some ladies in 1895, and in 1900 it was incorporated, and is now styled " The Incorporated Society of Trained

Masseuses." A long list of members of the medical profession have signified their approval of the aims and objects of the Society. The founders were Mrs. Arthur, late matron, Firs Home, Bournemouth (trained masseuse); Miss E. Buckworth, late instructor of massage to St. Bartholomew's Hospital, King's College Hospital, and Royal National Hospital; Miss Fynes-Clinton, late assistant-matron, London Hospital (trained masseuse, L.O.S. Cert.); Miss Florence Dove (trained masseuse); Miss Griffiths, late matron, Lambeth Infirmary (trained masseuse, L.O.S. Cert.); Miss C. F. Maclean (trained nurse and masseuse); Miss Manley, late sister, London Hospital (trained masseuse); Miss G. Manley (certified nurse, trained masseuse and teacher of massage); Miss Molony, late sister Guy's Hospital, and matron, Institute English Nurses, Paris, and St. Mark's Hospital, Dublin (trained masseuse); Miss Rosalind Paget, late inspector of nurses, Queen Victoria's Jubilee Institute (trained masseuse, L.O.S. Cert.); Mrs. Palmer, instructor of massage, and masseuse to the London Hospital (L.O.S. Cert.); Miss Robinson (trained masseuse, L.O.S. Cert.).

The offices of the Society are at the Trained Nurses' Club, 12, Buckingham Street, Strand, and the honorary secretary is Miss Grant. The organ of the Society is *Nursing Notes*.

The objects of the Society are to improve the status and training of masseuses; to provide for the examination of and granting of certificates of qualification to masseuses; to keep a roll of members; to establish a registry for members and a centre of information for the public on matters connected with massage; to arrange lectures, provide a reference library and afford opportunities for the discussion of subjects of interest and importance to masseuses; and to provide an organization to which members have a right to apply for advice and help in professional difficulties. The members of the Society are masseuses over the age of twenty-one who hold the Society's certificate, and who have been elected by the Council. Associates are trained masseuses who have been or are in practice, and who have been elected by the Council. Honorary associates are persons other than masseuses who are interested in the objects of the Society, and have been elected by the Council. All members and associates, residing within a radius of fifty miles, pay an annual subscription of seven shillings and sixpence, which carries with it membership of the Trained Nurse's Club. Country members pay an annual subscription of two shillings and sixpence. Members must work under the direction of a registered medical practitioner. The Society neither fixes nor controls the working fee of its members. Fees for massage vary from three shillings and sixpence to ten shillings and sixpence per hour. The Society holds two examinations each year in the theory and practice of massage, and grants certificates to successful candidates. The fee for examination is one guinea. There is a registry for members.

The founding of the Incorporated Society of Trained Masseuses was the first attempt made to organize the profession of massage, and the society remains the only representative body of masseuses. It has granted already 1043 certificates. Of the holders of these 338 are members of the Society, and 35 associates.

Instruction in massage can also be obtained from hospitals for epilepsy and nervous disorders, from many of the Poor Law infirmaries, and some of the general hospitals teach massage in their ordinary curriculum. At Guy's Hospital the Raphael Gold Medal is awarded for massage. Some medical men take pupils in massage, and there are qualified masseuses who are professional teachers. Fees for a course are from ten guineas upwards, and the period for training from three weeks to three months. There is an increasing advance in the employment of massage, and it affords a lucrative field for the really skilled worker.

CHAPTER XXI

INDIAN AND COLONIAL NURSING

The nursing problem in India—Lady Canning's work during the Mutiny—
The women of India without medical help—Pioneers in the Zenanas—
Queen Victoria receives Miss Beilby, a medical missionary—Lady Dufferin
founds her Fund—Its objects and Organization—Report of work, 1905—
Lady Curzon founds the Victoria Memorial Scholarship Fund—Nurse
Training School, General Hospital, Madras—The Cama Hospital Nurse
Training School—No standard of training in Indian institutions—Recommendations of Colonel C. H. Joubert—Difficulties of nursing and training
—The Up-Country Nursing Association—Lady Minto's new scheme—
The Indian Military Nursing Service instituted at the suggestion of Lady
Roberts—Work of Miss Katharine Loch—Miss R. A. Betty, senior
superintendent—Lady Roberts's Fund—Nursing in the self-governing
Colonies—Canada—Australia—New Zealand—Tasmania—Cape Colony
—Natal—South African training-schools—Its military service—The
Crown Colonies and Protectorates—Lady Piggott founds the Colonial
Nursing Association—Its work and progress.

THE problem of organizing a system of trained nursing for the countless millions of our fellow-subjects in India is one before which the most intrepid reformer may well stand aghast. There is a country to be dealt with as large as Europe, with languages and dialects as numerous, and a corresponding variety of customs and religious observances, while the fetters of caste cripple social progress. The density of the population may be judged from the fact that there are on an average in British India two hundred and seventy-nine people to the square mile. The women of the country are only just beginning to emerge from long centuries of ignorance and seclusion. If in our own land fifty years ago many excellent people were shocked at the idea that educated women should become nurses, what must be the feeling of Hindoo ladies, trained to regard the nursing of the sick as work only fit for the lowest caste woman ? It is not surprising that as yet little advance has been made towards providing India with trained nurses native to the country.

The Indian Mutiny, following immediately on the interest in nursing roused at home by the Crimean War, first turned attention to the subject of nursing in India. Lady Canning, the wife of the Governor-General, during that terrible period, was indefatigable in her efforts to provide succour for the sick and wounded soldiery. Florence Nightingale, recruiting her shattered health, scented the battle from afar, and wrote to Lady Canning, offering to come out to India at twenty-four hours' notice, if there was "anything to do in her line of business." Lady Canning did not encourage such a sacrifice on the part of the heroine of the Crimea. One of the outcomes of the nursing spirit of that time was the founding of the Calcutta Hospital Nurses' Institution in 1859, with which is associated the Lady Canning Home, Calcutta, institutions doing valuable work to-day in supplying nurses to hospitals, and in the training of a skilled private staff. There was, however, nothing accomplished for bringing medical aid and good nursing to the people of India until after the advent of the medical woman.

Even twenty years ago, the women of India were practically without medical assistance. In sickness they were tended by the lowest type of native women, who were ignorant, superstitious, and frequently barbarous in their methods. When in case of extremity the doctor was summoned, he entered the zenana with his head in a bag, or remained outside the purdah, feeling his patient's pulse, and without any opportunity for observation. While the stronger sex had medical provision for all their aches and pains, the so-called weaker sex, who, in addition to the sickness to which all flesh is heir, were burdened by the perils of maternity, were left without skilled medical aid.

The first step towards bringing relief to the sick and suffering women of India was to provide them with doctors of their own sex, trained in modern science, and as a natural consequence, the trained nurse followed in the wake of the woman doctor. The medical women missionaries got in the thin edge of the wedge. Amongst pioneer workers there are the honoured names of Mary Seelye, M.D., who was sent out by America, and worked alone as a doctor in Calcutta, and Mrs. Janet Colquhoun Smith, who, in 1860, aided by the municipality and the Baptist missionaries, got an entrance into the zenanas of Serampore, and her sad experiences led to the foundation of the Medical Mission to Women. The Ladies' Association for Zenana Work was formed in 1867 by the Baptist Missionary Society, and in 1880 the Church of England Zenana Society was started. By means of missionary reports, public feeling was roused as to the neglected condition of the sick women and children of India, and great interest was taken in zenana work.

When, in January, 1877, in the historic spot outside the walls of Delhi, Queen Victoria was proclaimed Empress of India, a new era dawned for the women of the Eastern empire. With true womanly solicitude, the Queen-Empress was desirous of bettering the education and social condition of Hindoo women. She saw with heartfelt thankfulness the barbarous suttee abolished, and her influence inspired the rapid spread of zenana work.

In July, 1881, Queen Victoria received in private audience Miss Beilby, a medical missionary from India, and after listening to her account of the sufferings of Hindoo women for need of doctors, her Majesty turned to her ladies and said, " We had no idea that things were as bad as this." Miss Beilby then took from a locket, which she wore round her neck, a folded piece of paper, containing a message to the Queen from the Maharanee of Poonah. " The women of India suffer when they are sick," was the burden of the dark-eyed queen's appeal. The Queen-Empress returned a message of sympathy

and help to her subject in that far-off land, and to the
women of her own country said, " We desire it to be
generally known that we sympathize with every effort
made to relieve the suffering state of the women of
India."

When in 1884 the late Marquis of Dufferin and Ava
was appointed Viceroy of India, Queen Victoria sent for
Lady Dufferin before she left England, and asked her to
take a practical interest in the condition of the women of
the country. The commission could scarcely have been
entrusted to more capable or sympathetic hands. Immediately after her arrival Lady Dufferin took pains to learn
all that she could of the medical question in India as
regards women, and found that, although certain great
efforts were being made in a few places to provide female
attendance, hospitals, training-schools, and dispensaries
for women, and although missionary effort had done
much by sending out pioneers into the field, the women
of India as a whole were without that medical aid which
their European sisters have. With the idea of forming
a National Association, Lady Dufferin wrote to Mrs.
Grant Duff, Lady Reay, Lady Aitchison, Lady Lyall, and
Lady Rivers Thompson on the subject, and received their
cordial support. " The National Association for Supplying Female Medical Aid to the Women of India " was
started in 1885, a prospectus was published in various
languages all over India, appeals were made, and the
money collected was credited to " The Countess of
Dufferin Fund."

The objects of the Dufferin Fund are threefold—

1. *Medical tuition*, including the teaching and training
in India of women as doctors, hospital assistants, nurses,
and midwives.

2. *Medical relief*, including (*a*) the establishment,
under female superintendence, of dispensaries and
cottage hospitals for the treatment of women and
children ; (*b*) the opening of female wards under female
superintendence in existing hospitals and dispensaries ;

(c) the provision of female medical officers and attendants for existing female wards, and the founding of hospitals for women where special funds or endowments are forthcoming.

3. *The supply of trained female nurses and midwives* for women and children in hospitals and private houses.

Branch associations were established in different parts of India, each working under its own committee. Lady Dufferin desired to make the organization popular with the people, and each committee adopted measures to meet the religious feelings and customs of its locality. During the time that she remained in India, Lady Dufferin had the satisfaction of seeing the work firmly established, with most successful results. Some of the finest hospitals were built and are supported by native princes, and the Fund was augmented from all parts of the country. On her return home in 1888 Lady Dufferin became the very active president of the United Kingdom branch to promote all the objects of the National Association, and still continues her valuable work. Queen Alexandra is patron.

The work of the Association in India has been successively carried forward by Lady Lansdowne, Lady Elgin, and the late Lady Curzon, in their position as Vicereines, and Lady Minto is now devoting herself to it with great enthusiasm. The visits paid by the Princess of Wales to many of the Dufferin Fund hospitals during her recent tour in India was a great pleasure and encouragement to the doctors, nurses, and patients. The Princess, at the request of the Nizam of Hyderabad, laid the foundation-stone of the Victoria Zenana Hospital, Hyderabad, which will accommodate sixty purdah patients.

The reports of the work of the Association up to 1905 show that there are now forty-two lady doctors of the first grade, *i.e.* persons qualified for registration in the United Kingdom (special scholarships or grants-in-aid are made by the Association to students who, having

commenced their medical studies in India, proceed to
England to pass for the higher degrees in medicine),
eighty-seven assistant-surgeons or practitioners of the
second grade, who have been trained in India and hold
Indian qualifications, and two hundred and seventy-four
hospital assistants or practitioners of the third grade.

The female students in the principal medical colleges
and schools in India are ninety-nine European and native
ladies training as assistant surgeons, one hundred and
fifteen as hospital assistants, and three hundred and
twenty-three as nurses, *dais* (native midwives), and compounders. This latter total does not include a hundred
and seventy-two *dais* who are being trained under the
Victoria Memorial Scholarship Fund.

This Fund was initiated by the late Lady Curzon in
1901-02 during her husband's viceroyalty, for the purpose
of keeping in perpetual remembrance the name of the
Queen-Empress, and with the object of stimulating the
training of the *dais* or indigenous midwives, by offering
scholarships for proficiency. These practitioners are the
"Gamps" of India, only considerably worse than the
immortal "Sairey." Already the Dufferin Fund was
educating midwives of a superior class, but as the
standard required that these must be able to read and
write, understand lectures, and study text-books, the
number was restricted until female education had spread
amongst native women. Lady Curzon's idea was in the
mean time to get hold of as many of the *dais* as possible,
and instruct them at the Dufferin hospitals and dispensaries,
and by lectures in the country districts, and by enlightening their understanding, induce them to abandon the
cruel and barbarous practices to which they were accustomed. The teaching is at first oral, and conveyed in
the colloquial language familiar to the class of women,
and by degrees it is hoped to lead up to a higher form of
education. The practice of midwifery has been terribly
degraded in modern India. In the fourth century A.D.,
India had the ***Susruta Samhita*, a** treatise on midwifery

which has been described by a well-known specialist as
"a thoroughly rational system of medico-surgical teaching
based upon accurate observation of nature." The barbarous modern treatment is ascribed in part to caste
prejudices.

Since the formation of the Victoria Memorial Scholarship Fund, four hundred *dais* have passed through a
regular course of training, and of this number a hundred
and thirty-seven were instructed during the past year.
One hundred and seventy-two women are now attending
classes in various districts. Training in midwifery and
in gynæcological nursing is afforded at the Eden
Hospital, Calcutta, the Maternity Hospital, Madras, and
the Motlibai Hospital, Bombay. There are also institutions for the training of midwives only, the principal
being the Dufferin Hospital at Rangoon.

There are now in India two hundred and sixty
hospitals, special wards, and dispensaries of various kinds,
for the treatment of women, and officered by women,
governed by, or affiliated to, the National Association.
Many of these institutions afford training for nurses.
The length of training considerably varies.

We may take, as an example of Indian nursing regulations, the training-school of the General Hospital, Madras.
The nursing staff is under the immediate supervision
of the matron superintendent, and the assistant matron
(having English qualifications), and under the general
control of the senior medical officer of the hospital. The
duties consist in nursing patients, in the male and in the
female European and native wards, both night and day.
The day nurses are on duty from 6.30 a.m. to 6 p.m.,
and the night nurses from 5.55 p.m. to 6.45 a.m., with
intervals for meals. All the nurses are with
quarters in the hospital. The pupils ofptheidediining-
school are divided into (1) lady nurse probationers,
(2) special nurse probationers, (3) Government nurse
probationers, and (4) private nurse probationers, trained
at the cost of the Dufferin Fund, or of local bodies. Of

the first class, not more than two are admitted at a time. They receive a six months' course of training in sick nursing, and are required to pay a fee of Rs. 100 a month towards the cost of their board and tuition. Of the second class, not more than six special nurse probationers are received at a time, and their period of training covers a year. They pay Rs. 30 a month for their board, and are housed and trained free. The Government nurse probationers, are trained with a view to their ultimate employment in the hospital; not more than six are entertained at a time, and they are trained for a year. They are required to wear the nurses' uniform, and are allowed, in addition to free board and lodging, money and clothing to the value of Rs. 15 per mensem. The nurse probationers of all classes are required to do a certain amount of duty in the wards, and at the end of the period of their training, those that pass an examination are granted by the board of examiners certificates of qualification as sick nurses.

Nurse candidates are required to read and write well, and produce certificates of good character. They must be between the ages of twenty-one and forty, and only single women, widows, or women who have been permanently deserted by their husbands, are eligible for employment. The term of engagement is in the first instance for two years, after which, if their services are retained, they come on to the permanent pensionable establishment. The training-school supplies the nurses for the hospital, and for private work.

The following table shows the public nursing staff of the hospital, and rates of payment:—

1 Matron superintendent	on Rs.	300—20—400.
1 Assistant-matron superintendent	,,	300—20—300.
1 Head nurse	,,	70 per mensem.
1 Assistant head nurse	,,	60 ,,
8 First grade nurses	,,	55 each per mensem.
10 Second ,, ,,	,,	45 ,, ,,
10 Third ,, ,,	,,	35 ,, ,,

Each nurse, from the head nurse downwards, receives a ration allowance of Rs. 20 a month, and uniform at a cost of Rs. 30 a year.

The Cama Hospital, Bombay, has a training-school where the pupil nurses are instructed in their work on the lines of an English hospital. Lectures are given in a good lecture-room in the nurses' bungalow. The courses are sick-nursing, midwifery, elementary anatomy, and physiology. The lectures are given by the members of the medical staff in English, and also in the vernaculars. A dispensing class is held by one of the medical staff, when there are five or six pupils of sufficient intelligence in arithmetic to attend. The first acting physician of the hospital is Miss E. B. Meakin, M.D. The training school has sustained a great loss in the death of Miss Edith Atkinson, who had been lady superintendent since 1886, and had accomplished valuable pioneer work. The length of the course of training at the Cama has now been raised from eighteen months to three years. A new wing is being added to the nursing quarter.

The nursing problem of India has only just been touched. Nurses are very difficult to obtain, and women holding only midwives' certificates practise nursing on their own account in all branches, charging fees from three to ten rupees a day, and in many of the institutions the women under training as midwives nurse the sick. British trained nurses hold the superior posts in the big Government hospitals, but the difficulties of language and religion largely disqualify Europeans from nursing in the homes and native institutions of the country. Trained Hindoo and Eurasian nurses are greatly needed. Nursing has not yet become popular amongst the educated class. The modern Indian girl is more ambitious to use her new-found wings of learning to soar into the medical or some other profession rather than that of nursing. The supply of medical women is now greater than the demand. The Central Committee of the Dufferin Fund feel that their main duty lies, not so much in the erecting of new hospitals, but in

promoting the wider education of hospital assistants,
nurses, and midwives, who may be enabled to carry relief
to the outlying districts and villages.

At present there is no standard for training, and
unqualified nurses are, it seems, frequently turned out as
certificated nurses from the smaller local training and
licensing centres, and claim the same fee as the highly
trained English nurses from home. Colonel C. H.
Joubert, Inspector-General of civil hospitals in the United
Provinces, has made a strong protest on the subject in his
Government Report. "I consider," he writes, "that
small scattered training and licensing centres are a mistake,
though of course they are better than nothing. Women
should not be certified as trained nurses, except by one
examining board for each province. In each province
there should be only one centre, where probationers
receive a year's theoretical and practical training from a
competent instructor or an instructress, who should be an
English trained person. After this, the women should
be sent for six months' further practical work to certain
selected hospitals, where European patients are admitted,
and at the end of that time should be required to appear
for examination by the Provincial Board." Colonel
Joubert is of opinion that there is plenty of material in
India for producing good and efficiently trained nurses
and midwives, and instead of bringing so many nurses
from England at great expense, efforts should be directed
towards training women of the country, European and
Eurasian, in the existing hospitals where European
patients are treated, and that a few highly trained women
should be brought from England for the purpose of
instructing and teaching.

The nurses in the Zenana hospitals are largely recruited from the girls of the native Christian Mission
Schools. It is difficult to induce them to perform some
offices for the sick, which they have been taught to
consider degrading. As they are Christians, the patients
will not take food from them, but a Brahmani cook is

employed. At meal times all Christians, whether native or English, must keep at a discreet distance, lest their shadows fall upon the food and pollute it. Such are the difficulties of nursing in India. Yet when one thinks of the appalling ravages of plague and cholera, and the sufferers from famine and attendant sickness, it seems that no people in the world are so much in need of a system of good nursing as these millions of our Eastern Empire.

The nursing of Europeans in India has been met to some extent in the large towns by the Clewer, Wantage, and All Saints' Sisterhoods and kindred private institutions, but the dwellers up-country were for many years left totally unprovided with trained nurses. Hundreds of our country people, suffering from typhoid and malarial fevers, dysentery, and such complaints particularly dependent on good nursing, had to battle through sickness alone, or attended only by their kind but inexperienced friends.

To meet this want, the Up-country Nursing Association for Europeans was started in 1892. The special business of the Association was to engage nurses in England, pay for their outfit and passage to India, and place them at certain central stations where their services would be readily available. Upwards of thirty nurses have been sent. Applicants must be over twenty-five years of age. The term of service is five years. The honorary secretary is Mr. H. M. Birdwood, Dalkeith House, Twickenham, and Mrs. Sheppard of 10, Chester Place, Regent's Park, supplies information to nurses as regards rules and application forms.

The Countess of Minto, wife of the Viceroy, soon after her arrival in India devised a scheme for a wide extension of the provision for the nursing of Europeans and by the newly founded Indian Nursing Association, with which the Up-country Nursing Association is to be amalgamated, hopes to establish a system which will bring trained nursing within the reach of Europeans in every part of British India. Lady Minto's appeal in the *Times* for the starting of a fund has been favourably received.

The military nursing service of India was instituted in 1888, when Sir Frederick, now Lord Roberts, was commander-in-chief in India. Lady Roberts drew attention to the need of skilled nursing for the British soldier, and the Government of India consented to the formation of an Indian Nursing Service. In March, 1888, the little band of eight nursing sisters from England arrived at Bombay, under the superintendence of Miss Katharine Loch and Miss Oxley. Miss Loch and five sisters went to the military hospital at Rawal Pindi, and Miss Oxley and three sisters to Bangalore. A period of arduous work followed before any approach to the modern system was established. The sisters had to deal with untrained orderlies, unteachable native ward boys, and to overcome medical prejudice in some quarters. But perseverance and a kindly, tactful spirit helped the pioneers in their task. Miss Nightingale took great interest in the work, and sent cheery letters of encouragement to Miss Loch, who, as senior superintendent, bore the responsibility of initiating the service.

Miss Loch was the daughter of George Loch, Esq., Q.C., and of Catharine Brandeth, and was born in 1854, at Worsley Old Hall, Manchester. Born in the Crimean year, it seemed as though the spirit of military nursing had come with her into the world, and destined her to be the Florence Nightingale of India. Miss Loch was a nurse probationer at the County Hospital, Winchester, and in 1882 became night superintendent at St. Bartholomew's Hospital. She received the Royal Red Cross in 1891, in recognition of her work in organizing the Indian service. At Rawal Pindi, the memory of "Lady Loch," as the soldiers called her, is still green. She had great personal charm, was bright, witty, and vivacious; a good administrator, and a tactful disciplinarian. In 1902 her health gave way, and she was invalided home, to her keen sorrow and disappointment. It was a consolation to her in the last years of her life to be able still to render some service to India, as a member of the committee of the India Office, who deal with the appointment of ladies to the Indian service. Miss Loch died, July 1, 1904. A memoir, together with her letters home from India, has been published by General Bradshaw, the medical officer at Rawal Pindi, with an introduction by Lord Roberts.

Miss R. A. Betty, R.R.C., the attached friend and fellow-worker of Miss Loch, is the present senior superintendent of the Indian service, and has completed its organization as Queen Alexandra's Military Nursing Service for India. Miss Betty recently received the Royal Red Cross in recognition of her work. In its early years, the service consisted of four lady superintendents, nine assistant superintendents, and thirty-nine nursing sisters. In 1903 it was named the Queen Alexandra's Military Nursing Service, and the establishment has been increased to four lady superintendents, fifteen senior nursing sisters, and sixty-five nursing sisters. The rules of the service are furnished to applicants by the India Office, Whitehall. Nursing sisters are received between the ages of twenty-five and thirty-five, and must have a three years' hospital certificate and be medically certified as fit for service in India.

Lady Roberts continues to take a deep interest in the army nursing in India.

Lady Roberts' Fund for Nursing Sisters' and Officers' Hospitals was started with the object of supplying homes in the hills for the nurses working in the military hospitals of India, and also to provide hospitals for officers in connection with their homes, and to provide an auxiliary staff of lady nurses to work in those military hospitals to which the Government has not supplied nurses.

The Self-Governing Colonies.

The history of nursing in the self-governing colonies is practically a continuation of that of the mother country. As reforms were effected in our own institutions, they travelled across the water to our kith and kin, who began to set their nursing house in order, adapting the modern system to their peculiar requirements.

Early colonial nursing had the rough elements pertaining to the stalwart pioneers who dug the virgin soil and built their houses with primeval timber. The rough log house which served as a hospital for the little struggling colony, rose side by side with the primitive schoolroom and church, and was "nursed" by all and sundry who could give time to the work. Every colonial woman was credited with being "a born nurse." Wives and mothers nursed their husbands and families as a matter of course, and neighbour assisted neighbour in cases of extremity. The time-honoured remedies of the dear home land served most purposes—one can imagine a prairie farmer being persuaded by his family to ward off the effects of a chill by putting his feet in hot water and mustard, or an ailing youngster in the bush being dosed with Gregory powder and senna. Sometimes there would be a day's journey to borrow castor-oil from a neighbour. There were *sage femmes* who were fetched by anxious husbands in jolting ox-carts, and who presided over birth and death with characteristic equanimity, and ate buttered toast and imbibed spirituous liquors with a relish worthy of the old country. Counterparts of the Gamps and Betsey Prigs at home pursued their methods on snow-clad prairie or under the tropic zone.

There was no talk amongst those brave, hard-working settlers about fashionable cures, but they lived perforce the "simple life," and defied disease better than the old folks at home. Perhaps they would have been saved the expense of hospitals and the problem of a nursing question had things remained stationary. But the tiny settlements sprang up into towns and cities, the log hospitals were replaced by more pretentious institutions, and nursing staffs were organized out of such material as was available. The towns grew and flourished, disease increased, hospitals became unsanitary and overcrowded, and the patients fared no better than if they had been at " Bart's " or the " London " before the days of reform.

The advent of enterprising young doctors from the London schools seeking colonial appointments, brought the news to astonished ears that at home educated ladies were taking up nursing. The new-comers averred that they had seen some of the phenomena in the wards of King's College or St. Thomas's Hospital. Colonial committees pondered on these things, and the women were roused to action by the name of Florence Nightingale. As the colonial hospitals had adopted the easy methods of the old country, so they followed suit in matters of reform. Across the seas was wafted the Macedonian cry, "Come over and help us," and the home hospitals responded as soon as they had trained sisters to send. Graduates from St. Thomas's became matrons and superintendents of many colonial hospitals, and introduced the Nightingale system. When a new hospital was to be erected in Melbourne or Sydney, Montreal or Ottawa, the authorities generally sought the advice of the heroine of the Crimea. In her invalid's room she was a court of appeal for the colonies, and for the United States also, as well as for the mother country.

Florence Nightingale belongs to the British stock wherever it is planted, as do Elizabeth Fry and all those nursing pioneers who have built up the modern system in this country. Every organization and institution which has helped forward the work of reform in Great Britain is the equal heritage of the colonial men and women whose pluck, enterprise, and industry have made our Empire glorious.

In Canada the foundations of hospitals and of nursing institutions were laid nearly three centuries ago by the French settlers in Quebec. The Sisters of Charity were the pioneer nurses of the colony. They nursed the poor in hospital, and tended the sick in their own homes. Longfellow has made their ministrations immortal in "Evangeline"—

> "Thus many years she lived as a sister of mercy; frequenting
> Lonely and wretched roofs in the crowded lanes of the city,
> Where distress and want concealed themselves from the sunlight,
> Where disease and sorrow in garrets languished neglected.
> Night after night, when the world was asleep, as the watchman repeated
> Loud, through the gusty streets, that all was well in the city,
> High at some lonely window he saw the light of her taper.
> Day after day, in the grey of the dawn, as slow through the suburbs
> Plodded the German farmer, with flowers and fruits for the market,
> Met he that meek, pale face, returning home from its watchings."

As early as 1639 the Hospital of the Precious Blood was founded at Quebec by Mother Marie Guenet de St. Ignace, who was induced to come to Canada by the Duchess of Aiguillon, one of the ladies of charity assisting St. Vincent de Paul. The Hôtel Dieu, Pine Avenue, Montreal, was founded in 1642 by Mdle. Jane Mance, and nursed by the sisters of St. Joseph. Both these institutions still carry on their work of nursing the sick poor without regard to nationality or creed. There are now eight branches of the Hôtel Dieu, Montreal, in other dioceses. A number of other hospitals and nursing institutions in Canada have been founded by the Grey Sisters, the sisters of St. Joseph, and similar Orders. The Catholic sisters are showing some willingness to come into line with the modern trained movement. The Notre Dame Hospital, Montreal, managed by the Grey Sisters, grants certificates to the hospital sisters who have successfully followed the three years' course given by the staff doctors.

After the final settlement of the French and British colonies in Canada as a self-governing dominion of the British Empire, there was a great increase of immigrants, followed by the opening up of virgin territory, and many new hospitals were built by the Protestant community, and our French Roman Catholic fellow-subjects also followed up their early work by the starting of new institutions. There has been a rapid advance during the last twenty years. Nursing-schools are attached to the chief hospitals, and the regulations are similar to those of British institutions. At the Winnipeg General Hospital Training-School, there is an average of eighty pupil nurses, and the three years' course is a very thorough one in medical, surgical, and obstetric nursing. The Montreal General Hospital has seventy nurses in training, and the Royal Victoria Hospital, Quebec, has an average of fifty-four pupil nurses for a three years' course. The Canadian Nurses have two main associations—the Canadian Nurses' Association, Montreal, and the Trained Nurses' Association, Winnipeg. There are other smaller societies in various districts. The nursing journal is the *Canadian Nurse*. The movement for State registration is being vigorously promoted by the Ontario Trained Nurses' Association, which has a Bill before the Ontario legislature. The Bill provides for a governing body consisting of eleven nurses and four medical men.

District nursing in Canada was organized on a sound basis in 1897, when Lady Aberdeen, during Lord Aberdeen's viceroyalty, founded the Victorian Order of Nurses to commemorate the Diamond Jubilee of Queen Victoria. The headquarters are at 578, Somerset Street, Ottawa. There are training-homes at Montreal and Toronto, where nurse graduates of recognized training-schools receive a special four months' course in district work, after which they are given the diploma of the Order and assigned a district or hospital, as the case may be. The scheme of covering Canada, even to the furthest limits, with Victorian nurses is indeed a vast one.

Lady Minto, during her husband's viceroyalty, initiated the Lady Minto Cottage Hospital Fund in connection with the Victorian Order, and for the purpose of making grants to and establishing cottage hospitals in the sparsely populated districts. One of the most isolated of these hospitals is at Rock Bay, a lumbering camp on Vancouver Island. Here, where between three and four thousand loggers are employed, there was no medical aid at hand. It was a red-letter day for the toilers when a doctor and a staff of nurses, with medicines and dressings, arrived and "set up hospital" at the camp. The nurses are the only women within a radius of many miles.

The work which the Victorian nurses are doing in these rough and difficult places is beyond praise. In the towns they work on similar lines to our own district nurses. The work, begun eight years ago on a very small scale, now extends from the Atlantic to the Pacific, and includes seventeen hospitals and eighteen districts, making a total of thirty-five branches, and employing about ninety nurses. The next report will greatly increase this number. The work is indeed limitless. Miss Margaret Allen is the lady superintendent.

Australia, youthful and buoyant, profits by having been born when the nursing problem of the mother country was at the acute stage, and about to get a turn for the better. When the colonization of the great continent, discovered by Captain Cook, was beginning in earnest in 1840, Elizabeth Fry was founding our first institution for the training of nurses. At the back of the English reformers were long centuries of tradition to be overcome. Happy Australia to have no traditions!

All that the young colony had to do was to take warning from home institutions, and start well. The brilliant example of the Nightingale School was illuminating the Thames almost before Australia had had time to build hospitals. Still, the new continent has had to work out its own salvation from the nursing point of view. The people who rushed to its gold fields had to put up with such nursing as comrade gives to comrade. Then the towns arose; Sydney and Melbourne grew into beautiful cities, and with such a climate no one should have been ill; but, alas! the Australian colonists had to build hospitals, and have continued to go on building them. The nursing in the big general hospitals has been organized on the modern British plan, and in many instances by matrons and superintendents who came out from the home training-schools. In some of the larger hospitals of Australasia there is a highly organized nursing staff, classified into sisters, charge and ward nurses, nurses, assistant nurses, and probationers, with a training-school, systematic lectures, and certificates granted after examination by a medical board. In the smallest hospitals, the nursing staff may consist of the matron and wardsman only, who are frequently man and wife. Between these two extremes there are all gradations of nursing arrangements.

The largest training-school is, I believe, the one attached to the Royal Prince Alfred Hospital, Sydney, which has some fifty pupil nurses. The hospital beds two hundred and thirty-six. It was opened in 1882 on modern lines, and has rapidly progressed. Mrs. Murray was the first matron, and to her efforts the success of the nursing school is largely due. The hospital was built to commemorate the escape of the late Duke of Saxe-Coburg (then Prince Alfred), who was shot at by a madman in Sydney. Sir Alfred Roberts was the moving spirit of the enterprise, and devoted himself in a most thorough manner to making the hospital a model institution. The story is told that, one day, when on a round of inspection, Sir Alfred stopped on the stairs of C pavilion, and opening the small blade of his penknife, scraped in a corner for a short time, and then presenting to the matron an infinitesimal amount of dust sorrowfully said, "Mrs. Murray, this ought not to be."

Mrs. Murray began the organization of her staff at Maud Cottage in July, 1882, before the hospital was opened, and her experience presents an amusing picture of colonial work at this comparatively recent period. Nurses were advertised for in the local papers, and, "as there were but few applicants," writes Mrs. Murray, "we had to gather in the weeds and be thankful if we found a flower among them. They came with their hair flowing in ringlets to the waists; they came in wigs; they came in dresses up to their knees; they came in bed-gowns tied at the middle by a petticoat. We said we wished them from twenty-five to thirty years of age, but those who looked sixteen and those who looked sixty all declared they conformed to this regulation. I began to think Sapphira's descendants must have had an unfair allowance of daughters, who had all entered the nursing profession."

The matron's trials with the commissariat were on a par with procuring a nursing staff. When she asked where the patients' brandy was to come from, she was told, "Oh, you must get it from a public-house, until proper arrangements are made." "I did not like," continues Mrs. Murray, in her lively narrative of pioneer work, "to send any nurse for it, as I felt myself the guardian of their characters, so directly it was dusk I put on my longest cloak, and, looking this way and that, slipped across to the nearest public-house. I was too frightened to wait for paper, and seizing the bottle, I stowed it under my cloak and fled home again. Of course, it was soon all over the place, 'Such a shocking thing—the new matron drank so dreadfully.'"

Mrs. Murray raised a fund to build a Nurses' Home, which was opened in 1887, and by degrees she obtained nurses of a higher standard than the "Sapphira" band who first applied. A fourth year has been added to the usual three years' course at this School, during which midwifery, nervous and insane nursing, dispensing, and housekeeping are taught. There is no premium, and the salary for probationers is a rising one, from £5 to £15, nurses £36 to £44, sisters £50 to £60. Laundry and indoor uniform provided.

Great strides have been made in the status of Australian nurses since Mrs. Murray's experience, twenty-five years ago. Dr. Harvey, of the Perth Hospital, Western Australia, who has recently been visiting this country, gave me a glowing description of the Australian nurse. The domestic class have been largely weeded out, and the daughters of professional men and government officials now enter the profession in large numbers, and regard it as a most desirable and honourable calling. There is a very large number of trained nurses in private practice, and they are greatly esteemed by the community. Dr. Harvey, after twenty-six years in Australia, was surprised to hear on his return home the strictures passed on the private nurse in this country. In Australia she is popular, and receives from two guineas to five guineas per week. The private nurse enters the house as the servant of the doctor. If she has any complaint she makes it to the doctor, who arranges matters with the responsible head of the house, and so ructions are avoided. The nurse does everything in the sick-room, and everything is brought to the patient. The nurse does not look to the mistress of the house at all.

Homes for private nurses are kept by trained women who have been in active practice themselves. The nurse takes her own fees, and pays so much when she is in the Home and so much when she is not there. The superintendent of the Home is responsible to the doctor for the good conduct of the nurse she supplies.

District nursing in Australia has developed during the past few years, but there is no national organization corresponding to our own or to the Victorian Order of Canada. The Melbourne District Nursing Society was established in 1885, and the District Trained Nursing Society of South Australia, which has its headquarters in Adelaide, was established in 1894.

In Western Australia the reform in nursing set in about 1890-91. Ffteen years ago it was scarcely possible to get a trained nurse in West Australia. In 1894 the new Government hospital was built at Perth, nurses were procured from Sydney, Melbourne, and other hospitals, Miss Gordon became the first matron, and a central nurses' training-school for West Australia was established.

Dr. Harvey has been connected with it from the beginning and holds most progressive views with regard to the status and training of nurses. Judging from the impressions which he conveyed, the Australian nurses are practical, sensible women. The sentimental and hysterical girl is quite out of the running, and even the nice, good girl has no chance unless she is also sharp, keen, and intelligent. The nursing examinations are as hard as they can be made, and a thorough drilling by the matron in domestic economy is a prominent feature of the training. The nurses are well paid and well cared for, but not petted, and their quarters are refined and comfortable, though not luxurious. There is no pension system, as in Australia the idea is disliked as having a pauperizing element. The prudent nurse avails herself of the various insurance companies, which provide a very liberal scale.

Registration is a practical question in Australia, and organization is rapidly proceeding. In 1899 the "Australasian Trained Nurses' Association" was founded with the object of establishing a system of registration for trained nurses, and in 1901 "The Victorian Trained Nurses' Association" was founded in Victoria to establish a system of registration for trained nurses. The organ of the latter Association is *Una*. Recently a conference has been held between the two Associations, and a working basis for establishing a uniform system of training and examination throughout Australasia seems to have been arrived at. The first general examination for membership of the Australian Trained Nurses' Association was held this year, the centres being Sydney, Brisbane, and Fiji. It has been decided in future that examinations will be held simultaneously in each of the States.

There is a general feeling, and perhaps a natural one, amongst Australian nurses that Australia is for the Australian-born, and nurses from the old country are no longer needed. New-comers are required to pass an examination of fitness before taking up work.

In New Zealand great reforms have been effected

during the past year or two in the management of the hospitals and the organization of nursing, and judging from the Report of the Inspector of Hospitals, published in 1905, reforms were urgently needed. Sanitary arrangements in the majority of the smaller institutions are reported as all out of date, and the training of nurses almost entirely neglected. One reads of a small hospital or home for broken-down miners where the inmates were bathed *once a month*. At one hospital the matron is reproved for "extreme kindness, not to say softness;" the nurses did as they liked, and grave irregularities occurred. Another hospital persisted in appointing unsuitable matrons, and in rejecting first-rate applicants. Much of the trouble and unsatisfactoriness in the adversely criticized institutions seems to have arisen from having untrained matrons.

A very favourable report is given of the Wellington Hospital, and of the work there of Dr. Ewart, the medical superintendent, and of Miss Payne, the matron. A fine new Home has recently been opened for the nursing staff.

The Dunedin Hospital is also favourably reported upon. Miss Fraser, the matron, has been doing excellent work there for thirteen years, and was much gratified to find, after a recent visit to the hospitals in America and the Old Country, that her own hospital now compares most favourably with those she visited. "We possess," she writes, "a very progressive honorary staff; have also a medical school attached, consequently we aim at a very high standard and up-to-date system in all departments. Some of our wards and our operating theatre are comparatively new and on the most modern principles." Miss Fraser has a charitable word to say for the old untrained nurse, and does not think it fair that she should be criticized too severely when we remember the disadvantages under which she laboured. Miss Fraser was trained at the Edinburgh Royal Infirmary, later she was sister in the Western Infirmary, Glasgow; then she went to Australia, and was for two years night superintendent in the Melbourne Hospital, when she received her present appointment. She is a member of the Royal British Nurses' Association, and is a State registered nurse.

In 1901 the Legislature of New Zealand passed a Nurses' Registration Act, and in 1903 it was further enacted by the Public Health Act of New Zealand that all Nursing Homes in the colony should be registered and inspected by the Public Health Department. The effect has been a steady improvement in the nursing staff of the hospitals, and in other branches of the profession, by the weeding out of the unfit. Mrs. Neill, the nursing inspector, reports favourably on the work of the Act, as also the medical inspector. The Registration Act of New Zealand provides that, "every person who has attained the age of twenty-three years, and is certified as having had three years' training as a nurse in a hospital, and who passes an examination from time to time held by examiners appointed under this Act, is entitled to registration on payment of a fee of one pound." When a nurse is duly registered, she receives a certificate, together with a badge bearing her name and the date of registration. Registration may be cancelled for misconduct. The Act came into operation January 1, 1902.

Tasmania is well to the front in its nurse training-schools. At the Hobart General Hospital, lectures and instruction to nurses have been given by the honorary medical officers, the resident house-surgeon, and matron for the past thirty years. Its training-school was therefore started prior to many of those in connection with large hospitals in the home country. The period of training for nurses at the Hobart Hospital was originally two years, but in 1893 it was increased to three years, and in 1904 it was further extended to four years. Accepted candidates have now to undergo three months' trial duty. After passing the third year's examination, nurses take their senior gynæcological work, which includes three months' duty as operating theatre nurse.

In July, 1900, the Hobart Hospital was enrolled as a hospital recognized by the council of the Australian Nurses' Association, and in joining that modern Association pointed out with pardonable pride that for the past sixteen years the nurses trained in the Hobart Hospital have received practical, oral, and demonstrative training in all such subjects, as well as others not mentioned in the curriculum adopted by the Australian Trained Nurses' Association. The first matron of the Hobart Hospital was Miss F. Abbott, and the present lady superintendent is Miss Nancy Johnstone Turnbull, who has held the post since 1896.

The Launceston General Hospital, Tasmania, has also a good training-school, which was started and has been admirably developed by Miss J. H. Milne, who was appointed matron in 1886, and still occupies the position. Miss Milne was trained at the Royal Infirmary, Edinburgh. When she first came to Launceston, one of the sisters could not even read, and could hardly sign her name. The chief function of the nurses was to keep the ward clean and the beds tidy; the medical officers took the temperature and administered necessary enemata. She gradually substituted trained for untrained nurses, and established a proper curriculum and course of training. Miss Milne was successively assisted in building up the school by Dr. L. G. Thompson and Dr. F. J. Drake, surgeon-superintendents, who organized lectures, and by Dr. J. Ramsay, medical superintendent. On the death of William Barnes, Esq., chairman of the Visiting Committee, who had taken a keen interest in the welfare of the nursing staff, his widow invested the sum of one hundred and fifty pounds for the purposes of a prize— the "William Barnes Prize," to be awarded annually to the most successful nurse of each year. In 1893 the term of training was increased from two to three years; and finally, in 1905, the period of training was fixed at four years, the fourth year being devoted entirely to practical work in the wards. There are now twenty-six probationers in training. A new Nurses' Home on the hill above the hospital was erected in 1897. The Queen Victoria Hospital for Women at Launceston trains nurses, and grants a certificate for midwifery and obstetrical nursing.

A united effort is now being made by the trained nurses of Tasmania to have a "Trained Nurses' Registration Bill" introduced into Parliament that will safeguard their interests, provide for State registration, and for a uniform standard of examination throughout the State of Tasmania by a central examining body. The Federated States of Australasia seem all uniting in the demand for the State registration of nurses, and New Zealand has led the way.

South Africa is at present a land of problems and experiments, and nursing is, like other matters, in a state of being organized. British colonization in South Africa began at the Cape of Good Hope about 1814. The first general hospital established in Cape Colony was the Somerset Hospital, named after Lord Charles Somerset, and founded in the year 1816 by Dr. Bailey, a naval surgeon, who established himself about that time in private practice in Cape Town. Then came, in 1856, the Grey Hospital, King William's Town, designed to serve a certain purpose amongst the natives by educating them, and weakening the hold of witchcraft upon them. These two hospitals remain entirely under Government control. Next followed the Provincial Hospital, Port Elizabeth, the Albany General Hospital, Grahamstown, and, sixteen years later, the Kimberley Hospital. Within the past ten years the number of hospitals in Cape Colony has been doubled, and now stands at twenty-four. The nursing was first of all of the old order, and bad at that. Some trained nurses then began to be recruited from the home country, and finally, in 1891, the registration of trained nurses and of midwives was enforced in Cape Colony under the Medical and Pharmacy Act, Cape of Good Hope, promulgated August 21, 1891. The Medical

Council decides whether a nurse or a midwife is a fit person to be put on the register, and grants certificates of competence, with the approval of the Government. In 1899 Natal followed suit, and its nurses were registered under the Medical and Pharmacy Act.

A very small number of probationers are trained in the Cape hospitals; the largest training-school is that of the Provincial Hospital, Port Elizabeth, where there are upwards of thirteen probationers. Certificates are granted upon the satisfactory completion of the three years' course of training. State examinations are held every six months, and all nurses passing the examination are registered by the Government. Probationers receive a rising salary from eighteen pounds to forty-five pounds per annum; staff nurses, fifty pounds per annum; sisters, seventy-two pounds per annum. The Victoria Nurses' Institute, Cape Town, was established in 1897, and supplies private and district nurses.

South Africa having only recently been accorded the dignity of a self-governing colony, it is for the present chiefly dependent on the home country for its nurses, a number of whom are sent out by the Colonial Nursing Association. The Johannesburg Hospital has a training-school with upwards of fifty probationers, who are received for three years' training. There is a Nurses' Co-operative Society at 72, Jeppe Street, Johannesburg. Candidates must have had three years' hospital training and experience in private nursing.

Since the war, Queen Alexandra's Military Nursing Service for South Africa has been organized, with headquarters at Pretoria. Miss Keer, R.R.C., now matron-in-chief at the War Office, organized the new service, and has been succeeded by Miss Addams-Williams, R.R.C., as principal matron for South Africa. The position involves the general supervision and inspection of all military hospitals in the country, including the hospitals of women and children at the various military stations. A reserve of nurses is always maintained at Pretoria to meet emergencies. There are also district nurses employed.

Nursing in South Africa presents many difficulties, owing to the unsettled state of the country, and the work in many parts is rough and hazardous. British nurses are, however, plucky pioneers, and the latest self-governing colony added to the Crown will not want for volunteers.

The Crown Colonies and Protectorates.

Until ten years ago, little attention was given to providing trained or, indeed, any kind of nursing for the British communities in the Crown colonies and protectorates, a large number of which are in tropical or subtropical regions, where our people are particularly exposed to disease. The families of the resident officials, and of those engaged in business enterprises, were often in great straits in time of sickness, and many valuable lives were lost for need of nursing. Young men who went out to these deadly climates often died in remote regions untended and uncared for, save by the ignorant efforts of native servants. The more important Crown colonies have for many years had good Government hospitals, with English-trained nurses; but these were of no avail for people stricken with sickness in isolated districts.

Mrs. Francis, now Lady Piggott, the wife of a distinguished member of the Colonial Service, while living in the island of Mauritius, had the need of a provision for trained nursing in that colony brought home to her by some painful facts. Three young Englishmen died on one plantation alone, and it was evident that each life might have been saved by proper nursing. Another case was that of the young wife of an officer lying seriously ill, her child at death's door, and only an ignorant native woman to attend them. Often Lady Piggott went to the assistance of friends in similar distressing circumstances, and she was made keenly sensible of the fact that the services of a good nurse were not procurable, even for money, and that, too, in a colony with many well-to-do people.

Lady Piggott extended her inquiries to other colonies, where it was found the same state of things prevailed. When she returned to England in 1895, Lady Piggott laid the matter before influential friends, and also obtained the support of the Colonial Office." A fund of several hundred pounds was raised, and two private nurses were sent out to the Mauritius, at salaries of sixty pounds each per annum and their passage paid. Such was the nucleus of the Colonial Nursing Association, which is now carrying the boon of trained nursing even to the most remote dependency.

The Association held its first general meeting in the summer of 1896. The Rt. Hon. Joseph Chamberlain, Secretary of State for the Colonies, gave the imperial seal to the scheme by sending an official notice to the governors of the Crown colonies, recommending it to their consideration. Mrs. Chamberlain is a warm friend of the Association, and has greatly helped it by her pen and by her influence.

Her Royal Highness Princess Henry of Battenberg consented to become patron, and Lord Loch, chairman of the Association. A small committee of management was formed with Lady Piggott as honorary secretary. In 1899 more formal rules were adopted, and the work divided between three sub-committees—colonial, finance, and nursing. The colonial committee was the medium for arranging for local committees at the centres requiring nurses, the finance committee dealt with money matters, and the nursing committee selected candidates to be sent out as nurses.

The original idea was to provide private nurses, but the Government requested that the Association would relieve them of the task of selecting nurses for the Crown Colony hospitals, and so the work of the Association has proceeded in two main lines. It selects and sends out nurses to the Government hospitals in the Crown colonics, and provides private nurses in centres where the British inhabitants have formed a local committee. The Association has no financial responsibility regarding nurses whom it selects for the Government hospitals, who are under the regulations for Government servants, and are paid by the colony in which they are employed. The private nurses, however, come under the rules of the Association, and sign an agreement to that effect, and bind themselves to obey the rules of their local committee.

Colonial nurses are paid not less than sixty pounds per annum, board and lodging being provided by the local committee in each colony. For hospital appointments the salaries vary from seventy pounds to one hundred and fifty pounds. The nurse's second-class passage out and home is paid. The usual term of engagement is for three years. Candidates must be fully trained, and preferably gentlewomen. They must in almost every case possess midwifery training. Very few vacancies occur where this is not an essential. The limit of age is twenty-five to thirty-five. All nurses must conform to regulations regarding uniform, and wear the silver badge of the Association. As the work of colonial nurses largely lies in climates where tropical diseases prevail, special grants are given to those who attend the course held at the schools of Tropical medicine in London and at Liverpool. The committee have recently passed a resolution that in the future they will give grants to nurses who, having done well during their terms of agreement abroad, would like to bring their nursing knowledge up to date by a course of three months at one of the large general hospitals in this country. There is a small Sick Pay Fund attached to the Association, worked by a separate committee, which gives grants to the colonial nurses who are invalided home from abroad, sending them for a treatment and change of air to Convalescent Homes. Owing to the fact that the nurses serve in dangerous climates, there are many invalided home, and the Sick Fund has proved most useful. The headquarters of the Association are at the Imperial Institute, S.W. The secretary is Miss M. E. Dalrymple Hay, to whose practical and business-like methods much of the success of the Association is due.

Good progress has been made during the ten years that the Association has been at work. Two hundred and fifteen nurses have been selected for the Government hospitals in the Crown colonies, and ninety nurses have been sent out for private work. It is a study in geography to note the places where colonial nurses are serving. The Association now selects the matrons and nurses for twenty different Crown colonies and protectorates in Central, East, and West Africa, the Transvaal, the Eastern Crown colonies, the Mediterranean colonies, and the West Indies, whilst the private nurses are working in Bangkok, Ceylon, Costa Rica, Cyprus, Hong Kong, India, Japan, Lisbon, Mauritius, Oporto, Singapore, South Africa, Teheran, and Rhodesia. Recently a nurse has been selected for work with the South African Church Railway Mission, which is doing such useful work in ministering to the large British and Dutch population scattered along the South African railways; and another nurse has been sent to the lonely and wind-swept Falkland Islands in the South Atlantic. She is the only nurse in the colony. Interesting particulars of the work, received from the nurses themselves, are published in a special column in *Nursing Notes.*

Many are the dangers faced by the colonial nurses, and difficult is the nursing which they are often called upon to undertake. In Uganda they are battling with that strange devastating epidemic, the sleeping sickness, which has not only decimated the native population, but has also begun to attack Europeans. At Zanzibar, emergency nurses have been dealing with the outbreak of plague. The nurse sent out to Teheran in October, 1905, just when the troubles in Russia were at their worst, had to encounter many difficulties and dangers. She had the advantage of travelling under the escort of the late

Dr. Odling (Physician to the British Legation, Teheran) and Mrs. Odling, but the journey was rendered more than usually adventurous by the railway strike, which delayed the travellers for three days on the Russian frontier. Colonial British nurses, like colonial pioneers, meet bravely the day's work as it comes, and their services are held in grateful regard by the people at home, many of whom have sons out in lonely places exposed to sickness and disease.

Princess Henry of Battenberg continues her interest as patron of the Association, Lord Ampthill, G.C.S.I., has succeeded Lord Loch as president, the Rt. Hon. Sir Albert Hime, K.C.M.G., is vice-president, and Lady Piggott, honorary vice-president. The council and executive committee are composed of influential members. C. T. Bruce, Esq., is chairman of the General Purposes committee; Mrs. Weston Devenish is chairman of the Nursing committee; Lady Ommanney, chairman of the Sick Pay Fund committee; Sir Edward Noel-Walker, R.C.M.G., is honorary treasurer; Miss Mowbray, honorary secretary; and Miss M. E. Dalrymple Hay, the secretary.

A Scottish branch has been organized with its own council and committees. The Lady Balfour of Burleigh takes an active interest in the work. She is president of the Scottish branch, also of the executive and of the nursing committee. The joint honorary secretaries are Charles F. Whigham, Esq., C.A., and Charles L. Dalzell, Esq., C.A. The headquarters are 46, Castle Street, Edinburgh.

Lord Elgin, the Secretary of State for the Colonies, is much interested in the work of the Association, and at the last annual meeting gave a stimulating and encouraging address. The meeting was held in the library of the Colonial Office, thereby testifying to the position of the Association as a branch of Government work. It has an invested fund, and is further supported by private subscription.

CHAPTER XXII

ORGANIZATION AND REGISTRATION

The nursing profession, the first profession for women incorporated by Royal Charter—Miss Catherine Wood suggests organization—A meeting in favour at the house of Sir Henry Burdett—Original plan abandoned—A meeting at the house of Dr. and Mrs. Bedford Fenwick—The British Nurses' Association inaugurated—Princess Christian consents to become president—Rules for members—Registration of its nurses—Is incorporated by Royal Charter—List of associates to whom granted—The purposes defined in the Charter—Government of the Association—Rules for membership—Its headquarters—The nurses' settlement—The Chartered Nurses' Society.—The Auxiliary Nurses' Society—Membership of the Royal British Nurses' Association. THE STATE REGISTRATION OF NURSES—History of the movement—A select committee of the House of Commons appointed to consider the question.—A resolution in favour of registration by the British Medical Association—Bill introduced into the House of Commons by Mr. Munro Ferguson—Thirty-four witnesses examined by the Select Committee—Views of the advocates for State registration—Views of the opponents to State registration—Conclusions and recommendations of the Select Committe—Deputations to the Lord President of the Council—Reply of Lord Crewe—The British Medical Association pass a resolution in favour of the principle of State registration—Active propaganda for Parliamentary Bills.

To the nursing profession belongs the distinction of being the first profession for women incorporated by Royal Charter. Since the early pioneer efforts in the forties nursing had been developing in the various branches dealt with in the foregoing pages. Nurses for the sick had grown into a large and rapidly increasing body. The changes in the treatment of disease had brought the nurse more and more to the front, and it was inevitable that the demands made upon her for superior training should result in her desire for a professional status. Throughout the Victorian era nurses had been developing from the uneducated into the trained and skilful workers, and with singular fitness the first steps towards organization took place in the jubilee year of Queen Victoria.

The 1887 marks an important epoch in the history of nursing. It saw the establishment of the first great nursing organizations, the Queen Victoria Jubilee Institute and the Royal British Nurses' Association. The Jubilee Institute has already been dealt with. It organized the trained women engaged in nursing the sick poor in their own homes. The nurses engaged in hospitals, infirmaries, and in private work were also many of them desirous of being banded together as an Association of trained workers, in order to differentiate themselves from the untrained or only partially trained nurse.

The idea of forming an Association of nurses originated chiefly with Miss Catherine Wood, then superintendent of the Great Ormond Street Hospital for Children. Miss Wood, in a letter to Sir Henry, then Mr., Burdett, of the Hospitals' Association, suggested that a nursing section might be formed in connection with that Association, to which he agreed, and a meeting of hospital matrons and others interested in the subject was held at Sir Henry Burdett's house, The Lodge, Porchester Square. This was the beginning of the movement for nursing organization. A basis of agreement was not, however, arrived at in conjunction with the Hospitals' Association.

On November 21, 1887, the ladies who had been interested in forming a nursing section met by invitation of Mrs. Bedford Fenwick at her house, 20, Upper Wimpole Street. Mrs. Bedford Fenwick had been well known in the nursing world as Miss Ethel Gordon Manson, the matron of St. Bartholomew's Hospital, and her marriage to Dr. Bedford Fenwick had recently taken place. At the preliminary meeting at her house it was resolved to form a British Nurses' Association, which it was hoped would in time include all nurses in the United Kingdom. An intimation was sent round to people likely to co-operate in such a movement, inviting them to a council. On December 7th a meeting took place, at which were present Dr. and Mrs. Bedford Fenwick, and the following representative matrons and superintendents :—Miss Catherine Wood, Great Ormond Street Hospital for Children ; Miss Isla Stewart, St. Bartholomew's Hospital ; Miss East, the National Hospital for the Paralyzed and Epileptic ; Miss Mollett, Chelsea Infirmary ; Mrs. Deeble, Royal Victoria Hospital, Netley ; and Miss Hogg, Royal Naval Hospital, Haslar. Mrs. Bedford Fenwick read a paper setting forth the objects of the proposed scheme, and with the concurrence of the ladies present an Association was founded to be called The British Nurses' Association, and an executive committee elected. On the suggestion of Mrs. Bedford Fenwick, it was decided to lay the matter before members of the medical profession, with the view of engaging their interest and support. It was also decided to ask Her Royal Highness Princess Christian to become president of the Association. Miss Catherine Wood undertook the duties of honorary secretary, which she discharged with characteristic ability until 1892, assisted by Miss Paul, secretary of the Association. Miss Catherine Wood, with her clear judgment and statesmanlike grasp of essentials, did most important pioneer work for the association, of which she still remains a member.

Her Royal Highness Princess Christian of Schleswig-Holstein consented to become president of the Association, and presided at the first council meeting. Throughout the various controversies which have arisen in the Association, Princess Christian has maintained a constitutional attitude as president now for close upon twenty years. Queen Victoria granted the Association the title of "Royal," and in 1893 it was incorporated by Royal Charter.

A bye-law provided that until January, 1889, the following should be eligible to become members on producing to the Executive Committee satisfactory evidence of professional attainments and personal character, and of having been engaged three years in nursing, viz. the past or present matrons or lady superintendents, sisters or nurses of any public hospital, or infirmary, or public or district nursing association in the British Empire, all trained midwives and women who have been engaged in private nursing. On or after January 1, 1889, the conditions of membership were to be determined from time to time by the Executive Committee, subject to the approval of the General Council.

In 1890 the Association began a system of registration of nurses analogous to that which has been for many years compulsory upon members of the medical profession. The idea of registering nurses as a safeguard for the public had been put forward many years before by the then president of the British Medical Council, but the British Nurses' Association was the first to put it into practice. The first meeting of the Registration Board was held March 7, 1890. During the first six months, in accordance with precedent, registration was open to women (whether trained in hospitals or not) who had been engaged for three or more years in nursing the sick, provided that their credentials and testimonials were satisfactory to the Registration Board appointed by the Association. At the end of that " period of grace," three years of hospital training was made an essential condition of registration, and has remained the rule. In 1891 the first register of trained nurses was published.

The application by the Association for a Royal Charter was the subject of an inquiry before the Privy Council, and caused powerful opposition. Members of the medical profession, and the authorities of many influential hospitals and institutions, opposed it. There was a similar battle over the Nurses' Charter that there is to-day over State registration, and the opposing camps contained equally distinguished members of the medical and nursing professions. The opponents feared that incorporation would place the nurse in too independent a professional position, and might militate against the interest of the medical practitioner and the best interests of the public, while the advocates desired to improve the status of the nurse, and promote her better training and education. The controversy was strenuous, and often heated, and to-day there is no need to revive the conflict.

Princess Christian was throughout a warm advocate for obtaining a Royal Charter, and her recommendations had influential weight in the highest quarter. In 1893 Queen Victoria, on the representation of "Our most dearly beloved daughter Helena, Princess Christian of Schleswig-Holstein, Princess of Great Britain and Ireland," so runs the document, granted a Charter of Incorporation to the Royal British Nurses' Association. The Charter was granted to the following associates :—Her Royal Highness Princess Christian of Schleswig-Holstein; Sir James Paget, Baronet; Sir Spencer Wells, Baronet; Sir William Savory, Baronet; Sir Richard Quain, Baronet; Sir Joseph Fayrer, Knight Commander of the Most Exalted Star of India; Sir Henry Thompson, Knight Bachelor; Sir James Crichton Browne, Knight Bachelor; Sir Dyce Duckworth, Knight Bachelor; Sir Edward Sieveking, Knight Bachelor; Sir Alfred Garrod, Knight Bachelor; Sir George Humphry, Knight Bachelor; Robert Brudenell Carter, Fellow of the Royal College of Surgeons of England; John Williams, Doctor of Medicine; William Bezly Thorne, Doctor of Medicine; Bedford Fenwick, Doctor of Medicine; Isla Stewart, Matron and Superintendent of Nursing of St. Bartholomew's Hospital; G. M. Thorold, Lady Superintendent of the Middlesex Hospital; Ethel Gordon Fenwick, late Matron and Superintendent of Nursing of St. Bartholomew's Hospital; Cassandra Beachcroft, Lady Superintendent of the Lincoln County Hospital; Margaret Breay, Acting Matron of the Metropolitan Hospital; Mary N. Cureton, Lady Superintendent of Addenbrooke's Hospital, Cambridge; Christina Forrest, Lady Superintendent of the York County Hospital; Louisa Hogg, Head Sister, Royal Naval Hospital, Haslar; R. F.

Lumsden, Honorary Lady Superintendent of the Royal Infirmary, Aberdeen; Henrietta C. Poole, Nursing Superintendent, Adelaide Hospital, Dublin; Gertrude A. Rogers, Lady Superintendent of the Leicester Infirmary; Georgina Scott, Lady Superintendent of the Sussex County Hospital; Maud G. Smith, Lady Superintendent of the Royal Infirmary, Bristol; Catherine J. Wood, late Lady Superintendent of the Children's Hospital, Great Ormond Street. The list, exclusive of the president, it will be noted, is composed of an equal number of representatives of the medical and of the nursing professions.

The purposes of the Corporation are thus defined in the Charter—

1. The founding and maintenance of schemes for the benefit of nurses in the practice of their profession, and in times of adversity, sickness, and old age.

2. The maintenance of an office or offices for supplying information to persons seeking for nurses, and to persons seeking for employment as nurses.

3. The maintenance and publication of a list of persons who may have applied to the corporation to have their names entered therein as nurses, and whom the corporation may think fit to enter therein from time to time, coupled with such information about each person so entered, as to the corporation may from time to time seem desirable.

4. The promotion of conferences, public meetings, and lectures in connection with the general work of the corporation.

5. The doing anything incidental or conducive to carrying into effect the foregoing purposes.

The Association is governed by a general council and executive committee. The general council consists of *ex-officio* members and elected members.

The *ex-officio* members are: The president, vice-presidents, vice-chairmen, treasurer, honorary secretaries, president of the Royal College of Physicians of London, president of the Royal College of Surgeons of London, president of the Royal College of Physicians of Edinburgh, president of the Royal College of Surgeons of Edinburgh, president of the Royal College of Physicians of Dublin, president of the Royal College of Surgeons of Dublin, president of the Faculty of Physicians and Surgeons of Glasgow, Master of the Society of Apothecaries of London, president of the British Medical Association, heads of the Navy and Army Nursing Departments, senior lady superintendent of the Indian Nursing Service, matron or superintendent of nurses of each of the hospitals or other institutions, which for the time being shall be on the list to be kept pursuant to bye-law 24.*

The elected members are ninety in number. Thirty are past matrons or superintendents of nurses of the hospitals or institutions which for the time being shall be on the list to be kept pursuant to bye-law 24, or present or past matrons or superintendents of nurses of any other recognized hospital or institution in the British Empire.

Thirty are sisters or nurses.

Thirty are duly qualified medical practitioners as defined by the Medical Acts.

Members of the general council retire in rotation.

The executive committee consists of *ex-officio* members and elected members. The *ex-officio* members are : The president, vice-chairman, treasurer, honorary secretaries.

The elected members are thirty in number, and are elected each year by general council, at the first meeting of the general council. After the annual general meeting of the corporation. The elected members are—

Ten duly qualified medical practitioners.

Ten present or past matrons or superintendents of nurses.

Ten sisters or nurses.

Those eligible for membership of the association are :

* " The general council shall keep and annually revise a list of the hospitals, infirmaries, and other institutions, which in the opinion of the general council are for the time being of sufficient importance to entitle the matron or superintendent of the nurses thereof for the time being to be an *ex-officio* member of the council."

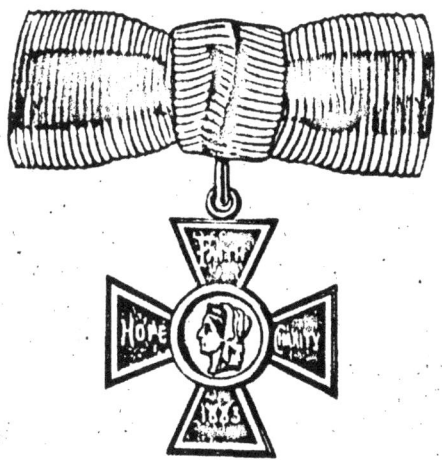

THE ROYAL RED CROSS.

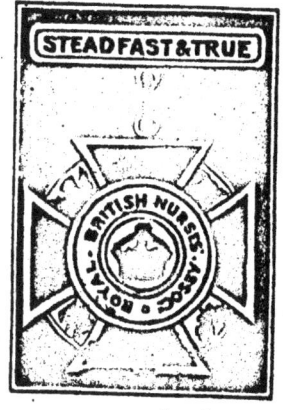

BADGE OF THE ROYAL BRITISH
NURSES' ASSOCIATION.

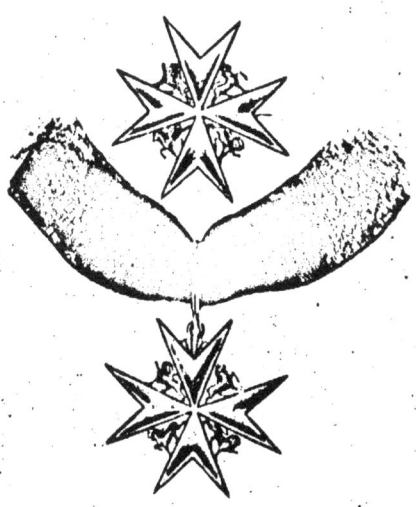

ORDER OF THE HOSPITAL OF ST. JOHN
OF JERUSALEM.

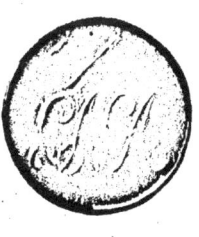

BADGE OF THE COLONIAL
NURSING SERVICE.

[*To face p.* 376.

All duly qualified medical practitioners; matrons of recognized institutions, and sisters and nurses whose names have been registered by the Board as having had three years' training in recognized hospitals, of which not less than twelve months has been spent in a general hospital, containing at least forty beds. Since April, 1905, it is required that not less than two of the three years shall have been spent in a general hospital.

The subscription for annual membership is five shillings, for life membership two guineas, and the nurses' registration fee is one guinea.

The names of all members, with particulars of their training and past experience, are printed in the roll of members, published by the corporation, a copy of which is sent to every member. A registration certificate and membership card, signed by Her Royal Highness the President, and with the seal of the Corporation affixed are issued to each member. The association, by publishing the names and qualifications of trained nurses, seeks to protect the public against unskilled and untrustworthy women. A bronze badge engraved with the owner's name and number can be obtained by each member, and a silver badge is reserved for past and present members of the General Council.

At the offices of the association, 10, Orchard Street, Portman Square, W., there is a commodious club-room where members can obtain light refreshments at cost price from 1 p.m. There is also a reading-room supplied with medical, illustrated, and daily papers. The organ of the association is the *Nurses' Journal*, edited by the secretary, Miss Annie J. Hobbs, who has worked indefatigably in furthering the interests of the association since her appointment to the post in 1902. She had formerly been secretary of the Auxiliary Nurses' Society, and now combines that with the secretaryship of the Royal British Nurses' Association.

There is a good medical and general library for the use of members, and various social gatherings and lectures take place during the year. The Helena Benevolent Fund gives grants to members in temporary distress. In 1904, a nurses' settlement was started at 20, Clapton Square, Hackney, for the benefit of members of the Association who are past work and in very straitened circumstances. They are allowed free quarters at the settlement provided they can pay for food and clothing. There are at present six nurses in residence.

In 1896, the Association being desirous of protecting its nurses against being exploited by private agencies, established the Chartered Nurses' Society on co-operative principles. It was founded and organized by Mr. I. Mark Hovel. Each nurse engaged in private work receives her earnings, less 7½ per cent., which is deducted to defray the working expenses of the office. Only nurses upon the register of the Royal British Nurses' Association are eligible for membership. There are at present one hundred and twenty-six nurses in the Society. The secretary is Miss Jackson, 24, Princes Street, Cavendish Square.

In 1900, another nurses' co-operative society was formed by some members of the Association and others with the object of finding employment for middle-aged members, under the name of the Auxiliary Nurses' Society. Candidates must be registered members of the Royal British Nurses' Society of thirty-six years of age and upwards, and possess the qualifications deemed necessary by the committee of management. They may be required to undergo medical examination as to fitness, and to produce a certificate of birth. No nurse may remain a member of the Society after the age of sixty without the special sanction of the committee. The Auxiliary Nurses are specially adapted for prolonged and chronic cases, which younger nurses often do not care to undertake. The Society serves the useful purpose of finding work for fully-trained women in danger of passing under the modern bane "too old at forty," and of supplying the public with a nurse suited to old people and chronic invalids on specially arranged terms. The secretary is Miss Annie J. Hobbs, 10, Orchard Street.

The membership of the Royal British Nurses' Association has not at any period, I believe, exceeded three thousand, and has sometimes fallen below. The number is not large when compared with the total number of trained nurses employed in the United Kingdom. Sir James Crichton Browne, one of the most influential and staunch friends of the Royal British Nurses' Association, from its initiation claims for the nurses that they are "the *élite* of the nursing world." Many reasons have combined to prevent the Association being the all-embracing institution which its founders designed it to be. Some important hospitals do not regard it with favour, and in consequence nurses employed in those hospitals do not join the Royal British Nurses' Association. There have, too, been critical periods in the history of the Association when matters of policy alienated many supporters. This leads up to the question of State registration, which may be more fittingly treated under a separate head. The Royal British Nurses' Association obtained the Royal Charter of Incorporation for nurses, and provided the first register of nurses. The badge of the Association bears the motto, " Steadfast and True."

The Royal National Pension Fund for Nurses.

The Royal National Pension Fund for Nurses was founded by Mr., now Sir, Henry Burdett in 1887, for the purpose of affording nurses a safe means of providing for their future at the lowest possible cost to themselves. Sir Henry Burdett had been superintendent of the Queen's Hospital, Birmingham, of the Seaman's Hospital, Greenwich, and secretary of the share and loan department, London Stock Exchange, so that his experience specially qualified him to deal with a financial scheme for the benefit of the nursing profession. Sir Henry is well known as an adept at statistics, and has published various books dealing with finance. He is the founder and editor of the *Hospital*, and the author of several works dealing with hospitals and nursing institutions and nurses. Very useful books of reference are his "Official Nursing Directory," and "The Nursing Profession: How and Where to Train."

Sir Henry Burdett was led to found the fund by the pathetic misfortunes of a nurse, which came under his notice at the Seamen's Hospital, Greenwich. A Swedish sailor suffering from a severe form of typhoid fever was received into the hospital. One of the attendants, Nurse Steer, wishing to make his bed, took him into her arms to lift him. The man was delirious, and resenting the action, spat in her face, and some of the saliva entered her mouth. Like a loyal nurse, she stuck to the patient until an assistant came to her help. Though she cleansed her mouth with a disinfectant, it was of no avail, the poison had entered into her system, and a virulent attack of typhoid supervened. She recovered, only to be a permanent invalid. The hospital discharged her with a gratuity, and by the help of friends she existed for a time. Finally, this heroic victim to duty was compelled to seek the shelter of the workhouse, and there she died.

Her case is not, unfortunately, an isolated one, and when it is remembered that a nurse's active money-earning life is, roughly speaking, from the age of twenty-five to that of forty-five, or at most to fifty, and that it is a very exacting life which leaves her with little energy to embark on fresh enterprises, the necessity for making a provision for the future is apparent. Sir Henry Burdett was much impressed by this, and formulated his scheme for a Pension Fund, to enable nurses to secure annuities for declining years.

The inaugural meeting was held at the Society of Arts, October 12, 1887, at which Sir Andrew Clark presided, and Mr. Burdett explained his scheme, which was to be "safe," to be "mutual," to be "self-helping," and to be "adequate." Mr. Burdett gave five hundred pounds towards the preliminary expenses of the enterprise, and collected one thousand pounds from his friends. A sum of twenty thousand pounds was required to be deposited in Chancery for the security of the Fund, and this was given by Lord Rothschild, Mr. Julius S. Morgan, Messrs. Anthony Gibbs and Sons, and Mr. E. A. Hambro, truly a princely gift. Mr. George King, F.I.A., on the death of Mr. Cornelius Walford, was appointed actuary to the Fund, and formulated the scheme. It was incorporated in February, 1888.

The promoters were fortunate in securing royal interest. The King, then Prince of Wales, became patron, and the Princess president. When the first thousand policies had been taken out, the Prince and Princess held a reception for the policy-holders at Marlborough House, July 4, 1890, the first of those delightful garden parties for nurses which have been given under the auspices of the King and Queen. The date was propitious, and July 4 has become known as "Independence Day" for nurses as well as for the American Republic. To show their appreciation of the Queen's great interest in their profession, the nurses offered a little gift on Her Majesty's birthday, December 1, 1891, consisting of a photograph screen, containing the portraits of six to seven hundred matrons and nurses belonging to the first and second thousand who had joined the Pension Fund. In the centre of the screen was a group of nurses sketched by Mr. Reginald Cleaver. The screen was designed by Miss Pritchard, secretary to Sir Henry Burdett.

The Pension Fund is not, however, a philanthropic venture or a merely benevolent scheme. It is a thoroughgoing business concern for enabling nurses to provide an annuity for declining years, just as the clergy have their annuity fund and other members of society insure for old age in companies offering special facilities to members of the profession to which they belong. The offices are in the heart of the city at 28, Finsbury Pavement. The

Fund is backed by some of the best-known financiers of the day, and its bankers are the Bank of England. Everard A. Hambro, Esq. (Messrs. C. I. Hambro and Son), is chairman, and Sir Henry Burdett, K.C.B., is deputy chairman. Upon the council are several distinguished members of the medical profession, while the nurse annuitants' representatives are eight matrons of important London and provincial hospitals. The secretary is Louis H. M. Dick, Esq., who is most courteous in explaining the scheme to intending annuitants who call at the office or who write to him upon the subject.

His Majesty the King remains patron of the Fund, and her Majesty the Queen, president. The patronesses are the Duchess of Beaufort, the Marchioness of Zetland, Alice Countess of Strafford, the Lady Rothschild, and Mrs. Walter H. Burns. The vice-presidents are the Earl of Aberdeen, Lord Rothschild, Lord Aldenham, J. Pierpont Morgan, Esq., Sir William Broadbent, Bart., M.D., J. Hutchinson Esq., F.R.S., and E. A. Hambro, Esq.

The invested funds amount to one million pounds sterling. Since the establishment of the Fund two hundred and twenty thousand pounds have been paid to nurses obliged, from one cause or another, to leave the Fund; over eighteen thousand pounds distributed in sick allowances, and over sixty thousand pounds in pensions. The popularity of the Fund is shown by the increase of policies issued during the past ten years. In 1895, the policies issued were eight hundred and twenty-two, and in 1905 the number issued was one thousand three hundred and four. The benefits of the Fund are open to nurses, attendants on the insane, and all responsible paid officials connected with hospitals and kindred institutions. In addition to a pension, nurses and hospital officials may insure for sick pay. During 1905, one thousand eight hundred pounds was paid by the Fund in sick pay. Only nurses may participate in the donation bonus fund. Many hospitals and institutions wishing to make a little provision for nurses who have served them faithfully for long periods affiliate themselves to the Royal Pension Fund, and one cannot but feel that money spent in that way is better disbursed than if devoted to very luxurious nurses' quarters, or, shall we say, to tessellated pavements in hospitals. At the annual meeting of the Fund, June 6, 1906, Miss Swift, matron of Guy's Hospital, made a very practical appeal to nurses to take advantage of the Pension Fund, and to matrons of hospitals, that they should encourage those under their charge in habits of thrift, and in taking care for the future.

The State Registration of Nurses.

In dealing with the question of the State registration of nurses at this juncture, one feels as an historian might have done, who, standing on the plain of Waterloo, began to describe the battle before the French cavalry had made their fatal advance to the treacherous fosse, or the approach of Blucher had been heralded. The nursing world is divided into hostile armies, the battle rages, and who shall say what may turn the fortune of war? Distinguished generals lead either side, and the rank and file have ranged themselves in opposing camps. Each professes to have the welfare of the nurse and the good of the public at heart, but holds conflicting views as to whether compulsory registration of nurses by the State will bring about those desirable results.

At present it is a battle amongst experts, and the "man in the street" is not concerning himself particularly as to who puts on his bandages or takes his temperature, providing she does not worry him too much. When, in due course, the question engages the attention of the legislature, the public will, as the employers, wake up to an interest in the matter, and parliamentary discussion may clear the air. The history of the controversy can scarcely be written while bullets fly and swords are unsheathed. A few years hence, when a treaty of peace has been signed, and the vanquished have gracefully capitulated to the voice of the majority, the story of the struggle for registration will be told more fittingly. In the mean time we may trace briefly the events which have led up to the present crisis.

When the modern movement for training nurses had fully set in, the question arose as to how the public were to distinguish between the woman who had passed through a course of training and the woman who had only spent a short time in a hospital, since both wore the uniform and called themselves qualified nurses. Some, indeed, donned the uniform who had served no apprenticeship whatever to their calling. The patient seeking a nurse could satisfy himself on this point by demanding the nurse's record from her hospital or institution. Still, members of the General Medical Council felt that some system of compulsory registration, with a fixed minimum standard for nursing education, would be a good method for every one concerned, and the matter was advocated, but no action taken until the formation of the British Nurses' Association in 1887. It issued, as we have seen, its first register of trained nurses in 1891. Still, the Association was a voluntary one, and there was no question of compulsory legislation by the State contained in its articles of incorporation.

Some of the more advanced founders of the Association considered that State registration was the ultimate aim, and sympathized with the action of the General Medical Council, which, in November, 1889, passed the following resolution: "That, in the opinion of the Council, it would be much to the advantage of the public, and particularly would it be of much convenience to the practitioners of medicine and surgery, that facilities, usable under proper guarantees in all parts of the United Kingdom, should be given, by Act of Parliament or otherwise, for the authoritative certification of competent trained nurses, who, when certified, should be subject to common rules of discipline." With the view of pressing forward the question and organizing sympathizers with State registration, Mrs. Bedford Fenwick founded, in 1894, the Matrons' Council of Great Britain and Ireland, which had for one of its objects "a uniform system of education, examination, certification, and State registration for nurses in British hospitals." This latter clause now runs, "for trained nurses in the United Kingdom." The Matrons' Council has vigorously continued to pursue its propaganda by means of conferences and discussions. The president is Miss Isla Stewart, matron and superintendent of nursing, St. Bartholomew's Hospital, and the honorary secretary, Miss Margaret Breay, 431, Oxford Street, London.

The years 1894-96 were fruitful in controversy on the registration question, particularly within the council of the R.B.N.A. In 1895 the British Medical Association, at its annual meeting, passed the following resolution, on the motion of Dr. Bedford Fenwick: "That, in the opinion of this meeting, it is expedient that an Act of Parliament should, as soon as possible, be passed, providing for the registration of medical, surgical, and obstetric nurses, and the Council of this Association are therefore requested to consider the matter, and to take such measures as may seem to them advisable to obtain such legislation." The following year a conference took place between the Parliamentary Bills Committee of the British Medical Association and representatives of nursing organizations. A resolution was put, "That a legal system of registration of nurses is inexpedient *in principle*, and injurious to the best interests of nurses, and of doubtful public benefit." This was carried by a majority of one, the representative of the Royal British Nurses' Association voting with the majority. This vote was protested against by the supporters of State registration on the executive committee of that Association, but was upheld by a majority. The controversy became acute. In 1899 the

Association substituted a roll of members for its original register of trained nurses.

Definite action for the formation of a society in favour of State registration was taken in 1902, when "The Society for the State Registration of Trained Nurses" was founded. The president is Miss Louisa Stevenson, Edinburgh ; the senior vice-president, Miss Isla Stewart, matron, St. Bartholomew's Hospital ; and the honorary secretary and treasurer, Mrs. Bedford Fenwick. The Report for 1906 shows that 1878 members have joined during the four years of the Society's existence. The object of the Society is " to obtain an Act of Parliament providing for the legal registration of trained nurses," and in 1904 a Bill was introduced into the House of Commons by Dr. Farquharson, Member for West Aberdeenshire. The organ of the Society is the *British Journal of Nursing*.

Meantime, in 1903, the Royal British Nurses' Association again took up the question of registration, and at a council meeting, the president, Princess Christian, being present, a resolution in favour of registration was passed. A Bill providing for the registration of nurses and nursing homes was promoted by the Association, and introduced into the House of Commons by the Hon. Claude Hay.

There were now two Bills on the question of registration before Parliament ; one promoted by the Society for State Registration, and one by the Royal British Nurses' Association.

A large and influential body in the medical and nursing world were entirely opposed to registration, and an opposition movement was organized by the Central Hospital Council for London, which passed a resolution in opposition to any State registration of nurses, and circularized Boards of hospitals, infirmaries, nursing institutions, and members of Parliament, inviting their co-operation. A Select Committee of the House of Commons was appointed to consider the question. In 1905 a resolution in favour of the principle of State registration was, on the motion of Dr. Langley Browne, carried by the British Medical Association meeting at Oxford. A bill in favour of registration was introduced into the House of Commons by Mr. Munro Ferguson, February 23, 1905. The Select Committee was reappointed, March 30, to consider the expediency of providing for the registration of nurses. It issued its Report, July 25, 1905.

Thirty-four experts, comprising distinguished men and women in the medical and nursing world, were examined before the Select Committee, and the evidence was conflicting. The ADVOCATES for State registration contended that it was desirable to establish a minimum standard of efficiency, determined by a Central Nursing Board, which would test whether the training received came up to modern requirements. At present each hospital and training institution has its own standard. Some are excellent, others deficient. The aim of registration was to bring all into line and make a one efficient portal entrance into the nursing profession. It was also believed that registration would raise the tone of nursing throughout the country, and serve as a test for training schools as well as for nurses, and would stimulate the appointment of matrons competent to educate their probationers up to the point required by the Central Board. The latter should appoint experts—doctors and nurses—to be its examiners. A public register should be kept of nurses who had passed the examination, and the efficiency and moral standing of the nurses would be kept up by their being required to report themselves at intervals to the Central Board. By such means it was hoped to do away with the untrained, semi-trained, and bogus nurses, and to protect the public from imposture, and also to place nursing on such a high basis that educated women would regard it as a desirable and honourable profession. Evidence was further adduced to show that State registration was working well in New Zealand, Cape Colony, and Natal; that the feeling in favour of it is strong in Australia; and that in America eight States had passed

Acts for registering nurses; while in France the training of nurses, having been taken out of the hands of the religious Orders, was entirely in the hands of the Government. It was further urged upon the Select Committee that private medical and surgical Nursing Homes should be registered and inspected by Government, it being pointed out that some Homes were not used for the purposes specified, and that grave scandals existed; while in others, where extortionate fees were charged, untrained nurses were put in charge of critical cases. Evidence was given of parlour-maids having been put into uniform and passed off as nurses. The patients naturally felt that they might have stayed at home and dressed up their own parlour-maids instead of paying for the interesting transformation in an expensive Nursing Home.

The OPPONENTS of State registration, who include some of the most honoured names in the nursing world and amongst the medical faculty, urged that the present system of hospital-nurse training-schools, each having its own curriculum and granting its own certificate of efficiency, created healthy rivalry. That by this means the modern system of trained nursing had been evolved, and had reached a high level. It was contended that each training school, whether hospital or private institution, could, by keeping a register of the trained nurses who had passed through its curriculum, satisfy inquiry on the part of the public, who could thus protect themselves against the untrained and spurious by demanding a nurse's record before they engaged her. Registration was further opposed on the ground that a State examination could not sufficiently gauge a nurse's fitness for her work. Something more than mere technical knowledge was needed. High character and personal fitness played an important part in constituting the really good nurse, who would be popular in the homes of the community. It was feared that the nurse, actuated by an anxiety to shine in her technical examination, would lose that fine and subtle art of sympathy and watchfulness—the "bedside qualities "—which make the ideal nurse. What was needed was not only a technically capable nurse, but a woman who was able to take her proper place in the household of her patient and be a comfort and help in time of sorrow and sickness. It was feared that an intensified professional consciousness engendered by the "hall mark" of the State would have the opposite result.

Some witnesses objected to making a three years' training compulsory for all nurses, on the ground that in a large hospital training school a nurse might, by having her work well distributed, gain adequate experience and training in a two years' course. Also, women with some knowledge of nursing, though not highly skilled, were useful for certain cases and acceptable to the public. It was contended that by prohibiting women nursing for gain, unless registered by the State, an injustice would be done to that useful and respectable class of person, "the woman to sit up," who is called in to relieve members of a family in time of sickness, by those who cannot pay the fees of a trained nurse. It was urged that much good work can be done by half-trained people provided that they do not attempt to pass themselves off as fully qualified.

Some objections were also made to a compulsory three years' training, on the ground that it retarded the turning out of a sufficient supply of trained nurses to meet the public demand. Figures were given showing that St. Thomas's, the oldest training-school, and the London Hospital, the largest training-school, had, in the course of forty-three years, only certified two thousand three hundred and seventy-seven nurses, nearly half of whom had had one year's training, and a little more than half had had two years' training. Had those two hospitals enforced a three years' course, the output of nurses would have been considerably smaller.

On the part of the general medical practitioner State registration was opposed, on the ground that, by giving an independent status to the nurse, she might become eventually a professional rival. In children's illnesses and the ailments of old people, a trained nurse might be employed to the exclusion of the doctor. The nurse might be encouraged to step outside her sphere and militate against medical practice.

Those who were in favour of the system of registration established under the Midwives' Act, objected to the registration of sick nurses, on the ground that they were not practitioners independent of the doctor, as were certified midwives. The nurse worked entirely under the order of the medical man, and had no separate status which needed to be registered by the State.

With regard to the registration and inspection of Nursing Homes, the OPPONENTS were much at one with the ADVOCATES of State Registration for Nurses. It was a matter for which the public required a legislative safeguard.

In the foregoing we have endeavoured to set forth the salient points of both sides, but the résumé is not exhaustive.

The Select Committee, amid many divergent views given in evidence, arrived at the conclusion that there was a general opinion in favour of some change in the conditions under which nursing is carried on. The Report sets forth in Clause 11, that " the Committee are agreed that it is desirable that a register of nurses should be kept by a central body appointed by the State, and that, while it is not desirable to prohibit unregistered persons from nursing for gain, no person should be entitled to assume the designation of 'registered nurse,' whose name is not upon the register." It is further recommended that "the central body should consist of matrons, nurses, and representatives of the medical profession, of training-schools for nurses, and of the public; that the central body should decide what constitutes a recognized training-school for nurses, should have the power of inspection, and that the examination be held at the training-school; that the minimum period for training should not be fixed by Act of Parliament, but should be left to the discretion of the central body (admitting, however, that the great bulk of evidence points to three years as the requisite period of training); that there should be an annual publication of the register of nurses; that the central body should make provision for striking off the register the names of those nurses who have died or who have ceased nursing, and also of those nurses who, in the opinion of the central body, have been guilty of serious misconduct in the discharge of their duty, or of moral delinquency; that existing nurses who can produce satisfactory evidence as regards efficiency and character should be placed upon the register on payment of the registration fee; that the latter should not exceed one guinea; that the central body, not later than four years after the passing of any Act for the registration of nurses, should submit a report to the Privy Council on the advisability of instituting a separate register of nurses, whose training is of a lower standard than that laid down for "registered nurses;" that a separate register of "registered asylum nurses" should be kept by the central body, to which should be admitted those who have received the certificate of the Medico-Psychological Association, and can produce satisfactory certificates of good character. Lastly, the committee recommended the licensing of Nursing Homes, where patients are taken for treatment, as highly desirable, and that the county, or county borough authority, should be empowered to draft regulations to be approved by the Local Government Board.

Deputations representing the advocates and the opponents of State Registration have since waited upon Lord Crewe, the Lord President of the Privy Council, to lay their views before him. On March 8, 1906, Mr. H. J. Tennant, M.P., late Chairman of the Select Committee, introduced an influential deputation in favour of registration to the Earl of Crewe at the Privy Council Office. On June 14th, a deputation * introduced by Mr. H. A. Harben and the Hon. Sydney Holland, chairman

* From the London Central Hospital Committee.

of the London Hospital, Sir Thomas Barlow, and Sir Frederick Treves, waited upon Lord Crewe to represent that the Government should not support State registration, as there was no concensus of opinion by medical men or the public on the matter. The Lord President of the Council—to summarize his replies to both deputations—said that the question of the State registration of nurses was a matter of national importance, and that it could not be long before the subject occupied the serious attention of Parliament, but that the Government programme was very full, and the matter could not be dealt with this session.

The British Medical Association, at its annual meeting, 1906, passed an almost unanimous vote in favour of the principle of State registration of nurses.

Meantime, the Royal British Nurses' Association and the Society for the State Registration of Trained Nurses have been redrafting their Parliamentary Bills to bring them more into line with the recommendations of the select committee, and their respective supporters are continuing their propaganda. The Central Hospital Council have also drafted a Bill which they propose to lay before Parliament, and in which they advocate the establishment of a nurses' register or directory to be kept by an official registrar, instead of State registration.

THE END